KV-512-278

This book is due for return not later than the last
date stamped below, unless recalled sooner.

REFRACTIVE ANOMALIES

RESEARCH AND CLINICAL APPLICATIONS

REFRACTIVE ANOMALIES

RESEARCH AND CLINICAL APPLICATIONS

Edited by

THEODORE GROSVENOR, O.D., Ph.D.
Professor of Optometry
Indiana University
Bloomington, Indiana

MERTON C. FLOM, O.D., Ph.D.
Professor of Optometry
University of Houston
Houston, Texas

With 27 Contributors

Butterworth–Heinemann
Boston   London   Singapore   Sydney   Toronto   Wellington

Every effort has been made to ensure that the drug dosage schedules within this text are
accurate and conform to standards accepted at time of publication. However, as treatment
recommendations vary in the light of continuing research and clinical experience, the reader is
advised to verify drug dosage schedules herein with information found on product information
sheets. This is especially true in cases of new or infrequently used drugs.

 Recognizing the importance of preserving what has been written, it is the policy of Butterworth–
Heinemann to have the books it publishes printed on acid-free paper, and we exert our best
efforts to that end.

Library of Congress Cataloging-in-Publication Data
Refractive anomalies : research and clinical applications / edited by
Theodore Grosvenor, Merton C. Flom ; with 27 contributing authors.
   p.   cm.
Includes bibliographical references.
Includes index.
ISBN 0-409-90149-0 (casebound)
1. Myopia.   2. Eye — Refractive errors.   I. Grosvenor, Theodore, P.
II. Flom, Merton C.
   [DNLM: 1. Myopia.   2. Refractive Errors.   WW 320 R332]
RE938.R43   1990
617.7'55 — dc20
DNLM/DLC
for Library of Congress   90-2443
                                                                        CIP

British Library Cataloguing-in-Publication Data
Refractive anomalies.
   1. Man. Eyes. Refraction disorders
   I. Grosvenor, Theodore   II. Flom, Merton C.
   617.755
   ISBN 0-409-90149-0

Butterworth–Heinemann
80 Montvale Avenue
Stoneham, MA 02180

10 9 8 7 6 5 4 3 2 1

Printed in the United States of America

This book is dedicated to the memory of
Frank W. Weymouth and Monroe J. Hirsch

CONTENTS

15 RETINAL FACTORS IN MYOPIA AND EMMETROPIZATION: CLUES FROM RESEARCH ON CHICKS 268
Josh Wallman

16 MECHANICAL CONSIDERATIONS IN MYOPIA 287
Peter R. Greene

17 ACCOMMODATION AND VITREOUS CHAMBER PRESSURE: A PROPOSED MECHANISM FOR MYOPIA 301
Francis A. Young and George A. Leary

CONTRIBUTORS

Frank W. Weymouth, Ph.D.   (1884–1963)

"Uncle Frank" Weymouth was an eminent vision scientist with an incredible range of interests — from composing poetry to writing books on crustacia, and from studying pilots' night vision to investigating the development of myopia in children. Trained as a zoologist, Dr. Weymouth was a member of the Stanford University Department of Physiology from 1916 until 1949, where he became Professor and Chairman of the department and Director of the Vision Laboratory. From 1950 to 1960 he was a Professor at the Los Angeles College of Optometry (now Southern California College of Optometry), and from 1960 until his death in 1963 he was a research scientist at the School of Optometry at the University of California, Berkeley. In 1960, he was elected Honorary Fellow of the American Academy of Optometry. While at Los Angeles, Frank collaborated with Monroe Hirsch on some outstanding papers, most notably "Notes on Ametropia — A Further Analysis of Stenstrom's Data" and "Relative Growth of the Eye."

Monroe J. Hirsch, O.D., Ph.D.   (1917–1982)

Monroe Hirsch served his profession in every capacity one might imagine — as practitioner, teacher, researcher, writer, editor, administrator, and diplomat — in addition to serving his community in many capacities, including as city councilman and mayor. Monroe practiced optometry while pursuing his graduate studies under Frank Weymouth at the Stanford University Department of Physiology. In 1949, he joined the faculty of the Los Angeles College of Optometry where he collaborated with Dr. Weymouth on research and writing on his favorite subject: myopia. He left Los Angeles in 1953 and started an optometric practice in Ojai, California, where he conducted his longitudinal study of refraction in schoolchildren. In his later years, Monroe served as Professor and Dean of optometry at the University of California, Berkeley. He will be remembered by many as editor of the *American Journal of Optometry and Physiological Optics*; as co-editor, with Ralph Wick, of *Vision of the Aging Patient* and *Vision of Children*; and as editor of *Refractive State of the Eye.*

*   *   *

Anthony J. Adams, L.O.Sc., Ph.D.
Professor and Assistant Dean, School of Optometry, University of California, Berkeley, California. First recipient of the Glenn A. Fry Award, American Academy of Optometry. Chairman, National Academy of Sciences Working Group on Myopia. Publications include: "Clinical Measures of Central Visual Function in Glaucoma and Ocular Hypertension" (with G. Heron, R. Husted); "Evidence for a Neural Basis of Age-Related Visual Field Loss in Normal Observers" (with C.A. Johnson, R.A. Lewis); "Adult Onset Myopia: Evidence for Axial Elongation Not Corneal Curvature Increase as the Basis."

William R. Baldwin, O.D., Ph.D.
President, River Blindness Foundation; formerly, Dean, College of Optometry, University of Houston, Houston, Texas. Principal area of research: myopia. Member, National Academy of Sciences Working Group on Myopia. Formerly, President, American Association of Schools and Colleges of Optometry. Publications include: "Factors in Myopia" (Ph.D. dissertation); "Clinical Research and Procedures in Refraction" (American Academy of Optometry Symposium); "A Longitudinal Study of Corneal Astigmatism and Refractive Astigmatism"; *Vision Science Symposium, a Tribute to Gordon Heath* (editor).

John C. Bear, Ph.D.
Professor of Population Genetics, Faculty of Medicine, Memorial University of Newfoundland, St. John's Newfoundland. Areas of research: human genetic variation as it relates to health and disease; the genetic structure of human populations. Publications include: "Ocular Refraction and Inbreeding, a Population Study in Newfoundland"; "Nearwork and Familial Resemblances in Ocular Refraction: a Population Study in Newfoundland" (with A. Richler and G. Burke); "Refraction, Nearwork and Education, a Population Study in Newfoundland" (with A. Richler).

Paul Erickson, M.S., O.D.
Contact Lens Division, Bausch and Lomb, Inc., Rochester, New York; formerly, Assistant Professor of Optometry, Northeastern State University, Tahlequah, Oklahoma. Areas of research: contact lenses; geometric optics. Publications include: "Visual Function with Presbyopic Contact Lens Correction" (with C. Schor); "Effect of Sampling Location on Data Sensitivity in a Three Compartment Model" (with E. Ackerman); "Complete Ocular Component Analysis by Vergence Contribution."

F.W. Fitzke, Ph.D.
Institute of Ophthalmology, Judd St., London. Areas of research: visual and clinical psychophysics. Publications include: "The Structural Organization of the Pigeon Retina," "A Morphological Analysis of Experimental Myopia in Young Chickens" (with W. Hodos, B.P. Hayes, A.L. Holden).

Pamela Flattau, Ph.D.
Staff Officer, National Research Council Committee on Vision and U.S. National
Committee for International Union of Psychological Science, Washington, D.C.
Co-director, Committee on Mandatory Retirement in Higher Education. Publi-
cations of the Committee on Vision include: "Myopia, Prevalence and Progres-
sion"; "Contact Lens Use under Adverse Conditions."

Merton C. Flom, O.D., Ph.D.
Professor and Dean, College of Optometry, University of Houston. Former president of the American Academy of Optometry and editor of the *American Journal
of Optometry and Physiological Optics*. Areas of research: binocular vision; amblyopia; strabismus. Committees: Vision Research Committee of the National Eye
Institute; Committee on Vision of the National Academy of Sciences/National Research Council. Publications include: "The AC/A Ratio and Undercorrected Myopia" (with E. Takahashi); "Visual Resolution and Contour Interaction" (with
Frank Weymouth and Daniel Kahneman); "Monocular Spatial Distortion in Strabismic Amblyopia" (with H. Bedell); "Issues in the Clinical Management of Binocular Anomalies" (chapter in *Pediatric Optometry*, edited by M. Morgan and A.
Rosenbloom).

Ernst Goldschmidt, M.D.
Head, Department of Ophthalmology, Frederiksborg County Hospital, Hillerod,
Denmark; formerly, Professor of Ophthalmology, Odense University, Odense,
Denmark. Area of clinical specialization: ophthalmic surgery. Major area of re-
search: myopia. Publications include "On the Etiology of Myopia, an Epidemio-
logical Study" (Thesis, University of Copenhagen); "Refraction of the Newborn";
"Myopia Workshop," (Copenhagen, 1987, organizer and co-editor). Formerly,
President, Danish Ophthalmological Society; Danish representative of European
Ophthalmological Society.

David A. Goss, O.D., Ph.D.
Professor of Optometry, Northeastern State University, Tahlequah, Oklahoma.
Areas of research: refractive errors, general optometry. Publications include: *Ocu-
lar Accommodation, Convergence, and Fixation Disparity*; "Progression of My-
opia in Youth, Age of Cessation" (with R.L. Winkler); "Prevalence and Pattern of
Adult Myopia Progression in a General Optometric Practice Population" (with P.
Erickson, V.D. Cox); "Meridional Corneal Components of Myopia Progression in
Young Adults and Children" (with P. Erickson).

Peter R. Greene, Ph.D., P.E.
Consulting Engineer, B.G.K.T. Consulting, Ltd., Huntington, New York;
formerly, Assistant Professor of Bioengineering, Johns Hopkins University, Baltimore, Maryland. Areas of research: applied mechanics, bioengineering. Publications include: "Scleral Creep vs Temperature and Pressure in vitro" (with T.A.

McMahon); "Mechanical Considerations in Myopia"; "Closed-Form Ametropic Pressure-Volume and Ocular Rigidity Solutions"; "Stress Amplification and Plastic Flow . . . Applications to Myopia."

Theodore Grosvenor, O.D., Ph.D.
Professor of Optometry, Indiana University, Bloomington, Indiana. Presented Monroe J. Hirsch Memorial Lecture on Vision Care, American Academy of Optometry. Areas of research: refractive anomalies; control of myopia progression. Publications include: *Primary Care Optometry*; "Decrease in Axial Length with Age: An Emmetropizing Mechanism for the Adult Eye?"; "Houston Myopia Control Study, a Randomized Clinical Trial" (with D. Perrigin, J. Perrigin, B. Maslovitz). "Silicone-Acrylate Contact Lenses for Myopia Control" (with D. Perrigin, J. Perrigin, S. Quintero).

B.P. Hayes, Ph.D.
Glaxo Research Group Ltd., Middlesex, England. Areas of research: anatomy of retina and visual pathways; ultrastructure of basement membranes; image analysis. Publications include: "The Structural Organization of the Pigeon Retina," "A Morphological Analysis of Experimental Myopia in Young Chickens" (with F.W. Fitzke, W. Hodos, A.L. Holden).

William Hodos, Ph.D.
Professor of Psychology, University of Maryland, College Park, Maryland. Areas of research: animal psychophysics; experimental myopia. Publications include: "Retinal Image Degradation Produces Ocular Enlargement in Chicks" (with W.J. Kuenzel); "Experimental Myopia in Chicks: Ocular Refraction by Electroretinography" (with F.W. Fitzke, B.P. Hayes, A.L. Holden); "Lower-Field Myopia in Birds: An Adaptation that Keeps the Ground in Focus" (with J.T. Erichsen).

A.L. Holden, M.A., D.Phil.
Institute of Ophthalmology, Judd St., London; Chairman, Academic Board and Academic Sub-dean. Area of research: the eye. Publications include: "The Structural Organization of the Pigeon Retina," "A Morphological Analysis of Experimental Myopia in Young Chickens" (with F.W. Fitzke, W. Hodos, B.P. Hayes).

Hanne Jensen, M.D.
Physician, Department of Ophthalmology, Odense University Hospital, Odense, Denmark. Principal area of research: pharmaceutical agents for the control of childhood myopia. Publications include: "Visual Acuity of Danish School Children" (with E. Goldschmidt); "Can Timolol Maleate Reduce the Progression of Myopia?" (with E. Goldschmidt, D. Marushak, I. Ostergaard); "Timolol Maleate in the Control of Myopia, a Preliminary Report" (Myopia Workshop 1987).

I. Knox Laird, Dip.Opt., M.Sc., Ph.D.

Optometric practitioner specializing in the areas of binocular vision and pediatric optometry, Manurewa, New Zealand; Academic Associate, Optometry Department, University of Auckland, Auckland, New Zealand. Areas of research: binocular vision, pediatric optometry, color vision, anisometropia. Publications include: "Monitoring the Home Training of Fusional Reserves." Developments in clinical instrumentation: variable stereogram for use in fusional vergence training; tests for color vision anomalies.

George A. Leary, F.B.O.A.

Refracting optician (optometrist); former member of Professor Arnold Sorsby's research team; Washington State University Psychology Department, and Primate Research Laboratory. Areas of research: the optical system of the eye; ocular ultrasonography; myopia and its development. Publications include: "A Longitudinal Study of Refraction and its Components During Growth" (with A. Sorsby); "Refraction, its Components in Twins" (with A. Sorsby, M. Sheridan); "Ultrasound and Phakometry Measurements of the Human Eye" (with F. Young).

J.C. Low, Ph.D.

Postdoctoral Fellow, Imperial College, London. Area of research: electrophysiology of vision. Publications include: "Refractive Sectors in the Visual Field of Pigeon Eyes" (with F.W. Fitzke, B.P. Hayes, W. Hodos); "Projection of the Visual Field upon the Retina of the Pigeon" (with B.P. Hayes, W. Hodos, A.L. Holden).

William M. Lyle, O.D., M.S., Ph.D.

Professor Emeritus, School of Optometry, University of Waterloo, Waterloo, Ontario, Canada; Editor, *Optometry and Vision Science*. Former optometric practitioner, Winnipeg, Manitoba, Canada. Areas of research: astigmatism; genetics; general pathology; pharmacology. Publications include: *Genetic Risks*; "Changes in Corneal Astigmatism with Age"; "The Unwanted Effects from Topical Ophthalmic Drugs, Their Occurrence, Avoidance, and Reversal" (with G.H. Hopkins).

Meredith W. Morgan, O.D., Ph.D.

Professor and Dean Emeritus, School of Optometry, University of California, Berkeley. Primary area of interest: binocular vision, clinical optometry. Recipient of the Apollo Award of the American Optometric Association, the Prentice Medal of the American Academy of Optometry, the Berkeley Citation of the University of California, and four honorary degrees. Publications include: *The Optics of Ophthalmic Lenses* and *Vision and Aging, General and Clinical Perspectives* (co-editor).

D. Alfred Owens, Ph.D.

Professor of Psychology, Whitely Psychology Laboratories, Franklin and Marshall College, Lancaster, Pennsylvania. Member, working group of National Research

Council Committee on Vision for "Emerging Techniques of Visual Assessment." Areas of research: visual perception, accommodation, binocular vergence, human factors; visual perception and performance. Publications include: "The Resting State of the Eyes"; "Perceptual and Motor Consequences of Tonic Vergence"; "Near Work, Visual Fatigue, and Variations of Ocular Tonus" (with K. Wolf-Kelly).

Jerome Rosner, O.D.
Professor of Optometry, University of Houston, Houston, Texas. Areas of research: pediatric optometry; links between visual and cognitive development. Publications include: "The Relationship between Clinically Measured Tonic Accommodation and Refractive Status in 6–14 Year Old Children" (with Joy Rosner); *Pediatric Optometry* (with Joy Rosner); *Vision Therapy in a Primary Care Practice* (with Joy Rosner); *Helping Children Overcome Learning Difficulties.*

Clifton Schor, O.D., Ph.D.
Professor of Physiological Optics, School of Optometry, University of California, Berkeley, California. Recipient of the Glenn A. Fry Award, American Academy of Optometry. Areas of research: binocular vision; ocular motility; space perception; infant vision. Publications include: *Vergence Eye Movements: Clinical and Basic Aspects* (editor, with K. Ciuffreda); "Disturbances of Small Field Horizontal and Vertical OKN in Amblyopia" (with D. Levi); "The Relationship between Fusional Vergence Eye Movements and Fixation Disparity."

Jacob G. Sivak, L.Sc.O., M.S., Ph.D., O.D.
Professor of Optometry, Director and Associate Dean for Optometry, University of Waterloo, Waterloo, Ontario, Canada. Recipient of the Glenn A. Fry Award, American Academy of Optometry. Areas of research: refractive development of the eye; cataractogenesis. Publications include: "Accommodation in Vertebrates," "Chromatic Dispersion of the Ocular Media" (with T. Mandelman); "Spherical Aberration of the Crystalline Lens" (with R.O. Kreuzer); "Optics of the Crystalline Lens."

Earl L. Smith III, O.D., Ph.D.
Greeman-Petty Professor of Visual Development, College of Optometry, University of Houston, Houston, Texas. Areas of research: normal and abnormal visual development. Publications include: "Binocularity in Kittens Reared with Optically Induced Squint" (with M.J. Bennett, R.S. Harwerth, M.L.J. Crawford); "Spatial Contrast Sensitivity Deficits in Monkeys Produced by Optically Induced Anisometropia" (with R.S. Harwerth, M.L.J. Crawford); "Effects of Optical Defocus on the Kitten's Refractive Status" (with J. Ni).

Josh Wallman, Ph.D.
Professor of Biology, City College, City University of New York, New York City. Presented Monroe J. Hirsch Memorial Lecture on Vision Care, American Academy of Optometry, 1988. Areas of research: control of the growth of the eye;

emmetropization; accessory optic system. Publications include: "Local Retinal Regions Control Eye Growth and Myopia" (with M.D. Gottlieb, V. Rajaram, L.A. Fugate-Wentzek); "Developmental Aspects of Experimental Myopia in Chicks: Susceptibility, Recovery and Relation to Emmetropization" (with J.I. Adams).

George O. Waring III, M.D., F.A.C.S.

Professor, Director, Refractive Surgery, Department of Ophthalmology, Emory University School of Medicine, Atlanta, Georgia. Area of research: corneal refractive surgery. Chief investigator, Prospective Evaluation of Radial Keratotomy (PERK) Study. Publications include: "Rationale for and Design of the NEI Prospective Evaluation of Radial Keratotomy (PERK) Study" (with S.D. Moffitt et al.); "Changing Status of Radial Keratotomy for Myopia"; "Three-Year Results of the Prospective Evaluation of Radial Keratotomy (PERK) Study" (with M.J. Lynn et al.).

Francis A. Young, Ph.D.

Professor and Director of Primate Research Laboratory, Psychology Department, Washington State University, Pullman, Washington. Founder and chairman, International Myopia Research Society. Areas of research: development of myopia in primates and humans; mechanisms of accommodation. Publications include: "The Effect of Restricted Visual Space on the Primate Eye"; "Reading, Measures of Intelligence, and Refractive Errors"; "The Pullman Study, a Visual Survey of Pullman School Children" (with R.J. Beattie, F.J. Newby, M.T. Swindal).

FOREWORD

Professors Theodore Grosvenor and Merton Flom have produced a book about refractive anomalies for both the vision-care practitioner and the vision scientist. They have brought together twenty-seven scientists, the majority of whom have degrees in optometry or medicine, to write this book. Despite this obvious clinical emphasis, the book differs from others on refractive anomalies by not stressing the aspects that are well understood by vision-care practitioners and applied in everyday practice, such as symptoms, detection, measurement, and management of refractive anomalies. The strength of this book lies in its reporting on research, both experimental and clinical, that tells us how, why, and under what circumstances refractive anomalies, particularly myopia, develop and change. It also reports on research concerning methods used to prevent and control myopia. Because this book relies so much on research, one might think it is a book for researchers. It is. But far more importantly, it is a book that vision-care practitioners will find interesting and valuable.

Practitioners typically attempt to solve the problems of their self-selected patients under uncontrolled conditions; over time, the apparent results can lead practitioners to make erroneous conclusions about the efficacy of specific forms of therapy. Clinical judgments based on outcomes for small numbers of patients need to be tempered by the experiences of others and by an understanding of the process involved in scientific research. Scientists, on the other hand, tend to deal with groups of subjects, selected randomly or for some specific attribute; their conclusions are about groups, not about individuals. A unique feature of this book is that it presents both points of view—that of the practitioner and of the scientist.

A clear aim of this book is to help the practitioner understand the basic underlying development of ametropia. The editors and their highly qualified collaborators obviously believe, and I concur, that only when we really understand the genesis of refractive conditions will we be able to invent ways to prevent or truly correct them rather than simply neutralize them with optical devices.

The editors have selected their contributing authors wisely. I especially appreciate their using unpublished original material of Frank Weymouth ("Uncle Frank" to those of us who knew him) and Monroe Hirsch for the foundation provided in the three introductory chapters for this book. Weymouth was a basic scientist with a deep interest in sensory physiology and psychology and with an uncanny understanding of the problems of clinicians; but, most of all, he was an inspirational teacher and humanitarian. Hirsch, a student of Weymouth, was a clinician and scientist. Through his findings reported in the Ojai Longitudinal Study, Hirsch provided new facts on when and how refractive anomalies appear and change in school-age children. Before this seminal publication of *longitudinal* data, most of our knowledge about refractive anomalies was based on *cross-sectional* data from normal populations or from selected clinical samples.

Continuing from the foundation built by Hirsch and Weymouth, John Bear further discusses the epidemiology of refractive anomalies with a strong interweaving of associated genetics. He expands and modernizes some of the concepts presented by Weymouth and Hirsch. Writing as a geneticist, he makes a strong case for *vision activity* influencing the development of myopia.

The six chapters devoted to different types of refractive anomalies comprise a self-contained set. Childhood and young-adult myopia are believed by Goss to have different mechanisms of progression, increased axial elongation in both forms, with the addition of corneal power increase in the latter. A chapter on young-adult onset myopia by Baldwin, Adams, and Flattau (based on a Working Group Report for the National Research Council's Committee on Vision) reports on the myopia that appears for the first time in about 20% of nonmyopes during the four years after entering college or a military academy. Hyperopia, especially of moderate degree, is emphasized by Rosner to have important consequences on learning and on oculomotor functions such as esophoria and esotropia. Grosvenor discusses the late-adult onset myopia resulting from nuclear lens changes and the *loss* of myopia that occurs in later adulthood; both have important clinical implications. Astigmatism (by Lyle) and anisometropia (by Laird) are logically discussed with emphasis on clinical matters.

Erickson makes a major contribution to the book in his chapter on the optical components that contribute to the refractive state. He reviews previous "model" eyes, indicates their shortcomings, and presents a new approach to optical component analysis based on clinical measures.

A series of four chapters describes studies of animal eyes in an attempt to further our understanding of how refractive anomalies develop in humans. Sivak reviews two prime environmental factors—terrestrial vs aquatic life and nocturnal vs diurnal vision—and shows how the vertebrate eye has adapted its optics in response to specific environmental needs. Although there are wide differences in the optics of vertebrate eyes, Sivak points out that, "This does not rule out the possibility that the same underlying molecular events that lead to myopia are fundamental to all species."

Hodos and his colleagues have shown that although the pigeon eye tends to be emmetropic for stimuli on the horizon or in the upper field, it is myopic for objects below eye level—a purposeful adaptation for a ground-feeding animal. This group also reports that, in chicks, if the entire visual field or just the lateral field of one eye is obscured for a matter of weeks, the eye elongates (to produce myopia) overall or selectively along the axis of obscured imagery, suggesting a local retinal mechanism involving a substance that modifies scleral growth in combination with heat generated by the optical devices worn. (Interestingly, Hirsch in 1957 postulated that the fever in febrile illnesses, such as measles, in combination with raised intraocular pressure from coughing could account for the common report of myopia occurring soon after having such childhood diseases.)

Smith's chapter tells the story of how image degradation in the neonatal cat, tree shrew, monkey, and man leads to the common result of myopia, the mechanism for which appears to involve local growth-regulating molecules—although central control, possibly through accommodation, may take place in one species of monkey. Wallman's chapter addresses two mysteries of eye growth: (1) how impaired form vision leads to increased growth in certain regions of the eye, resulting in myopia, and (2) how a normal eye can be "aware" of its own refractive error and grow to eliminate it (the process of emmetropization). All of these authors show the appropriate precautionary attitude needed in evaluating animal research with the aim of uncovering the mechanisms in man responsible for emmetropization and the development of refractive anomalies. The animal research described in these chapters points the way to designing the crucial experiments to be performed in humans.

Nearly everyone from the time of Helmholtz has been impressed by the apparent association between near vision tasks and the development of childhood and young-adult myopia. It seems apparent then that accommodation or convergence or both could be the triggering mechanism. These issues are raised in a set of four interesting chapters. Greene, an engineer, develops a mechanical theory for the development of myopia in humans and experimental myopia in animals based on *mechanical stress* imposed on the posterior sclera through the combined influence of the ocular oblique muscles and intraocular pressure. Young and Leary report that during periods of accommodation, their monkeys exhibited an *increase in vitreous chamber pressure*; since the sclera is plastic rather than elastic, such continuous pressure, they theorize, should result in scleral stretching and myopia. Schor takes a more expansive view of how sustained near work (in which the eyes accommodate and converge) can produce *adaptations in accommodation and vergence* that in the short term might temporarily alter the ocular refractive state and in the long term permanently change it. Owens discusses the evidence that an *increase in ciliary tonus* (as indicated by an increased resting state of accommodation in the dark) has an important role in the development of some types of myopia, such as the early-adult onset type. He points out that as more practitioners become familiar with the eye's dark focus and measure it with "dark retinoscopy," its role in myopia will become increasingly clear.

The control of myopia using clinical methods is evaluated in the concluding five chapters. First, Grosvenor systematically discusses numerous functional treatment methods: vision training, biofeedback, under- and overcorrection of myopia with lenses, bifocals, contact lenses, and orthokeratology. Clear evidence that any of these methods can control myopia is not available. Grosvenor stresses, however, that some methods for controlling myopia, such as bifocals, may be effective if they are begun early (based on predictions from risk factors) before the eye has elongated and its scleral tissue has stretched and thinned to the extent that its resiliency is lost and it continues to elongate even with lower intraocular pressure.

Jensen and Goldschmidt discuss the use of pharmaceutical agents for the treatment of myopia. Because of substantial problems in the design of the many studies on drugs for controlling myopia, it is not possible to make a clear claim for the therapeutic benefit of cycloplegic agents, adrenergic agents, or anti-glaucoma agents. Waring provides a classification of surgical methods used in the management of myopia. Grosvenor discusses the Prospective Evaluation of Radial Keratotomy (PERK) study conducted by Waring and colleagues in 1985 and presents the pros and cons of radial keratotomy as a clinical treatment of myopia. The last chapter covers the emerging technology of corneal sculpting with the excimer laser for the management of myopia. The early evidence, sparse as it is, suggests that direct reshaping of the cornea with the excimer laser gives better results than does indirect reshaping as with radial incisions (radial keratotomy).

This is a fascinating book that should, in the words of Hercule Poirot, stir up the little grey cells of every clinician and visual scientist so that some day in the not-too-distant future, we may truly understand the genesis of refractive anomalies and be able to correct or induce them rather than just neutralize them with lenses.

Meredith W. Morgan
Berkeley, California
June 1990

PREFACE

Although vision-care practitioners devote a large proportion of their time and attention to refractive anomalies, vision scientists have traditionally all but ignored refractive anomalies as an appropriate area for investigation. However, recent evidence that an animal's refractive state can be altered by lid suturing or by defocussing the retinal image has stimulated the imagination of clinicians and researchers alike: If refractive errors can be produced, it should be possible to prevent their occurrence or even to cure them.

The traditional reluctance to consider refractive anomalies as a suitable research area undoubtedly has been based on the widespread belief that the optical system of the eye is determined strictly by genetic factors: If an individual is destined to be a myope, a hyperope, or an astigmat, what value could there be in attempting to alter the eye's optical system? On the other hand, those clinicians and researchers who have taken a more functional approach to the visual system have consistently maintained that it should be possible to alter the refractive state of the eye; unfortunately, their efforts to do so have often been disappointing.

Newfound evidence that the refractive state is subject to manipulation has served to bring the "structuralists" and the "functionalists" together, in looking for ways to better manage refractive anomalies than prescribing lenses that provide best visual acuity with accommodation relaxed. Even before the reports of experimentally induced ametropia, there was evidence of a convergence of views of those who had previously taken extreme positions: Some structuralists have accepted the possibility that fever, in febrile illnesses, might result in a stretching of the scleral collagen to produce myopia, and some functionalists are willing to accept the possibility of a hereditary basis for ametropia, although stressing that environmental factors can play an additional role. Thus it seems that the old argument of whether ametropia is genetically or environmentally determined is no longer tenable; the issue today is the *relative roles* of genetics and environment.

In spite of the existence of strong evidence for the roles of both genetics and environment in the genesis of refractive anomalies, we were struck by the fact that many practitioners were nonetheless holding to their previous views and clinical approaches. It seemed to us that the time was propitious to begin thinking clinically about refractive anomalies occurring as a result of the interaction of hereditary and environmental influences, and further to begin developing a rational basis for interventions beyond lenses that provide clear vision. This book is our attempt to initiate this new clinical approach. However, we hasten to emphasize that the book makes no attempt to provide recipes (for example) for treating myopia. Rather, we have attempted to provide evidence from a variety of sources that will place the management of refractive anomalies—in particular, myopia— on a solid footing.

We are not the first to think of such a book on refractive anomalies. Frank W. Weymouth (chairman of the Physiology Department at Stanford University and later a professor at Los Angeles College of Optometry) and Monroe J. Hirsch (professor at the Los Angeles College of Optometry, practicing optometrist in Ojai, California, and dean of the School of Optometry at the University of California) developed a common interest in myopia when they worked together at the Stanford Vision Laboratory, and started writing their book in about 1952 after having spent some years reviewing more than 3,000 relevant articles and abstracts. In 1960, when Weymouth came to Berkeley to collaborate on a research project with one of us (M.C.F.) he would spend spare moments during the day and evenings revising and polishing the first five chapters that he and Hirsch had written. Unfortunately, due to Frank's death in 1963 and Monroe's prolonged illness prior to his death in 1982, their book was never completed.

Believing that the efforts of these two scholars should not have been in vain, and having access to their original manuscripts, we set out to complete their textbook. Our approach was twofold: (1) to excerpt those portions of the Weymouth and Hirsch chapters that we felt were still timely, although almost 30 years have elapsed since they were written; and (2) to contact those people currently conducting significant clinical or laboratory research on refractive anomalies, and to invite each to write a chapter relating to the area of his or her expertise. Many of these researchers were brought together in two symposia held at an Annual Meeting of the American Academy of Optometry. Following these very successful symposia, additional researchers were approached to write chapters that would help to round out the story we wanted the book to tell.

We hope this book will prove to be useful to all who are interested in vision, whether they be students, clinicians, teachers, or researchers.

Theodore Grosvenor and *Merton Flom*
June 1990

—1

Theories, Definitions, and Classifications of Refractive Errors

Frank W. Weymouth and Monroe J. Hirsch

☐

The problem of myopia is complex and, at present, unsolved. The optical basis of the anomaly — the focusing of the image of a distant object within the vitreous — is clearly understood; but the cause, prognosis, natural history, and best form of treatment are still obscure. Voluminous literature in itself attests to the complexity of the problem and forms the basis for the present discussion. So long as myopia is not fully understood, many contradictory concepts that might otherwise be discarded must be considered and evaluated.

Many reviews of the literature on myopia have served a useful purpose; however, we go a step beyond them and attempt a critical evaluation of the literature. Thus a review of the history of myopia is useful.

The history of myopia, especially during the early years, parallels that of refraction in general. Hirschberg (1912) began his historical introduction with a discussion of the Greek scientists and quoted Galen's definition of myopia as "that condition in which near objects are clearly defined, but not distant ones." Vision, until about the tenth century, was believed to be the result of the emanation of spirits from the eyes, and the interception of the spirit of the object perceived. Accordingly, the Greek concept of myopia was that of a condition in which too little spirit of vision poured out from the brain and hence was too feeble to extend to a distant object.

The concept that vision results from light entering the eye, rather than from a spirit leaving the eye, has been attributed to the Arabian physicists of the eleventh century. The science of refraction and the understanding of the effects of convex and concave lenses dates from the work of Johannes Kepler (1611). The views of Kepler on refraction, to a great extent similar to present day views, slowly gained acceptance. Concave lenses were prescribed for myopia with increasing frequency during the two centuries after Kepler.

During the period between Kepler and the beginning of the nineteenth century, refractive errors were to a great extent ignored by physicians (including oculists), and glasses were fitted by itinerant spectacle peddlers and by opticians. Duke-Elder (1949) in his historical review of refractive errors, cited a number of noted oculists (Franz, Mackenzie, Ruete) who in their writing either ignored refractive errors or, when mentioning them, advised sending patients to the optician's shop to try a series of lenses. Duke-Elder also stressed that during the first half of the nineteenth century oculists discouraged the use of spectacles. They were thought to aggravate the existing error of refraction (myopia, Mackenzie; hyperopia, Sichel) and to be harmful. The period was characterized by warnings from oculists rather than recommendations as to the appropriate prescription.

During the two decades between 1850 and 1870, a number of truly great advances were made. These twenty years represent perhaps the most fruitful period in the history of physiological optics in general and of refraction in particular. In 1851, Helmholtz invented the ophthalmoscope, which in addition to other uses, served as an objective method for determining the refractive state of the eye. In 1856, Arlt furnished anatomical proof that high myopia was due to an elongation of the globe and that the degree of myopia bore a direct relationship to the axial length of the eye. In 1864, Donders published his "On the Anomalies of Accommodation and Refraction of the Eye," and in 1866 Helmholtz completed his "Treatise on Physiological Optics." If the science of visual optics dates from Kepler, certainly the science and art of clinical refraction date from Donders. By 1866, the refraction of light, both by the eye and by lenses, was understood; an objective method of assessing the refractive state of the eye was available; and the clinical nature of refractive anomalies had been described.

------ ■ ------

USE-ABUSE THEORY OF MYOPIA

In the same year, 1866, a new era began. A kindly ophthalmologist, Herman Cohn (the father of writer Emil Ludwig), practicing in Germany had observed that myopia increased both in prevalence and in amount as children progressed from class to class in school. Cohn published the results of a study of the eyes of 10,000 children attending the schools of Breslau. Visual hygiene was poor in European schools during this period; the illumination level was neither controlled nor adequate; books were printed on paper that gave poor contrast, and the German script was difficult to read; children sat on benches, and when desks were used they were improperly proportioned for the comfort of the children. In the light of these conditions and noting the increase in myopia in the higher grades of school, Cohn arrived at what seemed to be a reasonable conclusion: namely, that use (and particularly abuse) of the eyes was what caused myopia. A crusade for better conditions of visual hygiene was begun, and Cohn's theory dominated the scene for the next 50 years. The literature on the subject of myopia increased rapidly.

In assessing the importance of Cohn's contribution, it is necessary to understand the period in which he lived. The statistician of today will quickly recognize that Cohn inferred cause and effect from association: He noted that two events, length of attendance in school and increased myopia, were associated, and he concluded that the former was the cause of the latter. In view of the obvious defects in school hygiene, such a conclusion, although not scientifically acceptable today, was in that period reasonable. Whether scientifically accurate or not, the philosophy of Cohn bore fruit. Badly needed reforms were instituted in European schools. Hours were shortened, illumination levels were raised and controlled, the size of type used in books (especially for the very young) was increased, and desks were designed for comfort. These changes were unquestionably necessary; a comfortable environment is helpful to successful learning. It is unfortunate, however, that such reforms had to be instituted on the basis of an unfounded assumption, that is, that the use of the eyes was the cause of myopia.

Before about 1890, most measurements of refraction were made by the use of the ophthalmoscope, by the use of test types, or both. Donders' fogging method, whereby plus lens power is placed before the eye and is reduced until maximum acuity is obtained, was used in some of the studies of this time. By the end of the nineteenth century, retinoscopy had replaced ophthalmoscopy as a rapid objective method for determining the refractive state of the eye. The principles of what we now call retinoscopy were first described by Bowman who, in 1859, found that when the ophthalmoscope was moved back and forth it was possible to see a light and shadow effect in the patient's pupil. Cuignet, in 1873, made use of this light and shadow movement to determine the refractive state of the eye; however, he mistakenly concluded that he was measuring reflections from the cornea. It was not until 1886 that the principles involved in retinoscopy were correctly described by Landolt.

Theories of myopia during this period were in keeping with Cohn's theory. It was obvious that during the period of time when children used their eyes for schoolwork, the prevalence of myopia increased. Theories were put forth as to the possible mechanism for such a correlation. The child looked downward when reading, and since Arlt had demonstrated axial lengthening as a correlate of myopia, the theory arose that the pull of gravity while reading caused a lengthening of the globe. Reading required accommodation, and the theory was put forth that the lens froze in its accommodated state. Convergence was also necessary in reading, so theories arose based on the pressure of the extraocular muscles on the globe. Theories based on a combination of these two factors were then propounded. Anatomical measurements of the orbit were taken, and an attempt was made to show that certain orbital measurements required different amounts and types of convergence. Many ingenious theories were propounded and many ingenious experiments were designed, but the final proof was always lacking. There were undoubtedly individuals who opposed these attempts to explain myopia on the basis of the use and abuse of the eyes, but they were neither vocal nor persuasive.

It is interesting to note the parallel between the history of myopia and that of science in general. Most of the conflicting theories during this period, all of which were stoutly defended by their proponents, were the products of German scientists. An example, which involved both Hering and Helmholtz, was the battle in psychology between the proponents of nativism and empiricism. It has been suggested that many of these battles had their foundation in the German university system, since the proponent of a disproven theory was likely to be replaced by his scientific opponent. For this reason, many scientists held to theories they had earlier proposed, even in the light of later contradictory evidence. Whether this was the case in the medical sciences and refraction, it is true that the period was characterized by a large number of publications on the subject of myopia together with the stout defense of rather weak theories.

BIOLOGICAL (STATISTICAL) THEORY OF REFRACTIVE ERROR

A strong rival to the Cohn theory did not appear until the second decade of the twentieth century. In 1913, Steiger published his text on spherical ametropia, a work containing a mass of data, a fine bibliography, and the formulation of what may be called the biological theory of refractive errors. Strangely enough, while the works of Helmholtz, Hering, Landolt, Hirschberg, and Cohn have all been translated into English, Steiger's work has not. Nonetheless, it has become one of the keystones of the biological theory. Steiger attempted to explain refractive errors on the basis of variation of one or more of the optical elements such as the lens, cornea, or axial length: Just as the height of individuals vary, so refractive state varies; and just as height is a combination of leg length, torso length, and head height, so refractive state is the combination of the opitical elements of the eye.

Since Steiger treated the eye in the same way as any other biological variable, the methods used in other fields of biometrics were used. Distribution curves of the variables were submitted to statistical analysis. Steiger himself accumulated a large amount of data on refraction of the eyes and of the cornea. Those who followed, Scheerer and Seitzer (1929), Kronfeld and Devney (1931), Sorsby (1932), Tron (1929) and others, all used what may be termed a statistical or biometric approach. Again, it is interesting to note the parallel in other sciences. During these early twentieth century years, a similar attack was being made on many biological problems by Pearson and his co-workers in Britain. All anthropometric variables were being subjected to similar statistical analysis, and information about these variables was being accumulated.

The problem of refraction, however, was not as easy to solve. Although it is relatively simple to measure height, bone length, and other anthropometric variables, it is difficult to measure such optical elements as the axial length or diameter of the living eye. Numerous ingenious methods were used to calculate values for these elements by Czellitzer (1927), Tron (1929), and others; but no direct measurement of axial length could be made. Thus, although statistical methods were used, the raw data were subject to criticism. In recent years, the statistical approach has received considerable impetus with the development of methods for the direct measurement of certain of these elements.

Using the retinal phosphene phenomenon described earlier by Helmholtz, many researchers, including Rushton (1938), Goldmann and Hagen (1942); Deller, O'Connor, and Sorsby (1947); and Stenstrom (1946) have been able to use X-rays to measure the axial diameter of the globe in the intact living eye. This approach to the problem is promising and, while all of the desired information has by no means been accumulated, rapid strides are being made.

The present role of statistics in science is twofold: The statistician first aids the scientist in describing a body of data and second enables the scientist to generalize within certain limits on the basis of the sample. The first type of statistical procedure is known as descriptive statistics, the second as the statistics of interference. It has already been stated that during the early part of the twentieth century those who followed the biological trend in studying refractive errors began to amass data on the various optical elements and to deal with these statistically. For the most part, these efforts would fall in the realm of descriptive statistics. On the other hand, the use of inferential methods to state the probability that certain observed phenomena could be due to chance has influenced the works of most authors, even today. The theories and hypotheses proposed have not been proven statistically.

Although refraction, like science in general, is of universal interest, certain national schools can be recognized. The beginning of the science of refraction was definitely a German and Dutch accomplishment. During the last half of the nineteenth century, data were accumulated by investigators in most European countries. Scientists in Russia, Scandanavia, France, and Britain, all under the influence of Cohn, investigated refraction in schools and proposed environmental improvements. Germany, however, was clearly the center of this activity. With the advent of Steiger's theory, there was a shift westward, for although Steiger was Swiss, a great deal of work on the biological approach to refraction centered in Britain. Steiger's theory found ready acceptance in England, to a great extent because of the influence of the statistician Pearson on British science in general.

Some of the larger studies in recent years have been American. Duke-Elder (1949) dedicated the section on refraction to Edward Jackson, and it seems reasonable to credit American authors with a good deal of recent work using a clinical approach. On the other hand, studies using the X-ray approach have been decidedly a European contribution, having been conducted by Swiss, British, and Swedish investigators. In recent years, a Russian group interested in the sociology of refraction has been active. Probably as a result of the two world wars, German contributions have fallen in both quality and quantity. This was particularly true during Hitler's regime when a good bit of nonsensical material, exhibiting a definite racial bias, appeared. The modern literature seems to be primarily British and American, with a strong base also in Scandanavia.

In summary, just as modern refraction dates from Donders, so the modern history of myopia may be said to have started in Donders' time. The first major theory, and one still followed today, was that proposed by Cohn in 1866 and more recently by Brown (1942), the use-abuse theory. Numerous subtheories attempt to explain how the use of the eyes can cause the development of myopia, but all have in common the basic tenet that myopia will develop if certain environmental conditions are present. The second major theory, for which Steiger is credited, did not receive any recognition until almost 50 years later. This theory, sometimes called the biological or statistical theory, states that myopia occurs as a result of biological variability. Here, too, there are a number of subtheories and minor differences, but those who adhere to the theory agree on one point: Factors other than environment are, for the most part, responsible for myopia.

DEFINING MYOPIA

The result of a discussion may be determined by a definition, which is, in a sense, the first assumption made in any hypothesis. Moreover, a definition reflects a theory or a short synopsis of a hypothesis. This section discusses a representative sample of definitions of myopia, and the reader is urged to carefully consider their implications.

Helmholtz (1856) described the myopic eye as "one for which the far point is a short distance away, sometimes only a few inches from the eye." The far point of the eye, it will be recalled, is the most distant point that is sharply focused (and, therefore, conjugate to the retina) when accommodation is relaxed. Donders (1864) described the myopic eye as "one in which the focus of the dioptric system lies in front of the retina; in other words, parallel rays derived from infinitely remote object units in the myopic eye focus in front of the retina when the eye is at rest." Numerous variations have emerged from this classical and, certainly most widely accepted definition. The definitions of both Helmholtz and Donders specify, or imply, the state of the vergence of light rays on the retina and the status of accommodation. These definitions make no assumptions about the cause of myopia, nor do they suggest how myopia might be assessed clinically.

A second type of definition attempts to explain how such a condition might be brought about — for example, "In the usual form of myopia the posterior principal focus lies in front of the retina because of an elongated eyeball (axial myopia)," and "that form of ametropia in which the axis of the eyeball is too long or the refractive power too strong, so that parallel rays are focused in front of the retina."

It will be noted that these definitions include both the elements of the earlier definitions and a statement of the possible cause of the condition as well.

A third type of definition or description of myopia is based on testing procedures, that is, an operational definition — such as, "myopia is a condition in which there is an acceptance of minus spheres . . . with a resultant improvement in vision." A difficulty with this definition is, of course, the lack of any statement about the status of accommodation. An operational definition might also be based not on subjective refraction (as is the preceding definition) but on retinoscopy. Myopia on such a basis would be defined as "that refractive state in which minus or diverging lenses are necessary in order to arrive at a point of neutral motion with the retinoscope while the subject fixates a distant object."

Operational definitions have the advantage that no assumptions need to be made, the definition being merely a description of the procedure used. Were it not for the fact that the optics of the eye are irrefutably established, such definitions might be highly desirable. However, since the optics are so well understood and firmly based, such definitions need not be used: Evidence in physiological optics overwhelmingly supports the view that blurred vision in uncorrected myopia and against motion in retinoscopy are due to the focus of the image of a distant object in front of the retina.

Two more recent definitions, those of Atkinson and of Laurance and Wood, are no more than well-worded variations of the original Donders and Helmholtz definitions. Atkinson (1944) defines myopia as "that condition of refraction in which the posterior principal focus of the eye lies in front of the retinal plane, so that neutral light waves, instead of focusing on the retina, come to a focus before they reach it, are reversed, and fall on the retina in diffusion circles of plus waves . . . the focal length of the refracting system of the eye is less than the anterior-posterior diameter of the eyeball." Laurance and Wood (1936) define myopia as "the condition of the eye in which, with accommodation suspended, parallel light comes to a focus in front of the retina, the latter being situated beyond the posterior principal focal distance of the refracting system."

CLASSIFYING MYOPIA

A major difficulty in classifying myopia is defining the question of degree that must be present before the condition is referred to as myopia. It is understood today that the spherical refractive states form a continuum, ranging from the greatest degree of hyperopia through emmetropia to the greatest degree of myopia. Sorsby has given Steiger credit for having been the first to clearly enunciate this concept. Those authors who have been interested in the statistical aspects of refractive errors (Scheerer and Seitzer, 1929; Betsch, 1929; Sorsby, 1932; Dunstan, 1934;

Stenstrom, 1946) have evaluated their data on this basis. Emmetropia on such a scale is an infinitesimally small classification, depending more on the accuracy of measurement and arbitrary criteria than on anything else. If the accuracy of measurement were 0.50 diopters (D), there would be more emmetropes than if it were 0.25 D, and if the degree of ametropia could be determined to the nearest 0.01 D there would be very few emmetropes.

□ Classification by Degree

One of the systems used frequently in the past involved three categories: emmetropia, hyperopia, and myopia. Three of the many methods that have been used to define points of demarcation among these three categories are shown in Table 1.1. Other systems have been used as well, but these will suffice to demonstrate the difficulties encountered. It should be obvious that an author using system A (Table 1.1) will find a greater percentage of emmetropes in a given population than will an author using system B, who, in turn, will find more emmetropes than an author using system C. Occasionally, an author will state what criteria were used in classifying ametropias; but all too often such a statement has been omitted, and the reader who attempts to compare the results of various studies cannot interpret the data.

Degree of refractive error also affects classifying refractive errors as low, medium, or high. For comparison, the classifications of myopia used by Jackson (1900), Hirschberg (1912), May (1949), and Duke-Elder (1943) are presented in tabular form. There are other arbitrary classifications, but these, shown in Table 1.2, illustrate the problem.

Because such categories as low, medium, and high myopia are arbitrary and because the concept of a continuum obviates the necessity of a term such as emmetropia, it would seem desirable to classify myopia in terms of numerical degree only. Although a system of low, medium, and high myopia may have certain clinical advantages, its impact on the thinking of those engaged in working with refractive errors makes it undesirable. It is just as simple to write "a 3.00 D myope" as "a myope of medium degree," and the meaning is much clearer because the reader does not have to concern himself with the writer's concept of "medium."

Table 1.1.   Classification of Ametropia and Emmetropia by Degree

System	Myopia	Hyperopia	Emmetropia
A	More than −1.00 D	More than +1.00 D	−1.00 D to +1.00 D
B	All minus lenses	More than +1.00 D	0.00 D to +1.00 D
C	All minus lenses	All plus lenses	0.00 D

Table 1.2. Categorical Classification of Myopia by Degree

Category of myopia	Degree of myopia			
	Jackson	Hirschberg	May	Duke-Elder
Low myopia	up to 2 D	up to 3 D	up to 3 D	up to 6 D
Medium or moderate	2 to 4 D	3 to 6 D	3 to 6 D	—
High myopia	4 to 10 D	6 to 15 D	over 6 D	over 6 D
Very high myopia	—	over 15 D	—	—

□ Classifications Involving Astigmatism

It was stated in the preceding section that emmetropia is only a theoretical concept and is more of an expression of the accuracy of measurement than of any other factor. Similarly, spherical refractive errors — myopia or hyperopia unaccompanied by astigmatism — are also only theoretical, as almost every eye has some astigmatism. Because the refractive power is different in the various meridians of the eye, the ideal method of presenting the data is unclear. Proposed methods include the following:

1. Some authors who use a three-category system (myopia, hyperopia, and emmetropia) have arbitrarily chosen the meridian of greatest power, whereas others have chosen the meridian of least power.
2. In some reports a fourth category, that of astigmatism, has been added. What degree of astigmatism has been included in this category differs with different authors: For example, in his commentary accompanying volume I of Helmholtz' *Treatise on Physiological Optics*, Gullstrand mentions that the limit of normal astigmatism should be given as 0.50 D.
3. Some authors classify astigmatic subjects into one of the three categories of spherical ametropia as well as into the astigmatic class. Thus, in some of Pearson's studies, the number of myopes, hyperopes, emmetropes, and astigmatic persons adds up to more than the total number of cases in the investigation, each case of astigmatism being listed twice — once as an astigmatism and once according to the spherical error.
4. Some authors use a three-category system and omit from their results all cases of astigmatism, the criterion for omission varying with different authors.
5. A method that the present authors and many other investigators have used is *spherical equivalent* refractive error, that is, averaging the power of the correcting lens in the two principal meridians.

It is obvious that the interpretation of statistics accumulated by other authors will depend on, among other things, the method of classifying astigmatism. In addition to using spherical equivalent refraction, the present authors have also used refraction in the horizontal meridian. Others have used the mean of the two principal meridians for both eyes, that is, the average of the spherical equivalents for the two eyes. Any of these methods will give results that can be handled statistically.

□ Descriptive Classifications

A number of adjectives have been used to describe myopia, and, as with definitions, these, too, represent assumptions. This concept may be demonstrated by considering one set of frequently used terms.

When it was observed that the prevalence of myopia was greater in the higher grades of school than in the lower grades, the term *school myopia* was introduced and was defined as "that myopia which comes on during the school years." With the general acceptance of this term, the concept that myopia was in fact *caused* by school work became firmly entrenched and is today a view held by many, although little evidence exists other than the increased prevalence of myopia in the higher grades. Such a definition, then, while inherently sound as a description of a phenomenon, is dangerous because of the emotional response it produces and because of the tendency to forget that it is only a description.

During the school years, the child is growing, so instead of school myopia this condition is sometimes termed *developmental myopia*. Such a term, while equally descriptive of the condition, immediately elicits a different emotional response, for now the reader concludes that the use of the eyes plays a lesser role and that the myopia is the result of a developmental process. Use of the still stronger adjective *maturation* would imply that the use of the eyes played a still smaller part in causation. If the cause of myopia were known, there would be no difficulty in choosing descriptive terminology, but in the light of present knowledge there seems to be no reason to adopt such terminology. Only those adjectives with little or no emotional tone and with the greatest descriptive power are desirable: Terms such as school myopia, developmental myopia, or maturational myopia, which suggest known causation, should be avoided.

□ Classification by Refractive Component

It has seemed logical to many authors to classify myopia as *axial, refractive, index, lenticular,* and so on, depending on which components of the eye must be altered to produce myopia. Such terminology, however, is undesirable for a number of reasons. For example, axial myopia would be present only if all other refractive components were held constant. However, there is no reason to assume that average values will be found in any individual eye, and hence the term axial is artificial. Essentially, such categorization assumes that one component differs from an arbitrary normal (or average) value, whereas all others are normal (or average). There appears to be no reason for such an assumption.

Optically, myopia results from a combination of various elements and their relationships to one another. An eye is not myopic because it is too long, but rather because it is too long for its particular refractive system or, conversely, because its refractive system is too strong for its axial length. Who is to say, then, whether a given myopic eye is axial or refractive? Moreover, simple calculations show that it is possible for a hyperopic eye to have an axial length in excess of "normal." In short, the terms axial, refractive, lenticular, and index seem to be of little real value other than as teaching aids for beginning students in optics. The distinctions made are highly artificial and lead to an undesirable mind set.

□ Classification by Other Criteria

Some authors have classified myopia on the basis of dichotomies such as primary vs secondary, simple vs degenerative, benign vs malignant, and congenital vs acquired. For example, Stansbury (1948) thought that there were two types of myopia and concluded: "A classification of myopia is essential in statistical and clinical research on this condition. The terms *primary and secondary* are suggested as simple and descriptive. . . . Differential diagnosis of these two types is of great importance clinically, in therapy and prognosis." Duke-Elder (1949) also has been troubled by this problem. He suggests the term *degenerative myopia* and introduces it as follows: "To find a suitable name to indicate the class of case described in this section has cost me some thought. The condition is frequently termed *progressive myopia*; but, as the habit of hypermetropia is to regress during development, so the majority of myopes — most of them of the simple type — progress. *High myopia* (for example above 6 D) is also inappropriate, for myopes should be classified not by retinoscopy but by ophthalmoscopy; low myopes, and indeed, eyes with an axial length less than normal, may show the degenerative changes characteristic of myopia, while cases over − 17.00 D may show no abnormal changes in the fundus (Harman, 1913). *Malignant*, as opposed to *benign*, myopia has too grave a connotation unless it is reserved for the worst cases — when, indeed, it is applicable. To complicate terminology, particularly in a well-known condition, is almost an unpardonable sin; but the term used here has the merit of describing what I mean. [p. 4313]"

The terms *congenital, hereditary*, and *acquired* are also used frequently in classifying myopia and certainly have some merit as descriptive terms. *Congenital* myopia is myopia present at birth; the only serious objection to its use is that refractive state is seldom measured at birth. Thus congenital myopia may be "early acquired myopia." *Hereditary* myopia is myopia present either at birth or later in a child whose ancestors exhibited a similar refractive error. The suitability of this term will depend on the strength of the evidence for hereditary transmission, a phase of the problem which will be discussed more fully in later chapters.

Acquired myopia is used to describe the myopic refractive state in a patient who did not have myopia at birth. This term is most undesirable since it implies an active process. The standard definition of the word acquire is "to gain, usually by one's own exertions." A term of this sort will obviously seem to support the theory that the use of the eyes is responsible for myopia. Until the evidence for an active acquisition of myopia is examined, we should be wary of this term.

The reader may wonder how so many terms came into use, especially since it has been stated here that many of the terms are undesirable. It should be understood that there are many theories of myopia causation: Duke-Elder (1949) lists eleven different theories. Each theory contributes certain terms; and many of these terms (such as *school myopia*, *developmental myopia*, and *maturational myopia*) describe the same condition but from the standpoint of different theories. Moreover, many of the terms are clinical in nature, for the clinician must classify the various disorders observed. Such classification often involves making assumptions or using working hypotheses. Clearly, the clinician cannot undertake a research project each time a patient is observed. On the other hand, the research investigator must make as few assumptions as possible. The reader, who will probably be both clinician and investigator, should realize this difference and adopt a different attitude reflecting both roles. The clinical approach will be to say, "This patient appears to have signs of pathological significance, so I'll call it pathological myopia." The investigative role will prompt the question, "What is the evidence that this myopia is really due to pathology?"

RECOMMENDATIONS

As stated earlier, a relatively satisfactory definition is that of Laurance and Wood (1936): "Myopia is a condition of an eye in which, when accommodation is suspended, parallel light comes to a focus in front of the retina, the latter being situated beyond the posterior principal focal distance of the refracting system." However, since accommodation is never completely suspended, a somewhat preferable phrase has been suggested, namely, "when acted upon only by normal tonus of the ciliary muscle."

The introduction of the concept of *tonus* is good, but the term "normal" seems unnecessary: The term "standard" best defines the conditions of the test. The following definition includes the best features of the others: "Myopia is that state of refraction in which the axial length of the globe is greater than the posterior focal distance of the refracting system when only that ciliary tonus which occurs under standard conditions is active." The suggested definition of standard conditions is as follows: "In refraction, standard conditions prevail when the eye is fixating a distant object that the individual is attempting to see through a fogging lens." This definition is equally applicable for the subjective method of refraction, using trial lenses and the test chart, or for retinoscopy, the two methods currently in use. Unusual situations, such as the refraction of the newborn, will require the use of some means for relaxing accommodation other than that suggested by the definition. Whenever such a method is used, it should be remembered that this alternative only approximates the proposed standard conditions.

Although many methods of classifying myopia have been discussed, all have been discarded as prejudicial. Although some of the terms used in these classifications may have pedagogical or clinical value, it is best to disregard them at the outset, with a view toward arriving at acceptable terms as the accumulated evidence allows.

REFERENCES

Arlt F. Die Krankheiten des Auges, Prague: Creder & Kleinbub, vol. 3, 1856.

Atkinson TG. Oculo-refractive cyclopedia and dictionary, 3rd ed. Chicago: Professional Press, 1944.

Bannon, RE. Use of cycloplegia in refraction. Am J Optom Arch Am Acad Optom 1947;24:513–568.

Betsch A. Uber die menschliche Refractionskurve. Klin Monatsbl Augenheilkd 1929; 82:365.

Bothman L. Refraction changes in the eyes of children under six years of age. Arch Ophthalmol 1932;7:294–296.

Brown EVL. Use-abuse theory of changes in refraction versus biological theory. Arch Ophthalmol 1942;28:845–850.

Cohn H. Unter der Augen von 10060 Schulkindern nebst Vorsehlangen zur Verbesserung der Augen Nachteilligin Schuleinrichtungen. Leipzig: Eine Atiologische Studie, 1866.

Cohn H. Die Refraction der Augen von 240 atropisieten Dorfschulkindern. Albrecht Von Graefes Arch Ophthalmol 1871;17:305.

Czellitzer A. Totalrefraktion und Horn-haut-refracktion mit besonderer berucksichtigung des physiologischen Linsenastigmatismus. Klin Monatsbl Augenheilkd 1927;79:301.

Deller JFP, O'Connor AD, Sorsby A. X-ray measurement of diameters of the living eye. Proc R Soc Lond, Series E, 1947;144:456–466.

Donders FC. On the Anomalies of Accommodation and Refraction of the Eye. London: The New Sydenham Society, 1864.

Duke-Elder WS. The Practice of Refraction. Philadelphia: Blakiston Co., 1943.

Duke-Elder WS. Textbook of Ophthalmology, vol. 4. St. Louis: CV Mosby Co., 1949.

Dunstan WR. Variation and refraction. Br J Ophthalmol 1934;28:404–421.

Goldmann H, Hagen R. Zur direkten Messung der Totalbrechkidff des lebendigen menschilichen Auges. Ophthalmologica 1942;104:15–22.

Harman NB. An analysis of 300 cases of high myopia in children, with a scheme for the grading of fundus changes in myopia. Trans Ophthalmol Soc UK 1913;33:202.

Helmholtz H von. Treatise on Physiological Optics, vol. 1, 1856. Engl transl, New York: Optical Society of America, 1924.

Hirsch MJ. Recent trends in thought in myopia. Opt J Rev Optom 1949;86:31–32.

Hirsch MJ. An analysis of inhomogeneity of myopia in adults. Am J Optom Arch Am Acad Optom 1950;27:S 562–571.

Hirschberg J. The treatment of shortsight (G. Lindsay Johnson, trans.). New York: Rebman Co., 1912.

Jackson E. Manual of the diagnosis and treatment of the diseases of the eyes. Philadelphia: Saunders, 1900.

Kempf GA, Collins SD, Jarman BL. Refractive Errors in the Eyes of Children as Determined by Retinoscopic Examination with a Cycloplegic. Public Health Bull No 182. Washington DC: Govt Printing Office, 1928.

Kepler J. Dioptrics. Augsburg: David Franke, 1611.

Kronfeld PD, Devney C. Ein Beitragzur Kenntnis der Refraktions Kurve. Albrecht Von Graefes Arch Ophthalmol 1931;126:487.

Landolt E. The Refraction and Accommodation of the Eye. Edinburgh: Young J. Pentland, 1886.

Laurance L, Wood HO. Visual Optics and Sight Testing. Chicago: Chicago Medical Book Co., 1936.

May CH. Diseases of the Eye, 17th ed. Baltimore: Williams & Wilkens, 1949.

Rushton J. Clinical measurement of axial length in the living eye. Trans Ophthal Soc UK 1938;58:136–140.

Scheerer R, Seitzer A. Uber des Auftreten von sogenannten myopischen Veranderungen am Augenhindergrund bei den verschiedenen Brechungszustanded des Auges. Klin Monatsbl Augenheilkd 1929;82:511. (Original not examined; cited by Stenstrom S, 1948.)

Sheard C. The comparative value of various methods and practices in skiametry. Am J Physiol Opt 1922;3:177.

Sorsby A. School myopia. Br J Ophthalmol 1932;16:217.

Sourasky A. The growth and development of myopia: a study in the changes of refraction during the school period. Br J Ophthalmol 1928;12:625.

Stansbury FC. Pathogenesis of myopia, a new classification. AMA Arch Ophthalmol 1948;39:273–299.

Steiger A. Die Entstehung der spharischen Refracktionen des menschlichen Auges. Berlin: S Karger, 1913.

Tron E. Variationstatisticke untersuchungen uber refracktion. Albrecht Von Graefes Arch Ophthalmol 1929;122:1–33.

2

Prevalence of Refractive Anomalies

Monroe J. Hirsch and Frank W. Weymouth

☐

The prevalence of myopia, like that of any anomaly or disease, may be considered with respect to four variables: (1) age, (2) gender, (3) ethnicity, and (4) environment.* Analysis of the prevalence of disease on the basis of these variables has proved useful and merits careful application to the problems of refraction. For example, the prevalence of diabetes among Jews and among persons of better than average economic status has called attention to the importance of dietary factors in the etiology of this disease. The greater prevalence of deficient color vision among males led to a study of its inheritance and to a genetic hypothesis of its transmission. The observation that scrotal cancer was found in an unduly large number of chimney sweeps led to the discovery of the carcinogenic action of certain coal tar derivatives.

Numerous other examples from the field of general medicine might be given, all serving equally to stress the importance of understanding the prevalence of an anomaly according to the suggested variables in the population. Clearly this subject is of more than academic interest, and the careful study of reliable data will lead not only to a better understanding of myopia but may suggest prophylactic measures deserving investigation.

The prevalence of refractive anomalies will be discussed in terms of 5 age groups:

1. The newborn.
2. Preschool children (from birth to 6 years).
3. Schoolchildren (from 6 to 18 years).
4. Early maturity (from 18 to 55 years).
5. Late maturity (over 55 years).

---

*The latter two variables are discussed in Chapter 4.

Although there is some physiological basis for this grouping, it is determined mainly by the accessibility of persons for measurement. Thus, refractive data on the newborn have come usually from maternity hospitals, from school visual surveys of schoolchildren, from military draft data, and from data on all groups from clinic and private practice records. Preschool children and persons in early and late maturity are of particular interest and importance as will be discussed later. Unfortunately, apparently because of their relative inaccessibility, these groups are poorly represented in the available data.

It should be clear that for valid generalizations about prevalence, the data must be drawn from random samples of the total population. The data most nearly approaching this ideal are those from school surveys and from draft examinations: Those from maternity hospitals, clinics, and private practices all represent varying degrees of selection. Infants measured in maternity hospitals often fail to represent the lower income groups; patients of clinics and private practices represent not the total population but that of those seeking relief from eye problems and, furthermore, differ from each other to the extent that they come from disparate economic groups. Some investigators, realizing that data from private practice are selected, have attempted to use a correction factor to make the data more truly representative. This practice cannot be too heartily condemned; the results are invariably worse than those of raw data, however much the raw data may have been biased.

Although data from the various age groups may be combined to furnish a picture of change in prevalence with age, the unequal representation and the differing types of selection make this a far from satisfactory procedure. The need for *longitudinal* studies, in which a single group of subjects, randomly selected, is reexamined periodically for a number of years, cannot be too strongly emphasized.

———— ■ ————

THE NEWBORN

Early data on the refractive state of infants are those of Jaeger (1861), who made ophthalmoscopic measurements without the use of cycloplegia. Callan (1875) in discussing this paper states that "as there are few, if any who excel him in the use of that instrument (ophthalmoscope) his results must be regarded as accurate." The infants examined by Jaeger were between 9 and 16 days old, and 78 of the 100 investigated were found to be myopic. This high percentage of myopia, according to Callan, was attributed to the great sphericity of the infantile lens and the incomplete development of the zonule of Zinn. Later authors, not finding the high percentage of myopia which Jaeger found, thought his results were incorrect because he did not use a cycloplegic.

The results of other early German authors may be briefly mentioned. Ely (1880), using atropine, found 11% of 100 eyes of children less than 2 months old to be myopic, whereas 33% of forty-nine eyes examined without atropine were found to be myopic (a value still much lower than that reported by Jaeger). To settle the dispute between Jaeger and Ely, Horstmann (1880) examined with atropine 40 eyes of infants under 20 days of age and found four myopes (two of − 0.50 D and two of − 1.00 D), or 10% of the number examined. Königstein (1881) found that only 2% of 600 eyes were myopic: the majority were hyperopic between 2.00 and 3.00 D, and many had more than 3.00 D of hyperopia.

Germann (1885) seems to have found a greater prevalence of hyperopia, together with a higher average value, than any other investigator. Three hundred consecutive cases yielded not one myope; later, two were found. One was a 3-month-old infant with myopia of 4.00 D, and the other was the child of a 12.00 D congenitally myopic physician. Germann found all of the 110 infants measured during the first 3 months of life to be hyperopic, some as high as 12.00 D, with an average hyperopia of 4.84 D. The percentages of the 220 eyes of the 110 infants showing varying degrees of hyperopia are given in Table 2.1, in which they are classified by age. These data indicate that hyperopia, high in degree at birth, declines markedly during the first 2 months of life.

All early investigators used the ophthalmoscope. With the exception of Jaeger, all used atropine. For this reason, Jaeger's results have been questioned.

The contribution of each to the total is indicated in Table 2.2. It is apparent, first, that the contributions are very unequal in number (Herrnheiser's data have over 20 times the weight of the data of de Vries). Second, the forms of the individual distributions are very different, that of Herrnheiser having a form that is very unusual for biological material, a fact noted by Wibaut.

Studies of the refraction of the newborn have for many years been neglected, probably because the data accumulated toward the end of the last century were considered adequate. The results of four of these studies were combined by Wibaut (1926), and his almost universally accepted data have been more widely quoted than those of any other author. The distribution of refractive states presented by Wibaut was characterized by a mean of about 2.50 D of hyperopia, a standard deviation of 1.52 (about the same as that for the adult), practically no myopia, and a distribution curve that is not significantly different from normal.

Table 2.1. Refraction of 220 Eyes of Newborns (Germann, 1885)

Degree of hyperopia	Number of eyes	Examined at 1 month	Examined at 2 months
0.00 to 1.00 D	8	2.3%	10.0%
1.25 to 4.00 D	95	36.3%	65.0%
4.25 to 8.00 D	98	50.0%	25.0%
8.00 to 12.00 D	19	11.3%	0.0%

Table 2.2.   Data on 3,938 Eyes of Newborn, Reported by Wibaut

	Herrnheiser (1,920 eyes)	Horstman (100 eyes)	Schleich (300 eyes)	de Vries (78 eyes)	Total (2,398 eyes)	Weighted Total*
−4.00 D	—	—	—	1	1	8
−3.00 D	—	—	—	2	2	15
−2.00 D	2	—	2	1	5	20
−1.00 D	—	—	—	1	1	8
0.00 D	—	—	10	11	21	145
+1.00 D	563	6	16	10	595	363
+2.00 D	683	26	16	15	741	478
+3.00 D	319	41	36	12	408	489
+4.00 D	251	68	14	12	345	390
+5.00 D	72	68	4	6	150	229
+6.00 D	30	58	2	5	95	176
+7.00 D	—	31	—	1	32	70
+8.00 D	—	—	—	1	2	10
Mean	+2.3 D	+2.4 D	+4.6 D	+2.4 D	+2.6 D	+2.9 D
SD	1.2 D	1.5 D	1.5 D	2.3 D	1.6 D	1.6 D
% Myopes	0.1 %	2.0 %	0.0 %	6.4 %	0.4 %	2.1 %

*Weighted by Hirsch and Weymouth (see text).

Data indicating that Wibaut's distribution was in error have appeared occasionally. Santonastaso (1930), for example, found that 25% of the newborns reported on by Wibaut were myopic. Nevertheless, a new study of the refraction of the newborn did not appear until 1951. The invalidity of Wibaut's long-accepted data rests on the method of examination (ophthalmoscopic determination) used by those whose results form the basis for his study, and on the inhomogeneity of the material of the four investigators.

Cook and Glasscock (1951), using atropine cycloplegia and a retinoscope (rather than an ophthalmoscope), determined the refractive state of 1,000 infant eyes at the Medical School Hospital of the University of Arkansas. Of this number, 625 were black and 375 were white. Because racial differences seem to exist, and because these data will be compared to other groups of whites, only the latter group will be discussed here. The frequency distribution for the refraction of the 375 eyes of newborn white infants is presented in Figure 2.1. The pertinent data for this frequency distribution are as follows:

Mean	+2.07 ± 0.14 D
Standard deviation	2.73 ± 0.10 D

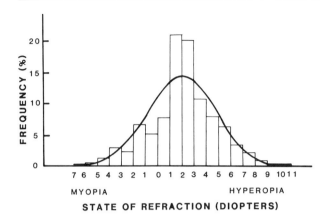

Figure 2.1.
Histogram and distribution curve for refractive state of 375 eyes of newborn white infants. (Data from Cook and Glasscock, 1951.)

g_1 (skewness)	-0.19 ± 0.13 D
g_2 (kurtosis)	$+0.41 \pm 0.25$ D

The values presented with each of the four major parameters are their respective *standard errors*. These figures, as well as the similar ones for the data of Wibaut (1926) and Kempf et al. (1928) (to be quoted later), were not given by the original authors but were calculated from their data by the present authors. The major parameters for the data of Kronfeld and Devney (1931) were calculated by Shyojiro Tom Taketa (a student of the authors) and the standard errors by the present authors.

In describing the frequency distributions of refractive states, use is made of certain statistical terms, which, although found in the common texts on statistics, may not be familiar to some readers. The four parameters of characteristic value of a distribution are as follows:

1. The arithmatic mean, or average, familiar to all.
2. The standard deviation, in the same units as the mean, measuring the scatter or variability and thus analogous to range.
3. The skewness, an abstract measure of asymmetry, which may be positive (long tail to the right, or high value) or negative (long tail to the left, or low value).
4. The kurtosis, an abstract measure of peakedness. For a particular standard deviation, the distribution may be normal, or mesokurtic (zero kurtosis); leptokurtic, or more peaked than normal and with longer tails (positive kurtosis); or platokurtic, or more flat-topped than normal, with shorter tails (negative kurtosis).

On the basis of these figures, we may make a number of observations with regard to the refraction of the newborn.

1. The average refraction, 2.07 D of hyperopia, conforms with that reported in most studies and requires no comment here.

2. The standard deviation of 2.73 D is considerably greater than the value of 1.52 D reported by Wibaut, and is a surprising finding. Because standard deviations reported for adults were 2.20 ± 0.05 D (Stenstrom, 1948) and 1.66 ± 0.03 D (Kronfeld and Devney, 1931), the standard deviation found by Cook and Glasscock (1951) is seen to be significantly greater (P_F = .001) than that of adults instead of being the same as indicated by Wibaut's data. If the data of Cook and Glasscock are accepted instead of those of Wibaut, considerable change in thinking will be necessary, and future theories will have to explain a decreased variability as the child grows instead of a lack of change in variability as was formerly thought.

3. The skewness does not differ significantly from that of a normal curve (g_1 = 0), a fact in agreement with Wibaut's data.

4. The distribution is slightly leptokurtic (excessively peaked compared with the normal curve). The value for g_2 of +0.41 borders on significance: Only five times in 100 (P = .05) would a value this high or higher be obtained by chance if the kurtosis were normal (g_2 = 0). This finding does not agree with Wibaut's data, as his distribution did not differ significantly from a normal curve. It is known that leptokurtosis characterizes the distribution of refractive states of the *adult*, but formerly it was believed (on the basis of Wibaut's data) that this characteristic of the distribution developed after birth.

Sato (1951) has written, "Judging from the fact that the distribution of the refractive state of the newborn does not show this special grouping (leptokurtosis) and that it is seen while they are growing up, the presumption is possible that the factors causing the change in grouping (increasing leptokurtosis) come from adaptation to external conditions." Thus, the absence of leptokurtosis at birth and its presence later in life is held by Sato as evidence for an environmental influence on the genesis of refractive state. However, the fact that leptokurtosis is present at birth would indicate that even if leptokurtosis *did* indicate environmental influence (a theory open to question), Sato's argument is invalid. This question will be discussed at greater length later in the chapter.

5. Examination of the figure shows the presence of a number of cases of myopia up to 6.00 D. There were seventy-two myopic eyes in the group of 375, or about 19%. This figure is in fair agreement with the 25% found by Santonastaso. Furthermore, as will be shown when these figures are compared to those for children entering school, this myopia found at birth disappears during early childhood (Santonastaso claims that it had disappeared completely by the end of the first year of life).

PRESCHOOL CHILDREN

Data for the refraction of young children are unfortunately lacking, probably because of difficulty obtaining a random sample of subjects during the first 5 years of life. The clinical data of Brown (1936) for children between the ages of 2 and 6 years who came to his practice suggest that the mean refraction becomes more hyperopic with age. However, because of the nature of Brown's data (clinical data) and the method of sampling, it is not possible to calculate the distribution curves for various ages.

The youngest children investigated by the present authors are 5-year-olds randomly selected from public schools. However, because these data were accumulated in a school survey and cycloplegia was impractical, it may be argued that they should not be compared with those of the newborn measured with use of atropine. Exact values obtained by the authors, therefore, will not be given, but trends observed will be discussed later. Fortunately, a study of 6- to 8-year-olds was made under conditions similar to those used in investigating the newborn. This study, by Kempf, Collins, and Jarman (1928), based on retinoscopic determination under cycloplegia and with random sampling, is ideally suitable for comparison with the similarly accumulated data of Cook and Glasscock.

The distribution of the refractive states of 333 children between the ages of 6 and 8 examined by Kempf et al. is presented in Figure 2.2. The characteristics of the distribution are as follows:

Mean	$+1.06 \pm 0.09$ D
Standard deviation	1.62 ± 0.06 D
g_1 (skewness)	$+0.73 \pm 0.13$ D
g_2 (kurtosis)	$+2.66 \pm 0.27$ D

The frequency polygon for the data of Kempf et al. is presented with the similar graph for the newborn data of Cook and Glasscock in Figure 2.3. On the basis of these two studies, certain general statements can be made about the changes in refraction that occur some time during the first 6 years of life. It is unfortunate that more precise year-by-year changes cannot be reported, but the present data give some indication of what is occurring. The following conclusions may be drawn:

The mean shifts about 1.00 D toward less hyperopia. Inspection of Figure 2.3 shows that most children's eyes seem to change by about this amount.

1. The standard deviation is significantly reduced, which is of considerable importance. Figure 2.3 shows that this reduction in variability during the early years of life is caused by the disappearance of both myopes and higher hyperopes. This

Figure 2.2.
Frequency distribution
for refractive state of
333 children between
the ages of 6 and 8
years. (Data from
Kempf, Collins, and
Jarman, 1928.)

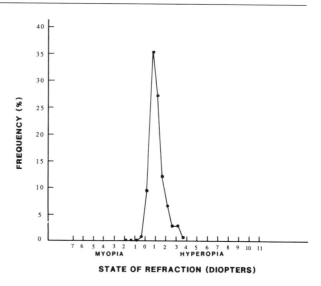

Figure 2.3.
Frequency distributions
for refractive states of
375 eyes of newborn
white infants (data from
Cook and Glasscock,
1951) and 333 children
between the ages of 6
and 8 years. (Data from
Kempf, Collins, and
Jarman, 1928.)

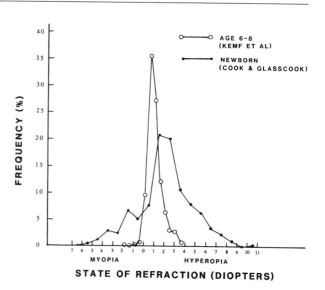

clearly indicates that during early growth a considerable degree of "emmetropization" takes place. The physical correlates of this phenomenon must assume an important place in any theory of the genesis of refractive errors.

2. The measure of skewness, g_1, which does not differ significantly from that for the normal curve at birth, is significantly greater than zero, indicating positive skewness or extreme deviation on the hyperopic side. Other studies made by the

authors, to be presented later, indicate that positive skewness exists at the age of 6 years, and that this value declines, reaching zero again at about the age of 9 or 10 years, and continuing on toward the negative skewness that characterizes the adult distribution curve.

3. The distribution curve, which was slightly leptokurtic at birth, is markedly so by age 6 to 8 years. Stenstrom (1948), who thought that the data of Stromberg (1936) were more representative of random sampling than were his own, calculated the degree of kurtosis for Stromberg's data, and found a value for g_2 of $+28.36$. We believe that this value is unduly high (Kronfeld and Devney, for example, found a value of $+4.56$), but all adult data yielded a value of g_2 in excess of $+4.00$. Thus, the distribution of refractive state becomes increasingly leptokurtic with age. However, it is important to note the significant variation from normality (in the direction of leptokurtosis) at birth, which increased considerably during the first 6 years of life. It is erroneous, therefore, to reason (as Sato did) that the development of leptokurtosis depends on environmental factors. It seems more likely that the phenomenon that leads to leptokurtosis of the distribution occurs during the entire period of growth (leading to increasing peakedness) but begins in utero. Such a mechanism could scarcely be due to the use of the eyes.

4. The higher degrees of myopia and hyperopia present at birth have for the most part disappeared by the time the child has reached the age of approximately 6 years.

SCHOOLCHILDREN

This period of life during the school years has been carefully studied by many authors, and an analysis of refractive data for a group of children in Ojai, California, was reported by Hirsch (1952). The data, accumulated by retinoscopy without cycloplegia, enable one to determine the changes occurring between 5 and 14 years. The results of this study may be summarized as follows:

Between the ages of 5 and 14 the mean refraction becomes about 0.50 D less hyperopic. However, since the median changes less than this amount, it may be concluded that the refractive state of most of the children changes little, while a few children are becoming distinctly more myopic.

The range between the seventh and ninety-third percentile increases with age between 5 and 14, and the standard deviation unquestionably does the same. In another study, conducted in Ohio in 1948, Hirsch found an increase of about 0.50 D in the standard deviation between the ages of 6 and 14.

The distribution is skewed toward the hyperopic side for 5-year-olds (as is that of Kempf et al.), becomes less skewed with increasing age, is symmetrical at about age 9 or 10, and then becomes increasingly skewed toward the myopic side (agreeing with the skewness toward the myopic side found by Stromberg [1936], Stenstrom [1946], and by Kronfeld and Devney [1931] and others who have analyzed adult data). This same trend was observed in the Ohio data, the skewness being toward hyperopia at the time of entering school, symmetrical at the age of about 10 or 11, and then becoming increasingly skewed toward myopia until puberty after which there is no appreciable change.

The kurtosis was not determined for the Ojai group; and the kurtosis found for the Ohio group may not be valid. Although kurtosis is a notable feature of the refractive distribution and, therefore, must be considered, its usefulness is questionable. It is greatly influenced by extreme values and, therefore, stable only for large numbers of subjects. In the Ohio data, for example, the value of g_2 was altered radically by the exclusion of a single case, a child with over 10.00 D of myopia. For the distribution of refraction of children of the ages being considered in which the range is small, yet in which extreme values may appear, the problem seems more difficult than in the data on the newborn or the adult. With reservations, the Ohio data may be considered. The value for kurtosis for the youngest group was about +15. (This value is markedly different from the value of +2.66 reported by Kempf, Collins, and Jarman [1928] for a similar group.) The value for the Ohio data then declined to approximately +6.00 for the oldest children (16 to 17 years). This value is close to the g_2 of +4.56 found by Kronfeld and Devney (1931).

The question of shifts in kurtosis between birth and maturity is of some importance. Unfortunately, the evidence is contradictory because sensitivity of this measure depends on the single odd case, and the problem will be solved only by the accumulation of large samples of the various age groups.

In summary, there is probably *some* leptokurtosis present in the distribution of the newborn, and the distribution of children entering school is *markedly* peaked. Whether this leptokurtosis declines during the school years, as the Ohio data indicate, or increases, as a comparison of the data of Kempf et al. to that of Kronfeld and Devney or Stromberg would indicate, must remain unanswered at present.

■

SUMMARY OF REFRACTIVE CHANGES DURING CHILDHOOD

The changes in refraction that occur during development can now be summarized. At birth, the refractive distribution is characterized by a mean of about 2.00 D of hyperopia and a standard deviation of about 2.75 D. The curve is symmetrical and three standard deviations on either side of the mean includes more than 99% of the cases, and this range is from about −6.00 to +10.00 D. There is a slight degree of leptokurtosis, that is, a piling up of cases around the mean. By the time a child enters school, almost all myopia has disappeared, as has most of the hyperopia above 4.00 D. This period of life, therefore, is characterized by a disappearance of the extremes of both sorts (probably during the first year of life) and a further clustering toward the middle (increased leptokurtosis). That both tails of the curve have pulled toward the mean indicates that during infancy and early childhood some children change in the direction of hyperopia, whereas others change in the direction of myopia. Because the curve is skewed toward the hyperopic side when the child enters school, the disappearance of the extreme myopes is more completely achieved than is the disappearance of the higher hyperopes.

During the school years, the refraction of the majority of the children changes little. For most people (more than half) the refraction has reached adult values by the age of 6 years. Skewness, however, now goes in the minus direction, as the number of myopes increases. We have stressed in previous papers that this increase in myopia seems to coincide with puberty, occurs between 1 and 2 years earlier in girls than in boys, and stops at the age of 14 to 18 years. The increased kurtosis of the curve from birth to maturity is due to one or both of two factors. It is due to the stretching out of the myopic tail, or to the further clustering of cases in the middle, or to both. The data (Hirsch, 1952) indicate that both phenomena are occurring. A considerable number of hyperopes between 1.00 and 2.00 D disappear, and there is an increase in the number of children within the range of −1.00 to +1.00 D. This increase is greater than is the number of cases in the myopic tail. During school years, then, most children change little in refraction. A considerable number of moderate hyperopes manifest a small decrease in hyperopia and add to the cluster near the center. A small number of children (especially at puberty) rapidly become myopic, increasing as much as 5 or 6 D and forming the myopic tail of the curve and also leading to an increased standard deviation.

It is impossible without a longitudinal study to state whether the very early changes are in any way related to those occurring later. For example, it is not known whether the infant who had 6 D of myopia and who became hyperopic or emmetropic during the preschool years is the same individual who at puberty again becomes myopic. In the absence of such a study, the early and later refractive changes must be treated separately, and one may only speculate about the true picture.

EARLY MATURITY

It is necessary to set the boundary between childhood and adulthood, or maturity, and between early maturity and late maturity. Neither longitudinal nor random studies are available at these boundaries, but data from private practice (Jackson, 1932) and from clinics (Tassman, 1932; Brown, 1942) cover the years from childhood to advanced age. These authors agree that changes at about 25 and 55 years may be considered to be these boundaries. It has been shown in preceding sections that between the ages of 6 and 18 there is a decrease in the prevalence of hyperopia and an increase in that of both myopia and emmetropia, while the average refractive state declines from +1.25 to +0.25 D. In the present section, the change between the age of 18 and 25, and that between 25 and 55, will be considered.

Brown (1942) found the average refraction at the age of 20 to be +0.50 D, and at age 29 to be +0.12 D. Data collected on West Point cadets indicate that one of every eighteen entering West Point Academy with emmetropia or low hyperopia developed myopia before graduation. Sixty-three percent of the students who entered with myopia showed some increase in the degree of myopia before graduation. Hirsch (unpublished data) has noted in university clinics that a number of students, emmetropic at the age of 17 or 18 when they enter college, develop low grades of myopia by the age of 22 or 23, the degree seldom exceeding 1.00 D. The prevalence of myopia between the ages of 18 and 25 does not increase as rapidly as it did during the school years, nor does the average refractive state change as markedly; the changes that occur are in the same direction, but of lesser magnitude.

The period between the age of 25 and 55 is characterized by stability, both of the average refractive state and of the prevalence of myopia. The recorded differences in the data of Brown, Tassman, and Jackson might well be due to chance. The percentage of young myopic adults will obviously vary with the criterion of myopia and with the method of measurement. For the ages 25 to 55 inclusive, the average percentage of myopia for Tassman's data is 14.6% and for Jackson's, 17.0%. Newcomb (1919), analyzing the first 1,000 officers, men, and civilians under 40 years of age examined by the Department of Ophthalmology of the U.S. Army, reports 20.4% to be myopic. These four studies average between 18 and 19%; if corrections of −0.25 D were classed as myopia, this value would rise considerably.

It may reasonably be estimated that between 8 and 14% of American adults have myopia in excess of 1.00 D; between 15 and 20% have myopia of more than 0.50 D, and between 25 and 30% have myopia of more than 0.00 D.

—■—————————————————————————————————

LATE MATURITY

The period after age 55 years, which may be called later maturity, has received less attention than other periods of life, but the information available deserves careful examination. During this period, many changes occur in the eyes, but those affecting the lens appear to be the most significant. The lens increases in refractive index and its elasticity decreases. These changes alter its refractive power and ultimately abolish accommodation, all latent hyperopia now becoming

Table 2.3. Numbers of Persons Showing Different Refractive States in Later Maturity*

Refractive state	Age 50–60	Over age 60	Total
Hyperopia of 7.00 D and over	9	9	18
	(11)	(7)	
Hyperopia 0.25 to 7.00 D	1,483	1,108	2,591
	(1,518)	(1,073)	
Emmetropia	324	141	465
	(272)	(193)	
Myopia 0.25 to 10.00 D	356	268	624
	(366)	(258)	
Myopia of 10.00 D and over	28	28	56
	(33)	(23)	
Total	2,300	1,554	3,754

*From Jackson, 1927. Numbers in parentheses represent those expected in each category on the basis of chance.

manifest. In a small proportion of eyes, poorly understood alterations eventuate in cataract.

The data of Jackson (1932) and Tassman (1932) show that after the age of 55 the percentage of both hyperopia and myopia increases, whereas that of emmetropia markedly declines. Table 2.3 presents Jackson's data for this period, and Table 2.4 presents Tassman's data. These have been presented in as nearly the same form as the classifications used by the two authors permit. We have calculated the numbers to be expected in the various categories by chance from the totals in the margin, and have placed these in parentheses in the tables. The two tables are in agreement. It will be noted that the proportions of both hyperopia and myopia increase with increasing age; that is, in the early decades there are fewer cases than expected by chance, but in the later decades, there are more; however, the differences are not great. The reverse is true of emmetropia. Here the numbers decline and fewer are found in the later decades than expected. The differences are, moreover, large, and the chi square test shows that for both tables such discrepancies between observed and expected numbers would occur by chance less than once in a thousand times.

In summary, the changes in later maturity, although less marked than those during childhood, are significant. After some 30 years during which the refractive state remains relatively constant, the following changes occur: (1) The percentages of both hyperopia and myopia increase; and (2) the change in prevalence of hyperopia is the reverse of that which occurs during childhood, while the increased prevalence of myopia is in the same direction. As might be expected from the fact that the prevalences of both types of ametropia increase, the percentage of em-

Table 2.4.   Numbers of Persons Showing Different Refractive States in Later Maturity*

	Age 50–60	Age 60–70	≥70	Total
Hyperopia over 3.00 D	318	203	69	590
	(214)	(191)	(57)	
Hyperopia 1.00 to 3.00 D	840	506	152	1,496
	(868)	(485)	(145)	
Emmetropia (+ 1.00 D to	545	220	46	(811)
− 1.00 D inclusive)	(470)	(263)	(78)	
Myopia 1.00 to 3.00 D	154	91	34	279
	(162)	(90)	(27)	
Myopia over 3.00 D	119	84	29	232
	(134)	(75)	(23)	
Total	1,976	1,104	330	3,410

*From Tassman, 1932. Numbers in parentheses represent those expected in each category on the basis of chance.

metropia decreases markedly during later maturity. In other words, the frequency distribution is less peaked in later than in early maturity.

------------- ■ -------------

PREVALENCE OF MYOPIA IN MALES AND FEMALES

Statements, often contradictory, have appeared in the literature that a higher prevalence of myopia occurs in one or the other sex. Part of this contradiction may be because the prevalence may be higher at one age for men and at another age for women. In recent years, there has been a tendency to think of two broad categories of myopia — one type of high degree, which is believed to be either congenital or pathological; and a second variety that appears for the most part during the second decade of life, seldom exceeds 6.00 D, and is thought to be based on biological variability. It may be that the prevalence is higher among men for one type and among women for the other.

□ Children

Boselli (1900) examined a number of schoolchildren in Italy (Table 2.5). These figures include cases of myopia and myopic astigmatism and all degrees of myopia.

Table 2.5. Relative Prevalence of Myopia for Females and Males, for Children in Grades 3, 4, and 5*

Grade in school	Sex	Percent myopic	Ratio F/M
3	M	13.20	2.0 / 1
3	F	26.56	
4	M	17.92	1.7 / 1
4	F	30.39	
5	M	19.03	1.8 / 1
5	F	33.37	

*From Boselli (1900).

Table 2.6. Percentages of Myopes Who Were Females

Age	Wilson (1935)	Hirsch (1948)
6–7	50	56 (age 6)
7–10	55	58
11–14	59	66
15–17	(boys higher)	53

This study, although not recent, is valuable because examinations were checked with the retinoscope according to Cuignet's method. The difference between boys and girls is statistically significant.

In the text of his article, Boselli quoted from Rochard (*Encyclopedie d' Hygiene, Tom. 4*) as follows, "School myopia is more marked among the boys than among the girls." Boselli stated that the majority of other authors had found a greater predisposition toward myopia and a greater number of myopes among the girls, which his data confirmed.

Nicholls (1940) determined the refraction of 521 Canadian rural schoolchildren between the ages of 5 and 20 years. He found myopia in 13.4% of girls and in only 4.6% of boys. Wilson (1935) concluded after an examination of 22,000 schoolchildren in Scotland that myopia was more frequent among girls. The data of Hirsch (1948), already mentioned, agree and are included with Wilson's data in Table 2.6.

Although Hirsch found a higher percentage of myopia among girls than did Wilson, the trend insofar as age is concerned is the same. For children less than 7 and greater than 15 years of age, the prevalence of myopia is approximately the same among boys and girls. However, between the ages of 7 and 14 years, the prevalence is higher among girls.

Table 2.7.   Relative Prevalence of Myopia in Girls and Boys*

Age	Percent myopia	
	Girls	Boys
6–8 years	1.7	2.7
9–11 years	4.4	6.4
12 years and over	8.6	10.7

*From Kempf, Collins, and Jarman (1928).

Table 2.8.   Percentages of Myopia in Girls and Boys
Between 6 and 18 Years Old*

Age	Girls (%)	Boys (%)
6	2.86	2.22
7	7.43	3.07
8	5.13	4.46
9	9.43	8.24
10	6.99	11.54
11	17.60	9.09
12	19.15	8.33
13	28.16	13.51
14	18.61	9.40
15	19.67	20.83
16	22.89	18.03
17	21.92	18.42
18	25.81	23.26
6–10	7.10	6.05
11–14	19.17	10.11
15–18	25.81	23.26

*From Hirsch (1948).

Kempf, Collins, and Jarman (1928) examined the eyes of 1860 white school-children in Washington, D.C. and found a greater prevalence of myopia among boys than among girls. The percentages of myopia found by these authors are shown in Table 2.7. These data do not agree with the conclusions of Boselli (1900) or Wilson (1935), nor is the reason for this lack of agreement apparent. The data of Hirsch (1948), presented in Table 2.8, however, do agree with those of Boselli and Wilson. These data include the refractive state of 3,127 schoolchildren in Ohio

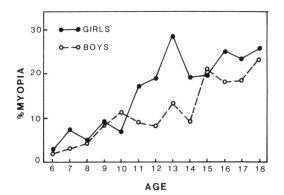

Figure 2.4.
Percentages of girls and boys found to be myopic, on the basis of age, taken from refractive data obtained by Hirsch on 3,127 Ohio children. (Data from Table 2.13.)

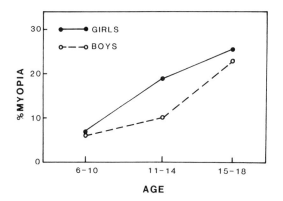

Figure 2.5. Data plotted in Figure 2.4, smoothed into three age groups. (Data taken from the lower part of Table 2.13.)

and were determined by retinoscopy as described in the preceding section. The study included between 75 and 200 boys and a like number of girls for each age group from 6 to 17 years, and a smaller number of 18-year-olds. The data presented in Table 2.8 are illustrated in Figure 2.4; so that trends might be seen more readily they have been smoothed by thirds (Figure 2.5).

Table 2.8 and Figures 2.4 and 2.5 demonstrate that between the ages of 6 and 10 years, the prevalence of myopia in boys and girls differs little. The prevalence does seem to be slightly higher among girls than boys, but this difference is not statistically significant. However, between the ages of 11 and 14 years, there is a marked increase in the prevalence of myopia among girls; a similar increase appears in the boys about 3 years later. This is seen quite acutely in the smoothed graphs. As a result, between the ages of 11 and 14 years, the prevalence of myopia is about *twice as high* among girls as among boys (19.17% among girls vs 10.11% among boys); this difference is highly significant statistically.

Between the ages of 16 and 18 years, an increase continues, but at a slower rate than before, both boys and girls now showing an increase of 1% per year. During these later ages, girls still have a higher prevalence (25.81%, as compared to 23.26% for boys between 15 and 18 years), but this difference, like that for the youngest group, fails to reach statistical significance.

The sharp rise followed by a decrease in prevalence found at about the time of puberty is seen in Figure 2.4 to be present primarily for girls. There seems to be a transitory myopia of puberty, which is characteristic of girls. The data illustrated in Figure 2.4 are in general very similar to the growth curves for many other anthropometric variables. The rapid increase in the prevalence of myopia associated with adolescence, coming 2 or 3 years earlier for girls than for boys, would seem to be strong evidence for a theory of the origin of myopia based on growth. It would be difficult to explain the sex difference here presented on the basis of the use of the eyes; and in view of the fact that puberty occurs earlier for girls than for boys, the difference becomes understandable.

Bruckner and Franceschetti (1931) have reported the refractive state of twenty-five children between the ages of 6 and 7 who had between 3.00 and 25.00 D of myopia. Two thirds of the cases were boys and one third were girls. Such a large difference could have occurred by chance one time in ten in a population in which no real difference existed. Bartels (1931) reported 17 cases of high myopia between 7.00 and 23.00 D. The ages of the children were between 2 and 9 years. Eight of these patients were boys and nine were girls, and the average degree of myopia was 12.75 D for the boys and 12.67 D for the girls. Among 2,025 children less than 12 years of age, Hirsch (1948) found only two children having more than 4.00 D of myopia — a 9-year-old boy with 14.00 D of myopia and an 11-year-old boy with 4.75 D. Clearly these data do not permit any generalization.

Knapp (1939), in a study of the effects of vitamin therapy, lists the degree of myopia as well as the sex of each child studied. We have reanalyzed these data (Table 2.9). The criterion of high myopia was an average refraction in the four meridians (two principal meridians of each eye) of −5.00 D or more. The chi

Table 2.9. Sex Differences in High and Low Myopia*

	Girls	Boys	Total
High myopia	12	6	18
	(9)	(9)	
Low myopia	12	16	28
	(15)	(13)	
Total	24	22	46

Numbers in parentheses are those expected if there were no difference in myopia between boys and girls.
*From Knapp, 1939.

square value is 3.29, and the probability is more than 0.5. In the Knapp study, there is some indication that high myopia is more frequent among girls than boys, but the difference is not statistically significant.

Bartels (1931) and Bruckner and Franceschetti (1931) stressed the distinct and different nature of high myopia among children. Bartels thought that there were two types of myopia: that usually described as "school myopia," and a type of congenital, high myopia, which could be considered a hereditary anomaly. Bruckner and Franceschetti call the latter condition "infantile myopia," and deny any hereditary influence. They thought that this anomaly was different from the myopia that develops during school years and pointed out that in infantile myopia visual acuity was never normal — the higher the myopia, the poorer the acuity. In some cases, the myopia remains stationary; for example, a 9.00 D myope showed no increase over an 18-year period. In other cases, there is considerable change, and a patient whose myopia increased 11.00 D over a 20-year period is reported.

The evidence suggests that there *is* a form of high congenital myopia that is found in a very small percentage of children (a fraction of 1%) with no predilection for sex. A hereditary nature has not been proven, nor has the rate of its progression been determined.

□ Adults

As reported by Witte in 1923, of 34,753 adult patients examined at the Greifswald Clinic (located in a rural district), 13.8% were found to be myopic (11% of the women and 16% of the men). As will be noted later, Witte found a larger percentage of *high* myopia among women than among men. On the other hand, Blevgard (1927), in reporting the refractive states of 53,000 Danish clinic patients, states that 3.58% of the men and 6.28% of the women were myopic. Stenstrom (1946) found 22.7% of the females examined to have myopia of more than 1.00 D, whereas only 13.3% of the males had a similar degree of myopia. The difference is significant at the .0004 level. However, the data were not based on a random sampling but rather on a group selected to approximate a normal sample. The subjects were all (1) patients at the clinic, (2) nurses and doctors, or (3) officer candidates in army and air corps. The large number of emmetropes that would be present in this last group may in part explain the lower prevalence of myopia among men in Stenstrom's sample.

Meyerhof (1914) has reported the following percentages based on his private practice in Egypt. The numbers refer to the percentage of his patients who had myopia.

	Women	Men
Egyptians	16.5%	32.1%
Europeans	16.3%	20.0%
Asians	9.8%	21.6%

This material, also, does not represent random sampling, a difficulty of which Meyerhof himself was aware. Trachoma is prevalent in Egypt and, due to corneal opacities resulting from this disease, refraction could not be determined in a large number of patients. Also, due to economic causes, it is possible that only those women with severe eye difficulties consulted the ophthalmologist.

There is little agreement among the four authors cited, two finding more myopia among women and two finding more among men. The prevalence varies from Blevgard's 3.58% for men to Meyerhof's 32.1% for Egyptian men. Undoubtedly, differing criteria of myopia played a part in causing such differences, and sampling errors also contributed. It is understandable that there should be a shortage of random sampling data among adults, since surveys among this age group are rare. The view that seems to have the greatest acceptance is that of Witte, namely that *moderate* myopia is slightly more common among men, and *high* myopia more common among women. However on the basis of the evidence here cited, the status of the problem insofar as moderate myopia is concerned is not at all clear.

The evidence for sex differences in adults is more clear-cut for high myopia than for myopia in general. Witte, in 1923, found a 16% prevalence of all myopia among men and 11% among women at the Greifswald Clinic, and stated that among those patients having myopia greater than 10.00 D, there is a greater percentage of women than men. Blevgard (1927) found that 1.14% of the men and 2.64% of the women at a Danish clinic had myopia above 6.00 D.

In an analysis of the records of 816 myopes who visited the Massachusetts Charitable Eye and Ear Infirmary between 1915 and 1916, Gage (1917) found that of the 1,632 eyes, 73 were blind, 11 were amblyopic, and 11 were not actually myopic; the remaining 1,537 eyes form the basis for her study. In the chi-square table (Table 2.10), the numbers without parentheses indicate eyes observed in each category; whereas the numbers in parentheses represent the values expected if there were no difference between the two sexes in regard to degree of myopia.

The value of chi square was 13.05, which for one degree of freedom yields a P value of $<.001$, the difference being highly significant. As is seen in the table,

Table 2.10. Number of Myopic Men and Women, by Degree*

	Women	Men	Total
Myopia of less than 6.00 D	559 (588)	650 (621)	1,209
Myopia of more than 6.00 D	188 (159)	140 (169)	328
Total	747	790	1,537

Numbers in parentheses are those expected if there were no difference in myopia between women and men.
*After Gage, 1917.

fewer women than expected have low myopia, whereas more than the expected number have high myopia. Among men, the reverse holds true. The data are perhaps more comprehensible if expressed as percentages; hence, it may be said that *among myopes visiting this clinic,* 17.7% of men and 25.2% of women had myopia in excess of 6.00 D. It should be noted that no statement can be made about the prevalence of myopia in the total population, but only about the percentage of high myopes among myopes visiting the clinic.

Rolett (1935) reported on 772 myopic patients who had visited the ophthalmic clinic at the University of Bern at least three times, enabling the author to classify cases as progressive or stationary. Progressive myopes are further subdivided into those with less and those with more than 6.00 D of myopia; the author calls the latter type *malignant myopia.* Rolett's data are presented in the chi-square table (Table 2.11).

Table 2.11. Number of Men and Women with Stationary and Progressive Myopia

	Women	Men	Total
Stationary myopia	85 (118)	122 (89)	207
Progressive myopia (under 6.00 D)	204 (196)	141 (149)	345
Progressive malignant myopia (over 6.00 D)	150 (125)	70 (95)	220
Total	439	333	772

Numbers in parentheses are those expected if there were no difference in type of myopia between women and men.
*Data from Rolett, 1953.

Table 2.12. Percentages of Progressive and Nonprogressive Myopes and Degrees of Myopia for Men and Women*

	Women	Men	Differences	P
Stationary myopes	19.4 ± 1.89	36.6 ± 2.78	17.2 ± 3.36	<.0001
Progressive myopes (less than 6.00 D)	46.5 ± 2.38	42.3 ± 2.35	4.2 ± 1.13	.26
Progressive malignant myopes (more than 6.00 D)	34.2 ± 2.25	21.0 ± 2.36	13.2 ± 3.27	<.0001

*Data from Rolett, 1935.

Table 2.13.   Relative Prevalence of Myopia in Women and Men

		Women	Men	Ratio W/M
Blevgard (1927)	Percentage of population with myopia > 6.00 D	2.6	1.1	2.3 / 1
Gage (1917)	Percentage of myopes > 6.00 D	25.2	17.7	1.4 / 1
Rolett (1935)	Percent with progressive myopia > 6.00 D	34.2	21.0	1.6 / 1
Witte (1923)	Myopes > 10.00 D	(greater percentage of women)		

The value of chi square is 33.80, which for 2 degrees of freedom gives a P value of <.0001. Thus, the greater proportion of males with stationary myopia and the greater proportion of females with progressive myopia of more than 6.00 D could have occurred by chance less than once in 10,000 times. The material may be further analyzed in terms of percentages. Table 2.12 expresses the percentages and their standard errors, the differences between males and females along with the standard errors of the differences, and the probability that the differences observed could have occurred as a result of sampling. Thus, among the myopes treated at this clinic, there was a higher proportion of stationary cases among males than among females, but the reverse was true for progressive myopia of more than 6.00 D.

Table 2.13 summarizes the cited evidence. It seems safe to conclude that in the general population as well as among populations of myopes, the prevalence of high myopia is greater among women than among men.

◾
SUMMARY

A sex difference in the prevalence of myopia is noted only when we consider (1) myopia of all degrees in children between the ages of 11 and 14 years, and (2) high myopia among adults. High myopia seems to be more common among women than among men, a fact which is of considerable interest when it is recalled that a similar difference could not be demonstrated among boys and girls. These findings would seem to indicate that high myopia is not all congenital: There may be a form of high myopia to which the female is more predisposed and which appears some time after early childhood. The marked difference between boys and girls of ages 11 to 14 strongly suggests that the basis rests on the earlier occurrence of puberty in girls. This interesting phase of the problem certainly deserves further investigation.

───■───

REFERENCES

Bartels M. Hohe Myopie in den ersten Lebensjahren. Klin Monatsbl Augenheilkd 1931; 86:536.

Blevgard O. Die Prognose der excessiven myopie. Acta Ophthalmol 1927;5:49.

Boselli A. La Ametropie Nelle Scuole Elementori di Bolona. Bologna: Regia Tipografia, pp 27–38, 1900.

Brown EVL. Apparent increase in hyperopia up to the age of 9 years. Am J Ophthalmol 1936;19:1006.

Brown EVL. Use-abuse theory of changes in refraction versus biological theory. Arch Ophthal 1942;28:845–850.

Bruckner A, Franceschetti A. Myopie in Kindersalter. Arch Augenheilkd 1931;105:1.

Callan PA. Examination of colored school children's eyes. Am J Med Sci 1875;69:331.

Cook RC, Glasscock RE. Refractive and ocular findings in the newborn. Am J Ophthalmol 1951;34:1407–1413.

Ely ET. Beobachtungen mit dem Augenspiegel bezuglich der Refraktion der Augen neugeborener. Arch Augenheilkd 1880;9:431.

Fletcher M, Brandon S. Myopia of prematurity. Am J Ophthalmol 1955;40:474–481.

Gage H. Myopia cases coming to the Massachusetts Charitable Eye and Ear Infirmary for the first time between January 1, 1915 and January 1, 1916. Arch Ophthalmol 1917; 46:154–163.

Germann T. Bciträge zur Kenntniss der Refractionsverhaltnisse der Kinder im Säuglingsalter sowie im vorschulpflichtigen Alter. Albrecht von Graefes Arch Ophthalmol 1885; 31:121–146.

Goldschmidt E. On the Etiology of Myopia. Copenhagen, Munksgaard, 1968.

Goldschmidt E. Refraction in the newborn. Acta Ophthalmol 1969;47:370.

Harman NB. An analysis of 300 cases of high myopia in children, with a scheme for the grading of fundus changes in myopia. Tr Ophthalmol Soc UK 1913;33:202.

Herrnheiser J. Die Refraktionsentwicklung des menschlichen Auges. Zeitschrift fur Heilkunde 1892;13:342–377.

Hirsch MJ. The refractive state of 3000 school children in Ohio. Presented at the Annual Meeting of the Am Acad Optom, 1948 (unpublished).

Hirsch MJ. The changes in refraction between ages 5 and 14 — theoretical and practical considerations. Am J Optom Arch Am Acad Optom 1952;29:445–452.

Horstmann E. Uber Refraktionsbestimmungen bei Heugeborenen unter 20 Tagen. Klin Monatsbl Augenheilkd 1880;18:495.

Jackson E. Norms of refraction. JAMA 1932;98:132–140.

McCoy LL. High myopia in a child. Am J Ophthalmol 1927;10:610.

Jaeger E. Uber die Einstellung des dioptrishen Apparates im menschlichen Auge. Wien, LW Seidel, UV Sohn. Wasson, 1861.

Jaeger E. Investigation de schulern Myopic. Klin Monatsbl Augenheilkd 1938;101:205.

Kempf GA, Collins SD, Jarman EL. Refractive errors in the eyes of children as determined by retinoscopic examination with a cycloplegic. Publ Health Bull No 182, Washington DC, Govt Printing Office, 1928.

Knapp AA. Vitamin D complex in progressive myopia: etiology, pathology and treatment. Am J Ophthalmol 1939;22:1329.

Konigstein L. Untersuchungen an den Augen neugeborenen Kinder. Wein: Medizinische Jahrbucher, 1881.

Koppe D. Ophthalmoskopisch-ophthalmologische Unter suchungen dus dem Dorpater Gymnasium, 1876.

Kronfeld PD, Devney C. Ein Beitragzur Kenntnis der Refractions Kurve. Graefes Arch Ophthalmol 1931;126:487.

May CH. Diseases of the Eye, 17th ed. Baltimore, Williams & Wilkens, 1949.

Meyerhof M. Study of myopia as a hereditary, racial disease among the Egyptians. Ann Oculistique 1914;151:257.

Newcomb JR. Refraction methods employed in the Department of Ophthalmology of the Attending Surgeon's Office, U.S. Army, Washington DC. Am J Ophthalmol 1919;2:326.

Nicholls JVV. A survey of the ophthalmic conditions among rural school children. Canadian Med J 1940;42:553–556.

Rolett DM. Is full correction of value in checking the progress of myopia? Arch Ophthalmol 1935;14:464–472.

Sato T. Summary of my various experiments in myopia (especially upon the cause of near work myopia). Yohahama Med Bull 1951;2:41–67.

Santonastaso A. The state of refraction of the eye during the first years of life (in Italian). Annali di Ottalmolgia e Clinica Oculista 1930;58:852.

Stenstrom S. Investigation of the variation and the covariation of the optical elements of human eyes, trans. D. Woolf. Am J Optom and Arch Am Acad Optom 1948;25(5):218–232; (6):286–299; (7):340–350; (8):388–397; (9):438–449; (10):496–504.

Stromberg E. Uber refraktion und achenlange des menschlichen auges. (Original not examined; cited by Stenstrom 5, 1948) Acta Ophthalmol 1936;14:281.

Tassman IS. Frequency of various kinds of refractive errors. Am J Ophthalmol 1932;15:1044–1053.

Wibaut JF. Uber die Emmetropisation und den Ursprung der spharischen Refraktionsanomalien. Albrecht von Graefe's Archiv fur Ophthalmol 1926;116:596.

Wilson JA. Ametropia and sex. Brit J Ophthalmol 1935;19:613–614.

Witte O. Zur myopie fraze. Zeitschrift F. Augenheilkd 1923;51:163–180.

3

Changes in Optical Elements: Hypothesis for the Genesis of Refractive Anomalies

Monroe J. Hirsch and Frank W. Weymouth

☐

Despite the existence of many theories, the causes of refractive anomalies are still not completely known. Realizing that an inclusive and fully developed theory will be many years in coming, we present an interim report and propose a working hypothesis. The chapter is organized so as to develop this hypothesis.

■

CHANGES IN THE OPTICAL ELEMENTS

Changes in overall refraction are relatively easy to measure and, as has been shown in Chapter 2, this variable has been measured at all ages. Refraction, however, is not a simple variable but rather results from the combination of a number of elements. Ideally, one would seek the solution to the problem by studying the changes in each of these elements during the period from birth to maturity; however, practical difficulties, sometimes insurmountable in the present state of technical knowledge, are encountered.

Although at least seven or eight elements contribute to overall refraction, the effects of three far outweigh the others: anterioposterior diameter or axial length of the globe, the refractive power of the cornea, and the refractive power of the crystalline lens. Only one of these, however, the cornea, may be readily measured in persons of all ages. Axial length is now measurable in the adult or older child, or may be roughly determined from an enucleated eye, which is the source of data for infants and young children. Lens power cannot be measured directly either in vivo or for the enucleated eye. Thus, not only have no longitudinal studies been made of the various optical elements, but even cross-sectional information for some ages is completely lacking. Despite these difficulties, knowledge about the three major optical elements is available from both direct measurement and from calculations based on measurements of other elements; these data will now be considered.

□ Corneal Refracting Power

Because corneal measurements may be made readily (and in fact are frequently made in the course of a routine vision examination), the distribution curve for this element is available, at least for the adult. Steiger (1913) among others has measured the cornea. Since all of the findings are in close agreement, the values of two authors only will be included. The figures of Tron (1940) and Stenstrom (1946) are given below:

	Tron	Stenstrom
Mean	43.41 D ± 0.08	42.84 D ± 0.04
S.D.	1.36 D ± 0.06	1.40 D ± 0.03

Although neither author gives the value for g_1 or g_2, both distributions, as well as those found by Steiger and others, did not differ significantly from the normal. It is then well established that the distribution of corneal power for the adult has a mean of approximately 43.00 D, a standard deviation of about 1.37 D, and is normal.

No distribution curve for corneal power for the newborn or the very young child exists. Thus it is only possible to treat this variable among the young in a sketchy fashion. Keeney (1951), in a summary of developmental changes in the eye, states that the cornea has reached adult size by no later than the age of 2 years, a conclusion not at variance with the views of others (Wolff 1933, Duke-Elder 1940). Mann (1950) states that the cornea at birth has a refracting power of about 50.5 D. Thus, the changes normally encountered in the cornea lead to a decreased radius of curvature during the first year or two of life, and then no further change during life. It is unfortunate that the distribution curves for this element at earlier ages are not available. In their absence, all that can be safely said is that thus far no evidence for lack of normality has been offered; it is reasonable to assume that normality is characteristic of this distribution at all ages.

□ Axial Length

Both Tron and Stenstrom have found that the distribution curve of axial length for the adult eye is skewed toward the higher values, and is leptokurtic. Stenstrom believes that the similar skewness and kurtosis in the distribution of overall refraction is merely a reflection of this phenomenon. The values found by Stenstrom for 1,000 eyes whose axial lengths were directly measured are as follows:

Mean	24.00 mm ± 0.035
S.D.	1.09 mm ± 0.024
g_1	+0.81 ± 0.777
g_2	+3.35 ± 0.154

Both the values for g_1 and g_2 differ significantly from zero, and hence from the value for a normal curve. Having stated that the skewness and kurtosis do not differ markedly in male and female subjects, Stenstrom (1948) concludes that "we must accept the conclusion that the distribution curve of axial length . . . arises from the addition of two or more types of subjects with different properties."

This view, namely that the skewness and kurtosis of the refractive distribution are for the most part a reflection of a similar phenomenon in the distribution of axial length, and further, that this distribution has this form as a result of the presence of two or more types of subjects, is today the prevailing one. The question of how these types shall be recognized and separated, however, is considerably more difficult and at present is addressed by three major hypotheses, each representing a different approach and each having certain advantages and disadvantages.

1. The view of Tron (1940) is perhaps the simplest. He pointed out that if all cases of myopia over 6.00 D were omitted, then the remaining distribution was normal. Today this is considered the weakest of the theories: The choice of 6.00 D as a point of demarcation is arbitrary, and Titoff (1938) has pointed out that if this procedure is followed insofar as the refractive curve is concerned, skewness and kurtosis differing from those of the normal curve still remain.

2. A second hypothesis is that used by Scheerer and Betsch (1929) and by Stenstrom (1946). This theory divides the group into two smaller groups on the basis of fundus changes. Scheerer and Betsch found that if cases with myopic conus are omitted, the distribution was symmetrical, although still decidedly leptokurtic. Stenstrom followed the same procedure and found that the resulting curve was symmetrical but leptokurtic, although less so than the curve for all cases ($g_2 = +1.54$ for the nonconus eyes). This concept has distinct advantages, in that the method of separating the cases is based on a variable (the fundus) not involved in any of the other calculations. It also has clinical significance, since the cause of the asymmetry may be sought in the cause of the conus.

3. A third solution rests on a mathematical treatment of the data to separate the overall distribution into a series of normal curves. It is clear to those who have worked with refractive data that the distribution cannot result from two normal ones, but must either include a greater number of normal distributions or two non-normal distributions. Curve fitting in such a problem is not capable of mathematical solution unless certain assumptions are made. If, for example, the means and standard deviations of some of the component curves are known or assumed, the problem has a precise solution. In the absence of such data, however, close approximations of the component curves may be made, as did Hirsch (1950) for

Figure 3.1. The refractive distribution curve may be explained by a series of four component curves. (Only three of the component curves — α, β, and γ — are shown here.)

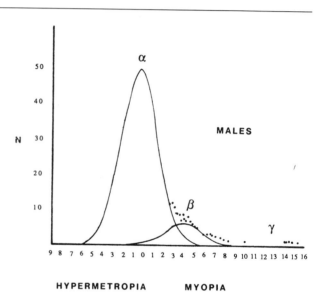

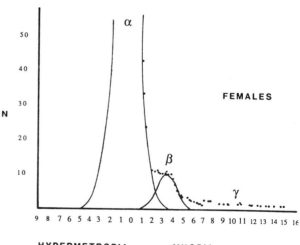

the refractive curve. It was demonstrated that the refractive curve could be explained by a series of four component curves (Figure 3.1) labeled as follows:

Alpha, the largest group includes both myopes and hyperopes of low and moderate degree.

Beta, a smaller group, was characterized by a normal curve with its mean between 3.00 and 5.00 D of myopia, and a range from about emmetropia to about 8.00 D of myopia.

Gamma, a very small group, included myopes of still higher degree and probably itself made up of smaller rare groups, but not capable of further analysis because of its small size. In this group would be such differing conditions as high congenital myopia, Marfan syndrome (lenticular myopia) and degenerative or progressive myopia with marked fundus pathology.

Delta is a small group that includes the markedly hyperopic cases, and particularly those marked by facial stigmata and other secondary signs described by many authors including Landolt (1886).

Hirsch (1950) pointed out that there was an overlapping of these component curves, and that a 3.00 D myope, for example, might fall within either the α group or the β group. Greek letters were used, to avoid prejudicial adjectives such as "pathological," "normal," or "school." According to this solution to the problem, the refractive distribution curve consists essentially of two normal curves, the α and the β, and two small residuals, one at each tail of the overall curve. In the original paper a table (shown here as Table 3.1) was offered that gave the approximate percentages of the types for varying degrees of myopia. By the use of these data and Stenstrom's correlation table for the refractive state and axial length, certain interesting calculations and speculations can be made.

Table 3.1.   Approximate Percentages of Possible Types of Myopia

Degree of myopia (D)	Males			Females		
	α	β	γ	α	β	γ
1.00	97	3	—	100	—	—
2.00	88	12	—	89	11	—
3.00	60	40	—	31	69	—
4.00	25	75	—	1	99	—
5.00	2	98	—	—	100	—
6.00	—	72	28	—	20	80
7.00	—	44	56	—	?	?
8.00	—	23	77	—	—	100
9.00	—	?	?	—	—	100
10.00	—	—	100	—	—	100

For each cell in the correlation table of Stenstrom, the proportionate number of β and γ cases was calculated. For example, Stenstrom found six cases with a refraction of −4.00 to −5.00 D and an axial length of 25.5 to 26.0 mm (midpoint 25.75 mm). According to Hirsch's data, about 94% of cases with this refraction will be in the β group and 6% will be in the α group. In making up the distribution of axial lengths, 94% of the six cases, or 5.64, was entered in the β group as having an axial length of 25.75 mm, and 6% (0.36 cases) was entered in the α distribution.

When this had been done for each entry in the Stenstrom correlation table, the distribution of axial length for each group was determined, and for the α and β groups a normal curve was fitted. The α distribution included 909 of the 1,000 cases and had a mean of 23.66 mm and a standard deviation of 0.83 mm. The theoretically determined normal distribution was tested for fit to the observed data by the chi square test, and the P-value was 0.13, indicating a good fit. The β distribution included sixty cases, and had a mean of 25.37 mm and a standard deviation of 1.01 mm. This too was tested by the chi square method and the *P* value was 0.90, indicating a very close fit. The remaining two distributions were too small to fit or to test for normality, but may be described roughly. The γ distribution included only about twenty cases, and had a mean of approximately 27.50 mm and a standard deviation of about 1.20 mm. The dozen or so more cases comprising the δ group had a mean in the vicinity of 21 mm, and the number is too small to permit further calculations.

The shape of the distribution curve of axial lengths for ages before the adult years is not known; only limited information about length at these earlier ages is available. The axial length at birth has been reported by Duke-Elder (1940) to be approximately 17 mm, and by Mann (1950) to be between 16 and 19 mm. Although it has certain dangers, the assumption of normality of the distribution at birth will have to be made until further information is available. During the first 6 years of life, axial length increases rapidly, reaching about 21 to 22 mm by the age of 6 years (Duke-Elder 1949). Unfortunately, the distribution at these ages has not been investigated, and once again assumptions must be made to arrive at any conclusions. Unfortunately, more complete data will have to await a method of measuring axial lengths as accurate as that used by Stenstrom, but suitable for use with infants and children. Until such methods become available, a great deal of important theory will rest on a few scattered observations.

□ Crystalline Lens Power

Because of its complicated structure and the presence of many variables (numerous refracting surfaces and different indices of refraction), the power of the crystalline lens has never been directly determined. Data for the adult lens has resulted from three types of investigations: (1) Tron (1940) measured four of the lens surfaces, made assumptions as to the lens indices, measured distances between the lens surfaces, and calculated the overall power of the lens; (2) Stenstrom

Table 3.2.   Refracting Power of the Lens*

	Stenstrom	Tron	Taketa
Mean	17.35 + 0.04 D	19.50 + 0.14 D	16.12 + 0.35 D
S.D.	1.48 + 0.03 D	2.00 + 0.10 D	3.88 + 0.25 D
g_1	X†	X	−0.013 + 0.33
g_2	X	X	+0.174 + 0.14

*From Stenstrom (1948), Tron (1940), and Taketa (1949).
†Value not given but stated not to differ significantly from the zero characteristic of the normal curve.

(1946), having measured overall refractive state as well as the power of the cornea, axial length, and anterior chamber depth, determined the lens power by calculation; (3) the authors, dissatisfied with the above methods, attempted a third solution. Work under their direction was carried out by Taketa (1949). Taketa analyzed a group of records of hospital patients who had undergone extraction of a cataractous lens. Records of the refractions of these patients many years before the development of the opacity were available, as were the postoperative refractive data; from this information it was possible to determine the power of the lens.

The findings of Tron (1940), Stenstrom (1948), and Taketa (1949) are summarized in Table 3.2. Values for Tron's study are the corrected values given by Stenstrom. Both Stenstrom and Taketa referred their values to the anterior vertex, a procedure which yields values that are about 3.00 D lower than the customary ones. For the adult, the mean value of the power of the lens seems to be between 16.00 and 17.00 D if the value is referred to the anterior vertex, and about 19.00 or 20.00 D if considered in its customary position. The findings of all of the authors were in close agreement. The slightly lower value found by Taketa may indicate a loss of lens power preceding the maturation of lenticular opacities and hence may be an artifact caused by the pathological process in the lenses of these patients.

No adequate data are available about the power of the lens for infants and children. However, the summary of Collins (1921) may be cited as authoritative. The period of growth from birth to maturity is characterized by a progressive flattening of the lens, accompanied by a decrease in refracting power. The distribution of lens power at various ages is not known, and once again the assumption of normality throughout seems to be the best guess.

In summary, the distributions for the most important elements insofar as their effects on overall refraction is concerned may be described as follows:

1. *Corneal power* is probably distributed normally throughout life, the cornea decreasing in curvature during the first few years of life and then remaining relatively constant throughout life.

2. *Axial length* is probably distributed normally at birth, but in the adult eye it is known to exhibit the same characteristics as the overall refractive curve for adults, being leptokurtic and skewed toward myopia (greater axial lengths).
3. *Lens power* is assumed to be distributed normally at birth and throughout life. The lens is more spherical at birth than in adulthood, and its growth is characterized by a loss of sphericity (and hence of power) during the growth period.

☐ Correlations between the Elements

Steiger (1913), regarded as the founder of the modern school of thought about the genesis of refractive errors, thought that each of the optical elements varied *independently*. Those who followed him, however, came to realize that this was not the case, and it is well established today that certain of the optical elements have variability associated with that of other elements. The establishment of the degree of correlation of the various elements began shortly after Steiger and reached its peak with the masterful study of Stenstrom (1946). The correlation coefficients found by Stenstrom form the basis for the present section.

Correlation between overall refraction and each of the elements is useful primarily to determine the *relative importance* of these elements. We (1947) have pointed out that the use of zero order correlations, which Stenstrom presented in this connection, tended to obscure the true condition. The correlation between refraction and lens power found by Stenstrom was 0.00, and this could not be interpreted as meaning that the lens power had no effect on overall refraction. Clearly an element as variable as the lens, and having its high refractive power, must play a part in determining the refraction of the eye. When the first-order partial correlations were extracted from Stenstrom's data, more meaningful results (in this connection) were obtained. On the basis of such calculation, the authors determined that at least 50% of the variability of the refraction of the eye was associated with variability of axial length; about 25% was attributable to the cornea, and about 20% to the lens.

Of perhaps greater importance than the correlation between the refractive state and each element are the correlations among the elements themselves, and particularly the major elements. The zero-order correlation coefficients between elements found by Stenstrom do not differ significantly from first-order partials, and hence the zero order coefficients are considered. These values, along with their interpretation, may be summarized as follows:

1. *Axial length and corneal radius.* The coefficient is +0.31, indicating that some relationship exists, the longer axial length being associated with a greater corneal radius and thus a lower corneal power (and, therefore, with less myopia or more hyperopia). The cornea and axial length, therefore, tend to counteract the effect of the other.
2. *Axial length and lens power.* The coefficient of −0.36 indicates a weak re-

lationship, with the greater axial length being associated with lower lens power (and hence less myopia or more hyperopia). Here again the effects of lens power and axial length tend to counteract each other.

3. *Corneal power and lens power.* Although cornea and lens power each tend to vary with axial length, the correlation between these two elements is very low, being − 0.12. The interpretation of this value is difficult. The effect of a decrease in either corneal power or lens power counteracts the effect of increasing axial length, whereas a decrease in both corneal power and the lens power combine to have a still greater counterbalancing effect on axial length. However, the cornea and lens tend to vary *independently* of one another. This would seem to indicate that in some cases the effect of axial length is counterbalanced by the lens, and in other cases by the cornea — an attractive speculation that unfortunately cannot readily be verified on the basis of Stenstrom's data.

A WORKING HYPOTHESIS FOR THE GENESIS OF REFRACTIVE ERRORS

Because of the lack of information, we hesitate to propose a theory concerning the genesis of refraction. This lack of knowledge also serves as a warning of possible weaknesses in any theory that may be propounded. With this in mind, an attempt may be made to tie together what information is at present available.

The work of Cook and Glasscock (1951) markedly changed the concept of refraction at birth. Most significant is its *extreme variability,* which must be explained. The distribution of refractive states found by Cook and Glasscock is characterized by the presence of a number of high myopes and high hyperopes, both extremes disappearing during the first year. Keeney (1951) reports the average length of the globe for the fetus at 7, 8, and 9 months as 14 to 15, 15 to 16, and 17 mm, respectively. These values agree with those of Weiss (1897) to whose data we (1950) have fitted our growth curve. Because the globe is growing rapidly between the seventh and the ninth month, a 2-month difference will account for a 3 mm difference in axial length. On the other hand, at the age of 1 year, a difference in development of 2 months accounts for less than 0.5 mm in length. The 3 mm difference between the axial length of the full-term and the 2-month premature infant can account for 8.00 or 9.00 D of difference in refraction.

The standard deviation of the Cook and Glasscock data was about 1.00 D greater than that of Kempf et al., and hence the range at the age of 6 years was about 6.00 D less than the range at birth. The phenomenon just described can adequately explain this decrease in variability. The status of the other variables at birth should be considered briefly. Mann (1950) states that two types of ciliary muscle can be recognized at birth, one with sparsely developed and the other with well-developed equatorial fibers. She concludes that this is suggestive because these types of ciliary muscle are seen in myopic and hyperopic adult eyes and may indicate that the ultimate refractive state has already been determined at birth.

Although this observation is interesting, the nearly normal distribution of refraction at birth would suggest normality of the distribution of the elements, as two types of lenses should lead to bimodality of the distribution of refraction. As has already been shown, lack of homogeneity in one element (axial length) in the adult eye is reflected as a similar lack of normality of the distribution of refraction. The evidence seems to point to the fact that each of the elements is normally distributed at birth, and that these elements combine in a more or less random fashion. The great variability of refraction at birth can be explained most simply on the basis of different periods of intrauterine life. This hypothesis should be checked in subsequent studies of the newborn. It is necessary to determine the relationship between the age of the fetus at the time of delivery and the refractive state of the eye at birth.

During the first year of life, two interesting phenomena occur: (1) the decreased variability of the axial length (and perhaps of the other elements as well) due to the events just described and (2) the growth of the eye from an average of about 17 mm to a little over 19 mm in axial length, accompanied by a decrease in the power of the cornea from about 50.00 to about 43.00 D. The increased length would make the eye about 6.00 or 7.00 D more myopic, whereas the corneal flattening would decrease myopia by about the same amount. Any net change in refraction would be due to a change in the power of the *lens*, but no reliable information about the lens is available for this period. By the end of the first year or shortly thereafter, the cornea has attained adult proportions and refraction. From this observation, an interesting inference may be made.

In the adult eye, there is a reasonable degree of correlation between corneal power and axial length. This may be ascribed to the fact that the longer globe is also a *larger* globe, as stressed by the authors (Weymouth and Hirsch 1950) and hence has a flatter cornea. However, as has almost been stated, the cornea has attained adult size by the age of 1 year; all authors agree that the cornea undergoes almost no growth after the age of 2 years. The basis for the correlation between axial length and corneal power, therefore, must be present by the age of 2 years. But the axis will continue to grow for many years after this time. Therefore, it must be inferred that the eye which is to become a big eye is already large at this early age and the eye that will remain small tends to be unduly small this early in the developmental period. This assumption, however, raises another problem because most children do not develop myopia until sometime around puberty. If the eye which is to become myopic is already large by the age of 2 years, then why is it not myopic at that age? The answer lies partly in the emmetropizing action of the cornea, which leads to the correlation. The only other answer is that the lens must counteract this excessive length. It should be stressed, however, that inferentially, at least, the length or size of the globe in maturity can be shown to be a result of its size at a very young age.

From the age of 1 or 2 years until the age of approximately 8 years, the growth of the eye is characterized by an increase from an axial length of about 19 mm to somewhere near the adult value of 24 mm, although the refractive state changes little. Since the cornea has already attained full size, this relative constancy of refraction is due mainly to *a flattening of the lens* and, to a lesser extent, to a deepening of the anterior chamber as the eye grows longer. This period is said to be characterized by a decrease in hyperopia of about 1.00 D (although this statement has never been satisfactorily authenticated). Whereas the increase in axial length is sufficient to cause an increased myopia (or decreased hyperopia) between 10 and 15 D during this period, the changes in the lens and anterior chamber normally compensate for all but about 1 D of the myopia that would otherwise develop. It is during this period of life that the correlation between axial length and lens power, and also between axial length and anterior chamber depth, occurs.

By the age of 8 or 9 years, it is claimed that the axial length has attained adult proportions. Keeney (1951) states that at the age of 8 years the "anterior-posterior diameter of the globe is established." The authors (Weymouth and Hirsch 1950), in fitting the limited data of Weiss (1897), also arrived at the curve for growth of the axis that became asymptomatic at about this age or even younger. However, this cannot be true in *all* cases because clinically it is observed that myopia (the major cause of which, from all data, is the axial length) for the most part develops after the age of 9 years. Furthermore, the overall refractive curve, whose shape has been shown to be a reflection of that of the axial length and whose kurtosis and skewness are believed to be due to two or more curves, is symmetric at the age of nine (Hirsch 1952). After the age of 9 years, the negative skew develops. The seeming conflict may be resolved by the inference that for most persons (but not all) the growth of the globe, especially in its axial length, is completed by the eighth or ninth year but that a small percentage of the cases (probably about 5 or 6% of the population) have globes that continue to increase in size for the years of puberty and a few years thereafter; these form a separate group whose eyes have continued to grow beyond the average period, the β group. If these conclusions are correct, it also means that the lens, which for the period from age 1 to age 8 or 9 years has been decreasing in power to counteract the effect of the length, must stop changing at somewhere about the age of 8 or 9 years.

On the basis of these theoretical conclusions, it is now possible to explain the various refractive anomalies, which are observed clinically. This discussion will serve to tie together the points discussed and it is again stressed that these classifications are tentative.

The high hyperope (in excess of 4.00 or 5.00 D) comprises 1% or less of the population and is characterized by an unduly small globe. These patients have an axial length of about 20 or 21 mm and exhibit high degrees of hyperopia throughout life. That the short anteroposterior diameter is the cause of the hyperopia is inferred from the fact that the distribution curve for axial length contains such a group, inhomogeneous with the main body of cases. That these cases are not lenticular or corneal is inferred from the fact that the distribution curves for these elements do not exhibit such inhomogeneity. Despite correlation between the elements, the lens and cornea never attain sufficient refractive power to counteract the effect of the small globe. Whether these cases also exhibit other signs of underdevelopment, such as facial stigmata, is a problem worthy of consideration.

The moderate hyperope and emmetrope constitutes the majority of the population. With regard to axial diameter, these patients have lengths that fall within the α group. These are the patients whose refraction changes little between the age of 1 or 2 years and maturity. This may be attributed to the fact that as the axis grows from infantile size to adult size, the myopia which would be produced is compensated for by decreased power, first of the cornea and later of the lens, and increased anterior chamber depth. It is noteworthy that overall refraction during the period from childhood to maturity always progresses in the *same direction*, that is, toward less hyperopia or more myopia. This may be explained on the basis of any one of three phenomena:

1. The growth rate of the lens is less than that of the axis, so that inevitably the effect of the axial length is not fully overcome.
2. The growth rate of the lens is in some way tied up with that of the axis. This relationship could be on the basis of mechanical factors or of chemical substances such as hormones, which serve as growth regulators. If this is the case, the evidence points to the axial length as the independent variable.
3. Growth has been completed at a very early age and refraction remains constant as a result.

To attempt to choose among these possibilities would be pure speculation, as the evidence does not seem to favor one possibility over the others.

It is sufficient to observe that little change in refraction occurs for the majority of the people over most of the period of growth. It may be argued that the act of seeing in some way influences the process, but the evidence is against such a view. For example, it might be supposed that as the axis increases in size, something concerned with seeing causes the lens to continue to grow less spherical when emmetropia was reached, and hence prevents the development of myopia. Such a concept, however, could not explain the maintenance of a moderate degree of hyperopia throughout the growth period, as frequently happens.

The myope of low degree constitutes between 15 and 25% of the population and is similar to the moderate hyperope and emmetrope. It is most probable that these are eyes whose axial length also falls within the α distribution but in which some growth in length occurred whose effect could not be counteracted by lenticular growth. If, as has been suggested earlier, the age of 8 or 9 years is taken as the age at which growth normally ceases, then it should be expected that by this age there will be a number of moderate myopes. That this is the case is demonstrated by the authors' data for children of school age (Hirsch 1952). By the age of 9 years, between 14 and 16% of the children have myopia of less than 2.00 D. It will be shown that the number who develop considerable degrees of this anomaly does not exceed 5 or 6%. Therefore, there is a considerable group of low myopes whose myopia has developed before the ninth year and does not increase markedly. One cannot help but wonder if much of the confusion about techniques for arresting myopia does not stem from this phenomenon.

By the age of 9 years, growth must be completed for the majority of cases. The curve for overall refraction is at this time (the only time other than at birth) symmetrical. The α curve of axial length for the adult probably does not differ markedly from the curve for axial length for all 8-year-olds. The presence of leptokurtosis at the age of about 9 years is due to the presence of a few cases at each extreme. We do not agree with the view that leptokurtosis is the manifestation of emmetropization. Rather, it is the result of combining a series of curves, namely a large central curve (α) and two smaller distributions of extreme cases at each tail. The combination of three such curves will give an overall distribution that is markedly leptokurtitic. The leptokurtosis at the age of 9 years, therefore, is due to a similar condition in the curve for axial length at this age. This in turn is due to the fact that while axial lengths of most of the children are normally distributed, there also exists a small number with very short axes, and a few with very long axes.

The moderate myope (between about −2 or −3 D to −6 or −7 D) is the individual whose myopia begins at the age of puberty, increases at a rapid rate for a period of months or even 2 or 3 years, and then becomes stationary. These patients are sometimes referred to as having "school myopia." We have shown that this anomaly comes on very close to the time of puberty and appears (as does puberty) a year or two earlier in girls than in boys.

It would appear that these children have axial lengths that fall within the β group. Such myopia, then, is not part and parcel of normal growth and development of the child, but rather represents a special anomaly. From the analysis of the axial length distribution of the adult, it was found that the β group includes about 6% of the population. The authors' data for schoolchildren (Hirsch 1952) indicates that about 5% of the children will have an increased myopia of more than a diopter at the age of 14 as compared to the age of 5 or 6. These figures, then, are in close agreement.

What is the cause of this anomaly? The evidence suggests that these are eyes that for some still undiscovered reason have an increase in axial length of 1 or 2 mm at a period (puberty) when the eyes of other children have ceased to grow. This extra growth leads to the development of the β distribution. It was shown in earlier calculations that the mean value for axial length of the adult was 23.66 mm for the α group and 25.37 mm for the β group. This difference of 1.71 mm will account for about 5 D of myopia.

Why does the lens that has successfully compensated for axial growth during the previous period not continue to do so? Perhaps, it occasionally does (a theory supported by the finding of Stenstrom and others that a small number of persons with large axial lengths are not myopic). For the most part, however, it must be assumed that the changes in refraction of the lens stop at the age of about 9 years. Although changes occur in the lens throughout life, this does not preclude the possibility that changes of refraction of this structure no longer occur beyond the age of 9 years.

Finally, the question may be raised as to whether this excessive length may not have been present for a number of years. For example, could it not be that a child had an eye of excessive length but manifested no myopia because the lens compensated until it stopped flattening at which time myopia manifested itself? The reason for rejecting such a hypothesis is that the distribution curve for refraction (and probably also the distribution curve for axial length) is still symmetrical at the age of 9 years.

The evidence all seems to point to the fact that both the lens and the axial length have achieved full growth by the age of 9 years. After this, for some reason still to be explained, about 6% of the eyes continue to grow axially. These eyes grow about an additional 2 mm over a period of 1 to 3 years. This rate of growth is more rapid than the rate before the age of 9 years; therefore, this group has a distinctly different anomaly than the myopes in the preceding section.

The higher myopes include those with degrees of myopia in excess of 6 or 7 D, and comprises no more than 1 to 2% of the population. The basic cause is an excessively great axial length (the γ group), and fundus changes are usually encountered in these persons. Duke-Elder (1949) discusses this group, calling them "degenerative myopes," and his treatment of the subject is admirable. Some of these myopes are high congenital myopes, but the number of these must be small because the degree of leptokurtosis at birth is not great. The authors (Hirsch 1953) have shown that there are about twice as many women as men in this group, and the group may be said to have a distinct anomaly (or anomalies) characterized by an unduly large globe. The anomaly is not common, the authors (1953) having found only 1% of women and 0.5% of men to have this refractive state. Therefore, the percentage in the population, randomly sampled, should be less. Percentages for European investigators seem to run higher, and it is possible, as Duke-Elder suggests, that this anomaly is more common in some countries and in some ethnic groups than in others.

SUMMARY

A working hypothesis for the genesis of refraction has been evolved on the basis of the statistical evidence accumulated by ourselves and other investigators. We are aware of the many uncharted areas in the field, and hence are aware that the hypothesis will in the future require revision and perhaps even complete discarding. However, in the present state of knowledge it adequately considers most of the evidence at hand. The salient features may now be briefly listed by way of summary:

1. The overall refractive state results from the combination of a number of elements, three of which are especially important.

2. The axial length is the dominating factor, changes in it being correlated with growth changes in the other elements in such a way that the resultant effect is a relatively stable refractive state.

3. The stable refraction and related growth of different parts may result either from mechanical factors (the large eye has the flatter cornea and the flatter lens) or from the response of various structures to the same substance (hormone or chemical growth regulator).

4. The distribution in refraction of the newborn develops into that of the adult in the following manner. During the first few years of life the extreme myopes and extreme hyperopes become less ametropic, with the result that the variability is distinctly reduced. The mean shifts about 1.00 D toward less hyperopia. Positive skewness develops, and we believe this is due to the fact that a small group of hyperopes, inhomogeneous with the majority of the cases, remain highly hyperopic. The symbol γ has been assigned to this group. Leptokurtosis increases, which is interpreted as being due to the presence of a large group, normally distributed, and a small group forming a tail. Between the first few years of life (present data preclude the possibility of stating an exact age) and about 9 years of age, there is a slight change in the mean (a shift toward less hyperopia) and little change in the variability. The positive skewness disappears, so the symmetry that characterized the curve at birth is again present at the age of 9 years, indicating the development of a myopic tail of similar value to the hyperopic tail.

This development eventually leads to an increased leptokurtosis. For most people, refraction is stable after the age of 9 years. However, a small percentage of individuals becomes more myopic at puberty, from 1.00 to 5.00 D. These cases (estimated at about 6% of the population) form a normally distributed group with a mean of 3.00 to 4.00 D of myopia. This leads to a further increase in leptokurtosis and the development of negative skewness that characterizes the adult curve. To the main body, that is, those who remained stable after the age of 9 years, the symbol α has been assigned, whereas this group of myopes is referred to as the β group. Finally, a very small percentage of the population becomes highly myopic, and to this group, who seemingly has a degenerative process, the letter γ is assigned. This leads to further negative skewness, increased leptokurtosis, a small increase in variability, and a slight shift of the mean toward less hyperopia. All of these changes in the distribution curve do in fact occur between the age of 9 years and maturity.

5. The distribution of refraction for the adult has a mean of about $+0.50$ D and is negatively skewed and leptokurtic. This deviation from the normal curve characteristic of so many other anthropometric variables can be explained by postulating the existence of the four groups listed previously, each group being normally distributed.

6. The leptokurtosis and skewness of the adult refractive curve seem to result from similar phenomena in the distribution of axial lengths. The axial length is the only element whose distribution exhibits the same deviations from normality as the overall refractive curve.

7. With regard to the individual elements, the cornea appears to reach its final size by the age of 1 or 2 years; the axial length for most people reaches full size by the age of 9 years, whereas a small percentage of the population (about 6% exhibits a further growth of 1 to 2 mm in axial length between the ages of 9 and about 15 years. The crystalline lens grows throughout life with several different phases. Information about its refractive power is not available, and must be inferred. During the period of rapid growth, the lens shows marked changes (increased weight and decreased sphericity). The fact that axial length and corneal power are stable after the age of 9 years and overall refraction changes little after this time (except in the formation of the β and γ groups, which changes are believed to be associated with similar changes in axial length) should lead to the conclusion that the refractive power of the lens changes little after the age of 9 years. Unfortunately, this hypothesis is unconfirmed at this time.

8. The axial length is positively correlated with the other diameters of the globe so that an eye with a long axial length is in fact a large eye, whereas one with a short axial length is a small eye.

9. On the basis of the preceding conclusions, four patterns for development of refraction may be tentatively described.

- *High hyperopes:* This anomaly is due to a congenitally small globe that, during the growth period, did not attain a "normal" or near normal size. This group is not homogenous with the main body of the cases and, therefore, may be said to have an anomalous refraction.
- *High myopes:* This group, comprising 1 or 2% of the population, is characterized by excessively long anteroposterior diameters. It has been shown in another paper that this anomaly occurs twice as often among women as among men. The term degenerative has been applied by Duke-Elder.
- *Moderate myopes:* In about 6% of the population, the axial length (and probably the entire globe), the growth of which has been quite slow before puberty, increases markedly during this period. The lens at this age is seemingly no longer able to counteract such an increase, resulting in the development of marked myopia. The mean axial length for this group is about 1.7 mm longer than that for the bulk of the population. This entity, sometimes referred to as "school myopia," should more properly be called "developmental myopia," and merits further investigation in the light of the evidence cited. It is possible that a hormonal disturbance or an associated general disease may be the underlying cause of the sudden overgrowth.
- *Low myopes, emmetropes, and low hyperopes.* If the three groups just described are excluded, there remains a group of about 91% of the population. The distribution of the refractive state of this group is essentially normal, as is the distribution of each of the elements for this group. Differences in refraction occurring among individuals within this group result solely from biologic variability. Dur-

ing the first year or two, when increase in axial length is great, the effect of this growth is offset by growth of both the cornea and the lens. From this time until the age of 9 years, growth of the axis is offset by changes in the lens. At about the age of 9 years, the refraction of members of this group is for the most part stable and only slight changes (less than 1.00 D) take place thereafter.

REFERENCES

Collins ET. Changes in the visual organs correlated with the adaptation of arborieal life and with the assumption of an erect posture. Trans Ophthal Soc UK 1921;41:10.

Cook RG, Glasscock RE. Refractive and ocular findings in the newborn. Am J Ophthalmol 1951;34:1407–1413.

Duke-Elder WS. Textbook of Ophthalmology, vol 1. St Louis: CV Mosby Co, 1940.

Duke-Elder WS. Textbook of Ophthalmology, vol 4. St Louis: CV Mosby Co, 1949.

Hirsch MJ. Sex differences in the incidence of various grades of myopia. Am J Optom Arch Am Acad Optom 1953;30:135–138.

Hirsch MJ. The changes of refraction between the ages of 5 and 14 — theoretical and practical considerations. Am J Optom Arch Am Acad Optom 1952;29:445–459.

Hirsch MJ. An analysis of inhomogeneity of myopia in adults. Am J Optom Arch Am Acad Optom 1950;27:562–571.

Hirsch MJ, Weymouth FW. Notes on ametropia—a further analysis of Strenstrom's data. Am J Optom Arch Am Acad Optom 1947;24:601–608.

Keeney AH. Chronology of Ophthalmic Development. Springfield, IL: Charles C Thomas, 1951.

Landolt E. The Refraction and Accommodation of the Eye. Edinburgh: Young J. Pentland, 1886.

Mann I. The Development of the Human Eye. New York: Grune & Stratton, 1950.

Santonastanio A. The state of refraction of the eye during the first years of life. Ann Ottal Clin Ocul 1930;58:852.

Scheerer R, Betsch A. (Original not examined; cited by Stenstrom S, 1948). Scheerer R. Klin Monatsbl f Augenh 1929;82:511. Betsch A. Klin Monatsbl Augenheilkd 1929;82:365.

Steiger A. Die Entstehung der Spharischen Refracktionen des Menschlichen Auges. S. Karger, Berlin, 1913.

Stenstrom S. Investigation of the variation and the covariation of the optical elements of human eyes, trans. D. Woolf. Am J Optom and Arch Am Acad Optom 1948;25(5):218–232; (6):286–299; (7):340–350; (8):388–397; (9):438–449; (10):496–504.

Stromberg E. Uber refraktion und achenlange des menschlichen auges. (Original not examined; cited by Stenstrom S, 1948). Acta Ophthalmol 1936;14:281.

Taketa S. The Relation of the Crystalline Lens to the Refractive State of the Eye. M.A. Thesis, Leland Stanford University, 1949.

Titoff IG. The refraction curve in adults and in the newborn. Viestnik Opht 1937;11:591. (Original not examined; Abstract Am J Ophthalmol 1933;21:940).

Tron EJ. The optical elements of the refractive power of the eye. In: Ridley F, Sorsby A, eds. Modern Trends in Ophthalmology. New York: Paul B. Hoeber, 1940.

Weiss L. Uber das Wachsenden Auge. Anat Hefte 1897;8:193–248.

Weymouth FW, Hirsch MJ. Relative growth of the eye. Am J Optom Arch Am Acad Optom 1950;27:317–328.

Wolff E. The Anatomy of the Eye and Orbit. Philadelphia: P. Blakinston's Son and Co., 1933.

4

Epidemiology and Genetics of Refractive Anomalies

John C. Bear

☐

Refractive error is a *quantitative* trait. This determines the appropriate techniques for measuring epidemiological associations and familial resemblances. Many quantitative traits follow a more-or-less gaussian ("normal") distribution in the population: height is an obvious example (Harrison et al. 1977). In contrast, the population frequency distribution of refractive error has a marked excess of emmetropic and near-emmetropic eyes, long tails of hyperopic and myopic values, and relative deficiencies in low and moderate myopia and hyperopia (Sorsby et al. 1960, Sorsby 1980). In samples representative of the general population, the distribution has a single peak, and there is no indication of an additional peak of myopes (Sorsby et al. 1960), although in a series of clinical patients this may appear to be the case (Hirsch 1950, Sorsby et al. 1960).

Population variation in a quantitative trait can have public health implications. Blood pressure is a good example; persons with unusual values of the trait will benefit from clinical intervention. The same is true for refractive error. However, compared to other quantitative traits, it has been little studied. Therefore, the epidemiology and genetics of more extensively studied traits provides a framework for approaching the epidemiology and genetics of refractive error.

The anatomical variation determining clinically significant refractive error is relatively small, compared to clinically significant deviations in other quantitative traits. The average axial length of the adult eye is about 24 mm, and a deviation of 1 mm, or 4%, implies a refractive error of approximately 3.00 D (Duke-Elder and Abrams 1970, 115, 218–219). Uncorrected myopia of this degree would seriously impair vision, and errors corresponding to axial length deviations of 2% or even less would ordinarily be corrected. In contrast, diastolic blood pressure

Discussions with many people, particularly Avrum Richler, Ernst Goldschmidt, Gordon Johnson, and Clarke Fraser, have helped me develop the ideas outlined here. Financial support for this work is provided by the National Health Research and Development Program, Health and Welfare Canada.

would have to exceed 90 mm Hg before clinical intervention would be considered (Fodor 1980), and this value is 12.5% higher than the conventionally accepted population average of 80 mm Hg. As a nonclinical example, a person 4% taller or heavier than the average (6'1" vs. 5'10") would not be remarkable.

The fact that the population frequency distribution of refraction clusters around emmetropia, even though variation in refraction results from proportionately very slight anatomical variations, makes four things likely.

1. The excess of emmetropic values suggests that the genetic control of the development of refraction is very precise. Natural selection acts strongly against extremely high or low values of any metric trait to maintain the population at optimum values (Crow 1986, 144–147), and it is not difficult to imagine that in the earlier stages of human existence eyes that focused retinal images imprecisely must have placed their owners at a severe selective disadvantage (Post 1971).

2. The peaked distribution of ocular refraction is consistent with its determination by multiple genes. In general, evolution favors the determination of traits by numerous genes, the individual influences of which are small and additive, with none having a large effect on the value of a trait. The more genes that contribute to population variation, the more individuals will have optimum values of the trait and the greater the possibility for genetic fine tuning of trait values in response to environmental change (Crow 1986, 194); and the more genes that influence a trait, the more peaked will be the distribution of the trait (Vogel and Motulsky, 1979, 149).

3. Because the development of the eye must be so precise, it is likely to be extraordinarily sensitive to disruptions. Rare genes or environmental factors that do not greatly derange other aspects of development might confer a large refractive error; and commonly occurring environmental influences, though having only a slight influence on ocular development, might nonetheless contribute substantially to population variation in refractive error.

4. Because appreciable differences in refractive error result from very slight anatomical deviations, it is likely that much variation in refractive error may be unattributable to particular genetic or environmental influences, no matter how well these come to be measured and characterized.

It follows from these four points that population variation in refractive error may include not only components attributable to genetic and environmental variation, but also a component (possibly a large one) not attributable to any specific influence. Furthermore, emmetropia and low-to-moderate refractive errors may result from the combined influences of multiple genes, and be influenced also by both indentifiable and random environmental factors. Finally, it follows that high refractive errors may occur both as extremes of the "normal" variation in the population and as a result of a heterogeneous collection of causes including rare genes and specific environmental insults. These are simply plausible assumptions, but they provide a rational biological framework for epidemiology and genetic studies. It must be emphasized also that because individuals vary in their genetic makeup, they may respond differently to environmental influences (Vogel and Motulsky 1979, 259–262).

■ EPIDEMIOLOGY

The central historical question in the epidemiology of refractive error is whether the use of the eyes for close work can induce myopia. Kepler raised this possibility in 1611, only a few years after he gave the first correct description of the optics of the eye (Duke-Elder and Abrams 1970, 341); it was presented as an undoubted fact by Donders (1864, 343) in the first, and very influential, text on the anomalies of refraction and their correction. Subsequently, many studies have considered the question (Goldschmidt 1968, Duke-Elder and Abrams 1970).

□ Criteria for Causality

Using epidemiological data, it is generally difficult to demonstrate that an association between exposure and a disease is causal. For causality to be considered likely, several formal criteria are recognized (Mausner and Bahn 1974):

1. The association should be statistically significant and strong. A dose-response relationship strengthens the likelihood of causality — increasing exposure to the putative causal agent should increase the incidence or the severity of the disorder.
2. The association should be consistent in different populations. In any one population, the association might result from some systematic error in observation, or be spurious, reflecting covariation of the supposed influencing variable with the actual cause of the disorder.
3. The association should be temporally correct, the influence preceding the disorder by an appropriate interval.
4. The association should be specific and not attributable to other factors co-varying with the putative causal agent.
5. The association should be biologically plausible.

Studies of the association between refractive error and vision activity have not generally been conducted with these formal criteria in mind. For this reason, only recent, relatively well-designed studies of the association between refractive error and vision activity can be reviewed here, along with the evidence for associations between refractive error and other environmental influences.

□ Vision Activity: Indirect Measures

In industrialized societies, refractive error is convincingly associated with formal education. In a representative sample of young Danish male conscripts, Goldschmidt (1968) found that 30% of men educated to the university entrance level had myopia greater than 1.50 D and that this percentage decreased, with decreasing amount of formal education, to 3% for unskilled workers. Goldschmidt's study was carried out in 1964 and replicated that of Tscherning, carried out in 1882; findings of the two studies were essentially identical. In Tscherning's data, 32% of the most educated conscripts were 2.00 D myopic or more, 2% of the least educated men were 2.00 D myopic or more, and a graded decrease in myopia frequency was found in the groupings of men with intermediate amounts of education.

Sperduto et al. (1983) assessed the relation between the prevalence of myopia and the amount of formal education in the population of the United States, using the data of the 1971–1972 National Health and Nutrition Examination Survey of a representative sample of the population aged 18 to 54 years. Findings for all ages were very similar to those of the Danish studies. Among persons who had completed less than the fifth grade, 3 to 6% were myopes, and among persons who had completed more than 12 grades, 30 to 40% were myopes, with intermediate frequencies of myopia at intermediate levels of education.

□ Vision Activity: Direct Measures

Three recent studies have directly measured the statistical association between refractive error and measurements of vision activity.

Angle and Wissman (1980) analyzed data for 3,957 persons aged 12 to 17 years, with estimated refractive errors between -0.10 D and -8.00 D, from a representative sample of the U.S. population between 1966 and 1970. They found that the statistical association of myopia with vision activity measurements (grade in school, minutes spent reading per day, and a reading test score) explained its association with several sociological attributes (sex, race, region of residence, income, and age). However, the statistical association of myopia with vision activity explained only a small part of the variation of myopia in the population (5 or 6%, judging from their tables).

The populations of three rural Newfoundland communities were studied by Richler and Bear (1980a). Refractive error was measured for 971 persons (80% of the inhabitants over 5 years of age), and data were obtained by questionnaire on the amount of time spent in vision activities requiring focusing of the eyes at a distance of 20 inches or less. These persons were unselected, other than being over 5 years of age and resident in the study communities. The association of refractive error with nearwork was statistically significant and fairly consistent, at all ages between 5 and 60 years (Table 4.1). Formal education did not become compulsory in Newfoundland until 1949, and many subjects above middle age

Table 4.1. Statistical Associations of Refraction and Nearwork in Three Rural Newfoundland Communities†

Age interval	n	Partial correlation coefficient, adjusting for age, sex and education	Multiple regression coefficient
5–14	340	− 0.35**	− 0.43
15–29	269	− 0.26**	− 0.30
30–44	157	− 0.38**	− 0.29
45–59	125	− 0.21*	− 0.23
≥60	66	− 0.11	− 0.22

*$P<0.05$
**$P<0.01$
†Data from Richler and Bear (1980a)

had little or no education. Few subjects other than teenaged students did even moderate amounts of near work. Refractive error in this population shows usual age trends, toward minus values until the late teenage years and toward plus values thereafter (Richler and Bear 1980b). The persistence and consistency of the relationship between refractive error and nearwork is noteworthy because it spans a wide range of ages in this population who generally did little nearwork, and whose nearwork levels varied with age.

Ashton (1985a) analyzed the relation between refractive error and several measurements of vision activity in 925 persons, ages 12 to 33 years, from 723 Hawaiian families. The nearwork measures used, all self-reported, were books read per month, magazines read per month, hours spent on homework per week, and number of years of education completed. Refractive error measurements were adjusted for age, race, and sex, as well as for performance on tests of cognitive ability and school achievement. Ashton concluded that his results, taken together, did not support an association between myopia and nearwork because it could not be inferred that progression of myopia was related to measures of nearwork (although, as he points out, these data do not allow temporal associations to be measured directly but only inferred) and because only two of four nearwork measures were related to refractive error, although he considered each to be a good measure. It is noteworthy that Ashton's (1985a) data do show an association of refractive error with amount of formal education and book reading, consistent with findings in other studies reviewed in this section.

□ Ethnicity

In Japan, myopia is relatively common, and is considered a serious public health problem (Sato 1957). In population survey data, about 12% of 6-year-olds in rural

Japan were found to be -0.5 D or more myopic (Majima et al. 1960), compared to less than 4% of New Brunswick children of the same age (Woodruff 1986). In Japanese teenagers and young adults, myopia affects about 35% of high school students and 40 to 50% of university students, and the prevalence has apparently increased dramatically in this century (Otsuka 1967). Comparing Japanese to whites, a higher initial rate of myopia and a secular trend in myopia prevalence require explanation.

In populations following hunting and gathering modes of life, such as precontact Africans, Eskimos, and Australian Aborigines, reduced visual acuity for any reason was very uncommon and probably conferred a severe selective disadvantage (Post 1971); moderate and high refractive errors, and particularly high myopia, were rare or absent (Holm 1937, Skeller 1954, Taylor 1981). This cannot be taken to indicate an influence of vision activity on refractive error in white and Japanese populations; selective forces on these two types of population are different, and genetic differences may contribute to interracial differences in refractive error.

In Native American populations in Alaska and northern Canada, myopia, predominantly of mild degree, is unexpectedly common among persons born since World War II. Table 4.2 summarizes reports that allow intergenerational comparisons; the pattern is striking and consistent. By comparison, the U.S. white population shows little difference in myopia prevalence at different ages (Sperduto et al. 1983). Several studies included the great majority of their target populations and are in effect population surveys; in others, it is not likely that younger myopes would be more inclined to be examined than older myopes. The myopia increase affects the first members of these societies to be exposed to standard North American culture, including compulsory formal education, and an influence of vision activity on refraction would explain the increase. Alternative explanations are possible because a number of changes occurred simultaneously in the lives of these peoples; some observers have suggested that dietary changes are relevant (Cass 1973, and see references in Table 4.2). Presumably northern Native Americans are exceptionally susceptible to some environmental influences compared to whites, for in their older generations myopia is less prevalent than in whites of comparable age, while in younger persons it is often much more prevalent. Native Americans are of Asian extraction, and their current high rates of myopia bring to mind the secular increase noted in Japan (Otsuka 1967).

By contrast, in Vanuatu (formerly New Hebrides), a reasonably representative survey involving 977 of the native Melanesian schoolchildren aged 6 to 17 years found only 1.3% with myopia greater than -0.25 D, and no trend toward more myopic refraction with age (Garner et al. 1985). These students apparently took a conscientious attitude toward school attendance.

□ Nutrition

After vision activity, nutrition is the environmental variable most often considered as possibly influencing refractive error. In general, the eye is protected from

Table 4.2. Intergenerational Differences in Myopia Prevalence in Canadian and Alaskan Native Peoples

Reference	Date	Place	Ethnic group	Age interval in years	% Prevalence (no. tested)	Limit for myopia (measurement method)	% of Total population included in survey
Young et al. (1969)	1967	North Alaska	Inuit*	16–26 >26	70 (104) 14 (225)	−0.25D (c)†	25
Boniuk (1973)	1970–71	Northwestern Ontario	Indian	20–29 30–39	58 (ns)‡ 16 (ns)	−1 D (c)	~50
Morgan and Munro (1973)	1970–71	Yukon and Northwest Territories	Indian and Inuit	15–20 25–30	≈30 (ns) <10 (ns)	−1 D (c)	ns
Morgan et al. (1975)	1974	Northwest Territories	Inuit	15–29 ≥30	31 (112) 4 (186)	ns (c)	ns
Woodruff and Samek (1977)	1970–71	North Ontario	Amerind	21–22 61–70	61 (255) 11 (292)	−0.5 D (rs)§	32–70 in different communities
Johnson et al. (1979)	1977	Northern Labrador	Inuit	20–30 >30	37 (38) 14 (96)	−0.25 D (rs)	87
Alward et al. (1985)	1983	Southwest Alaska	Inuit	21–23	68 (252)	−0.5 D (c)	92
Sperduto et al. (1983)		United States	White	12–17 18–24 25–54	26 30 26 (with little variation in this interval)	screening methodology	probability sample

*Inuit peoples prefer this designation for themselves over the English term Eskimo.
†cycloplegic
‡not stated
§retinoscopy and subjective

growth retardation associated with malnutrition (McLaren 1980). High refractive error was found to be common among grossly malnourished African children (McLaren 1960); however, while marasmic Lebanese children were found to have a more myopic distribution of refraction than adequately nourished control children, this difference disappeared once the malnutrition was corrected (Halasa and McLaren 1964). These observations suggest that for adequately nourished persons any influence of diet on refraction is small or negligible and that only very comprehensive investigations could test for such an influence. Thus, it is not surprising that questionnaire studies comparing the food intake of hyperopes and myopes find no significant differences between them (Young et al. 1973). Reports claiming to show a relation between myopia and inadequate intake of animal protein and a slowing of myopia progression by dietary supplementation (Gardiner 1958) are uninterpretable because the subjects were clearly self-selected. More recent reports proposing complex relations between myopia and intake of calcium, chromium, protein, sugar, and vitamin C, as well as accommodative effort (Lane 1981a, 1981b), are also uninterpretable; they give no clear indication of the sources and selection of participants or of the numbers of statistical comparisons from which the significant results have been selected.

□ Illness

It has long been considered possible that myopia is sometimes precipitated by disease and debility (Duke-Elder and Abrams, 1970, 340), but there has been little specific investigation of this theory (Baldwin 1981).

Gardiner and James (1960) found that toxemia and other diseases occurred in 74% of pregnancies producing infants with congenital myopia (thirty-eight pregnancies), compared with 36% of a control series of thirty-nine pregnancies for infants suffering from other visual disorders. The possibility of prenatal influences on the subsequent development of refractive error seems otherwise not to have been investigated, although such influences can readily be imagined (see, for example, McLaren 1980).

Hirsch (1957) discussed the possible association between myopia and febrile diseases such as measles. He was not surprised that previous studies had failed to find an association, given that almost everyone has had measles at some time during childhood. He reported the results of a study in which the parents of a group of junior high school students were asked to complete a questionnaire, indicating whether the student had had measles and, if so, at what age. Comparing refractive state to the age of incidence of measles, Hirsch found a significant relationship between the presence of myopia from 1.00 to 6.00 D and the occurrence of measles at age 6, 7, or 8 years. Consistent with Hirsch's finding of a possible relationship between measles and myopia is the report of Maurice and Mushin (1966) that myopia was induced in immature rabbits by simultaneously increasing the intraocular pressure and increasing the body temperature. Hirsch argued that it was possible that myopia might be a consequence of a febrile disease, such as scarlet fever, whooping cough, or measles, in which coughing is likely to occur (causing a momentary increase in intraocular pressure) in the presence of fever.

□ Age of Onset

It cannot be assumed that all myopia reflects the same determinants. Grosvenor (1987) suggests that myopia can be classified as congenital, youth onset, early adult onset and late adult onset, without making assumptions about causation. Most myopia is youth onset; therefore, epidemiological associations result mainly from associations with this form of myopia, particularly if only the preadult population is considered.

About 2% of myopia is congenital (Grosvenor 1987), and some myopia is associated with low birth weight; this myopia of prematurity results from an undersized eye and a relatively highly curved cornea (Fledelius 1976). In Europe and North America the prevalence of myopia among premature births is 15 to 20%, and 6 to 7% of births are premature; therefore, this association should account for about 1% of myopia in these populations (Weale 1983) and should not obscure other epidemiological associations.

A small percentage of the population develops myopia in early adulthood (Grosvenor 1987), in some cases due to progressive changes in refraction continuing at an age when myopia progression has usually ceased (Goss et al. 1985) and, in some cases, due to progressive steepening of the cornea (Goss and Erickson 1987). Early adult-onset myopia may be associated with increased requirements for reading and studying; it tends to be noticed in students in professional schools and military academies (Dunphy et al. 1968, Gmelin 1976, Shotwell 1984). Presumably some individuals are susceptible and others are not because not all such students become myopic. If some early adult-onset myopia is induced by reading and studying, its prevalence may vary between populations depending on their usual levels of education. Late adult-onset myopia should not contribute much to differences observed among populations, however, because it is uncommon and because most studies do not include older adults.

□ Does Vision Activity Cause Myopia?

The evidence that vision activity influences the development of myopia is impressive, even though relevant investigations have not always been carried out according to stringent epidemiological criteria. The association of myopia with formal education is strong, remarkably consistent, and dose-dependent. A tenfold difference in myopia frequency between least and most educated persons is found for the Danish male populations of 1882 and 1964, and in the U.S. population for persons between the ages of 18 and 54 years (Goldschmidt 1968, Sperduto et al. 1983). These persons experienced widely differing noneducational environments, making alternative explanations for the association unlikely. If formal education indicates levels of reading and similar nearwork, these results suggest vision activity does indeed influence refraction in the populations studied. Three studies have examined the association of refraction with more direct measures of vision activity; two found convincing statistical associations (Angle and Wissman 1980, Richler and Bear 1980a) and the findings of the third (Ashton 1985a) are also suggestive of an association. Associations of refractive error with self-reported measurements of vision activity are less striking than associations with formal education, probably because such questionnaires give relatively imprecise measurements (Richler et al. 1986).

For U.S. myopes, Angle and Wissman (1978) estimated the regression of refraction on years of education as -0.22 D per year, implying a 1.5 D shift toward myopia associated with the 7-year difference between completing five and twelve school grades. For the rural Newfoundland study (Richler and Bear 1980a), regressions of refraction on years of education (adjusted for age and sex but not nearwork) are smaller, at -0.08 to -0.13 D per year in age groups from 5 to 44 years, perhaps reflecting lower educational levels. Also, the Newfoundland data include the entire range of refractive error, not just myopia. If the population frequency distribution of refractive error were shifted 1.00 to 2.00 D in the direction of minus errors, this would push at least 30% of persons from the emmetropic into the low myopic range (see for example Sorsby et al. 1960). It follows that the statistical association of refraction with education, found in measurements of individuals, is more than sufficient to account for the differences in myopia prevalence (approximately 30% vs 3%) between the most and least educated members of populations. Consistent with this is the finding in the Newfoundland study that the regression coefficients relating self-reported nearwork and refractive error (-0.43 to -0.23 D per hour of nearwork per day depending on age) indicate that usual levels of nearwork could have a clinically significant influence on refractive error (Richler and Bear 1980a).

These statistical relations highlight an interpretive paradox. The proportion of variation in refraction explained by its association with education is small (Angle and Wissman 1978, 1980; Richler and Bear 1980a), as is the proportion of variance in refraction explained by its association with nearwork (4 to 12% depending on age, in Newfoundland data [Richler and Bear 1980a]). Nonetheless, this statistically small association implies that vision activity can have a large influence on the prevalence of clinically significant myopia and the associated, more serious vision disorders, such as glaucoma and retinal detachment.

Available data are insufficient to indicate whether the vision activity-refractive error association meets the criterion of temporal correctness, as would be expected if vision activity influenced the development of refractive error. It may be argued that most formal education (and thus reading and similar nearwork) occurs after the late childhood years when myopia usually develops (Angle and Wissman 1978). On the other hand, among 11-year-old British children, myopes were found to have had higher levels of educational achievement than nonmyopes not only at 11 years of age, but also at age 7 years, before becoming myopic; the 11-year-old myopes did more reading than nonmyopes (Peckham et al. 1977). A Finnish study (Pärssinen 1987) reports that myopes recall doing more reading as children than nonmyopes. Such findings suggest that pertinent differences in vision activity are indeed present before myopia actually becomes manifest.

The intergenerational difference in myopia prevalence in northern Native Americans deserves more extensive study. The difference is too large and has occurred too quickly to be explained genetically. Vision activity changes (exposure to formal education, working in poor illumination) and dietary changes have been proposed as possible causes. The first possibility seems likely but the second unlikely, given observations in other populations. Dietary changes that have been blamed are increased consumption of refined carbohydrate and a parallel reduced consumption of animal protein (Cass 1973, see also the references to Table 4.2). Studies in North American and European white populations provide no convincing indication that diet influences refraction; if anything, the less educated members of these populations are likely to eat too much carbohydrate and too little protein, but these persons are less often myopic than more educated individuals, whose diets are presumably better. Although the data for native North Americans favor an influence of vision activity on the development of refractive error, the lack of an association of refractive error with education in Vanuatu (Garner et al. 1985) emphasizes the possibility that different racial groups may differ in the potential for refractive error to be influenced by environmental factors.

Observations on animals and humans (reviewed elsewhere in this volume) suggest mechanisms by which vision activity might influence the development of refractive error, but whether these are relevant to refractive error variation at the population level has yet to be investigated epidemiologically.

In summary, epidemiological observations suggest that vision activity influences the development of refractive error. The association of refractive error with education is strong, consistent, and dose-dependent. An association is found also with vision activity measured directly. The association seems temporally correct, and plausible biological mechanisms can be suggested for it. The strength of the relation between vision activity and refraction may well vary with race. An association with nutrition seems unlikely. Myopia is associated with premature birth, but this can account for little prevalence variation within or among populations. Epidemiological data on other possible associations are too few to permit conclusions. Available data are insufficient to allow exploration of interactions among environmental factors, which might influence refractive error variation within and among populations.

GENETICS

Genetic variation in quantitative traits must be characterized using methods that allow for the possibility that multiple genes and environmental factors influence trait values, and contribute to population variation. Refraction is a quantitative trait, and it is inappropriate to proceed as if myopia were an all-or-none trait, just as it would be inappropriate to analyze the genetics of height as if all persons were tall or not tall, on the unsupported assumption that tallness is a single-gene trait (Vogel and Motulsky 1979, 150).

☐ Single Gene Interpretations

The idea that myopia is a single gene trait is, unfortunately, remarkably persistent in the vision literature. Many pedigrees purporting to show particular refractive errors transmitted in families as single gene traits were collected early in this century, after the rediscovery of Mendel's work, when enthusiasm for genetics was great but quantitative genetic variation was not yet generally understood. Dominant, recessive, and X-linked pedigrees are reproduced side by side in standard texts on vision genetics (see, for example, Waardenburg 1963). Usually only the persons with "high" refractive errors are indicated, with no indication of their actual refractive errors, or of the refractive errors of other family members. This makes it impossible to get a complete picture of the variation in each family. The frequency of such pedigrees is unknown, so it is impossible to tell how much they contribute to total population rates of high refractive errors.

Ashton (1985b) presents more comprehensive data on the familial recurrence of myopia in the general population. The percentage of myopia among children when neither, one, or both parents were myopes was 10 to 11%, 16 to 25%, and 33 to 46%, respectively (the first percentage in each pair is for Hawaiian families of European ancestry and the second for Hawaiian families of Japanese ancestry). As Ashton notes, these values are not consistent with single-gene inheritance of myopia.

☐ Quantitative Genetic Analysis of Refractive Error

Fisher (1918) demonstrated that familial resemblances in quantitative traits could be explained in terms of mendelian inheritance by showing that quantitative variation would result if alleles (alternative forms of genes) at a number of genetic loci each had small, more-or-less identical influences on an individual's trait value. This has come to be called *polygenic* inheritance. Resemblances between two relatives are predictable from the proportion of alleles they have in common. For instance, a child is expected to receive half of the alleles that influence his or her trait value from each parent, and two sibs have half their alleles in common, on average. Assuming all variation in the trait is polygenic (and that no relevant genes are on the X or Y chromosomes), the predicted correlation coefficients between offspring and parents, and between pairs of sibs, are each 0.5. Similar predictions are possible for other pairs of relatives. If observed correlations are less, this suggests that some variation is due to randomly occurring environmental influences. Note that correlations among relatives may reflect influences other than polygenic inheritance and random environment, particularly single genes with large effects on trait values and environmental influences shared by family members. (For a more detailed discussion of quantitative inheritance, see Falconer 1981, the standard reference and an excellent textbook, or Spivey 1976).

Table 4.3 summarizes the findings of studies that have evaluated both offspring-parent and sib-sib resemblances in refraction. Findings of studies that report only offspring-parent or sib-sib resemblances are similar (Young 1958, Keller 1973, Hegmann et al. 1974, Johnson et al. 1979). The pattern of resemblances found is fairly consistent. Correlations of offspring with parents and correlations between pairs of sibs are moderate. There is no correlation between the parents of the children studied to suggest that people prefer spouses with similar refractive errors. (Such a parental correlation would act to increase the similarity of sib pairs and would have to be taken into account in analyses.) If population variation in refraction were determined only by polygenic inheritance and random environmental variation, the polygenic component of variation would be twice the offspring-parent or sib-sib correlation, and these studies would suggest that about half of population variation in refraction is due to polygenic inheritance. In most studies, sib-sib resemblances exceed offspring-parent resemblances, which may be explained in at least two possible ways. First, resemblances among relatives may be influenced by shared environmental factors: Sib pairs might share envi-

Table 4.3.   Resemblances between First-degree Relatives in Refractive Error

Reference (ethnic group)	Offspring-parent	Sib-sib	Father-mother
Sorsby et al. (1966) (English)	0.23 (100)*	0.36 (24/22)	−0.12 (28)
Young et al. (1969, 1972) (Alaskan Inuit)	0.23 (258)	0.45 (100)	(ns)†
Alsbirk (1979) (Greenland Inuit)	0.07 (159)	0.25 (160)	0.03 (108)
Bear et al. (1981) (Newfoundland)	0.23‡	0.29 (714/215)	0.04 (123)
Ashton (1985b) (European and Japanese, in Hawaii)	0.25 (1564)	0.37 (782)	0.01 (378)

*Values are correlation or regression coefficients, with numbers of pairs or pairs/families in parentheses.
†(ns) – not stated
‡See Table 4.4.

ronmental experiences that increase their resemblance, environmental differences might reduce the resemblance of offspring to their parents, or both. In view of the evidence that vision activity influences the development of myopia, such environmental possibilities cannot be ignored. Second, among the alleles influencing refraction, some might be dominant; this also would cause sib-sib to exceed offspring-parent resemblances.

Three studies of familial resemblances in refraction have considered the possible influences of environment.

Bear et al. (1981), using the refractive error and vision activity data from the rural Newfoundland population (described earlier) first evaluated offspring-parent and sib-sib resemblances for refractive error values adjusted statistically for covariation with age and sex only and then reevaluated these resemblances using refractive error values further adjusted for covariation with education and nearwork. (These were combined, as the best available measure of lifetime and current vision activity.) Table 4.4 summarizes the results. The additional adjustment consistently reduced the measures of resemblance, suggesting that vision activity, as

Table 4.4. Offspring-parent Regressions and Sib-sib Correlations in Refractive Error, before and after Statistical Adjustment for Vision Activity*

Age interval	5–14	15–29	≥30	All ages	Weighted average
Sib-Sib	0.29	0.26	0.39	0.29	
	0.25	0.16	0.36	0.24	
	(242)	(158)	(232)	(714)	
Son-Father	0.36	0.40	−0.06	0.33	
	0.19	0.20	−0.11	0.15	
	(75/107)	(43/62)	(18/22)	(111/191)	
Son-Mother	0.03	0.30	0.08	0.10	
	−0.02	0.27	0.09	0.06	0.23
	(112/167)	(49/70)	(32/43)	(161/280)	0.15
Daughter-Mother	0.22	0.46	0.18	0.28	
	0.12	0.51	0.13	0.25	
	(94/131)	(71/111)	(31/55)	(164/297)	
Daughter-Father	0.08	0.31	0.26	0.22	
	0.03	0.21	0.18	0.15	
	(60/85)	(56/85)	(21/36)	(106/206)	

Data from Bear et al. (1981).
*Upper value: Intraclass correlations (for sib-sib pairs) or regressions (for offspring-parent pairs), calculated on age-and-sex adjusted refractive error measurements.
Middle value: Correlations or regressions using measurements further adjusted for years of education and hours of nearwork per day.
Lower value (in parentheses): Numbers of sibships and pairs for each calculation.

an aspect of common familial environment, was inflating them. Even after statistical adjustment for vision activity, offspring tended to resemble their parents of the same sex more than their parents of the opposite sex; offspring-parent resemblances were relatively small for persons aged 30 years and up, compared to those for younger persons; and sib-sib resemblances generally remained larger than offspring-parent resemblances. This pattern parallels that of similarities and differences in education in this population and suggests that statistical adjustment did not entirely remove environmental influences on measures of familial resemblance. This is not surprising, considering that only an approximate measure of lifetime vision activity was possible. The extent to which measures of genetic resemblance remain inflated remains unknown.

Chen et al. (1985) studied 238 monozygous and 123 dizygous Taiwanese twin pairs, children aged 10 to 15 years, to determine whether their concordance for refraction (whether twins' refraction differed by less than 0.5 D) was influenced by their concordance in studying and reading habits (whether twins' average times spent per day in these activities differed by less than 1 hour). As expected, monozygous twins were more often concordant than dizygous twins. Moreover, twin pairs not concordant in studying and reading habits were less often concordant in refraction, indicating that both genotype and reading habits influence refraction. Further analyses suggested an additive interaction, that is, that genetic differences determine the amount by which vision habits influence refractive error.

Ashton (1985b) analyzed resemblances in refraction in two samples of Hawaiian families, 185 with both parents of Japanese ancestry and 192 with both parents of European ancestry. Using techniques of complex segregation analysis (Lalouel et al. 1983) too elaborate to summarize here, Ashton concluded that influences of familial environment determined the familial resemblances found. Measures of vision activity were not actually analyzed. This conclusion was reached by a process of elimination designed into the analysis, and is favored because it accounts for the patterns of resemblances exhibited by the families better than do a variety of plausible genetic models. The results of this study are not inconsistent with those of Bear et al. (1981) and Chen et al. (1985).

□ Dominance Variation

The possibility that part of population variation in refractive error could be due to genetic dominance was assessed in the rural Newfoundland data by regressing individuals' refractive error values on their levels of inbreeding, determined from extensive pedigree data (Bear and Richler 1981). This revealed a slight trend to more myopic refraction with increasing inbreeding for persons aged 5 to 14 years, a stronger trend for persons aged 60 years and over, and no association at intermediate ages. These findings are consistent with some dominance in the direction of hyperopia. Findings for persons aged less than 60 years are consistent with those of similar investigations in Japan (Miller 1963, Neel et al. 1970); there are no comparable studies of persons aged 60 years and over. These analyses cannot reveal whether the relation between refraction and inbreeding indicates a small degree of dominance at a number of loci relevant to most persons' refraction, or larger dominance effects at a few loci relevant only in some families.

The association of refractive error with inbreeding is small, compared to that with vision activity, and would imply only about 0.5 D of excess myopia in the most inbred members of this Newfoundland population. The association is obscured in refractive error values not adjusted statistically for associations with education and nearwork; this might indicate that the relevant alleles influence refraction by influencing early ocular growth and development (Bear and Richler 1981). Inbreeding is associated with slightly reduced stature and weight (Schull and Neel 1972); perhaps this growth retardation extends to the eye. The under-development of the eye in persons with low birth weight may be recalled; myopia of prematurity is associated with an overall as well as an ocular growth retardation (Fledelius 1976). The relatively strong relation between refraction and inbreeding found among persons aged 60 years and over in the Newfoundland study may be due to their low nearwork and education levels leaving the relation unobscured, compared to that for the younger members of this population (G. J. Johnson, pers. comm., 1980).

If there is dominance of some alleles at the loci that determine population variation in a polygenically determined trait, the population frequency distribution of the trait should be skewed in the direction of the dominance effect (Falconer 1981, 94–96). The population frequency distribution of refraction, with an excess of low hyperopes, shows the shape expected were there some dominance in the direction of hyperopia. However, this is simply an observation consistent with the findings of inbreeding studies; dominance cannot be inferred solely from the shape of the distribution.

□ High Refractive Errors

Although in general, refractive error is a quantitative trait, high ametropia is sometimes transmitted as a single gene trait, accompanied by ocular anomalies that allow persons with the responsible gene to be distinguished from other family members. A good example is the combination of high myopia with night blindness (Nettleship 1912). Another example is high hyperopia due to cornea plana, inherited as an autosomal recessive trait (Eriksson et al. 1973); here an anomaly of the refracting system of the eye is actually determined by a single gene. A convincing pedigree of X-linked myopia, without accompanying anomalies, has also been described (Bartsocas and Kastrantas 1981). Goldschmidt (1968) surveyed nearly all the children aged 13 years attending school in Copenhagen in 1962 and found thirty-six with unilateral or bilateral myopia in excess of −6 D. For twenty-two children, neither parent had high myopia, and only one of their thirty-one sibs had high myopia. Eight children had one parent with high myopia, and three of their seven sibs were myopic. For one child, both parents were myopic, as was his single sib. The fathers of the other five children were not known, and their mothers were not high myopes. This representative series of families is too small to be interpreted with confidence; it does not suggest any single-gene mode of inheritance, but rather that high myopia is a genetically and etiologically hetero- geneous condition (Goldschmidt 1968).

A percentage of cases of high hyperopia and high myopia are probably due to single genes, for such refractive errors occur more frequently than expected, if all population variation in refraction were due to a single set of multiple genetic and environmental factors with small effects on individuals' refraction values. Put an- other way, high refractive error may often be analogous to single gene conditions resulting in unusual stature, such as achondroplasia. Single gene forms of high refractive error would confuse genetic analysis, unless such cases could be iden- tified and analyzed separately. Better characterization of the inheritance of high refractive errors might reveal molecular mechanisms relevant to variation in gen- eral (see next section, FUTURE DIRECTIONS).

□ Twins

For a number of reasons, it is practically impossible to quantify genetic and environmental variation in the general population by inference from the resem- blances between twins (Propping and Vogel 1976). There are influences on de- velopment unique to twin pregnancy. For instance, the placental circulation of monozygous twins can be unequal, making their development dissimilar even though their genes are identical (Benirschke and Kim 1973). As a particularly pertinent example, monozygous twins occasionally show mirror differences in re- fraction (Sorsby et al. 1962b). If a condition is etiologically heterogeneous, and in some instances due to the segregation of single genes (as high refractive error might be), such single gene forms will be disproportionately common among con- cordant monozygous twin pairs (Edwards 1963). Monozygous twins are more sim- ilar in refraction than are dizygous twins (Sorsby et al. 1962b, Sorsby and Fraser 1964, Chen et al. 1985), consistent with a genetic component in refractive error variation. However, Chen et al. (1985) found monozygous twins to be more similar than dizygous twins in vision habits as well as refraction, illustrating that the similarity of monozygous twins may not be due entirely to their being gene- tically identical; if unrecognized, the effects of such environmental similarities could inflate estimates of genetic variation in refraction. Similar and dissimilar twin pairs attract attention and tend to be reported in a highly selective fashion (Sorsby et al. 1962; Vogel and Motulsky 1979, 179–180), making genetic in- ferences from combined series of case reports (for example, Karlsson 1974) unre- liable.

□ Population Genetic Stratification

Population genetic stratification is a possible alternative explanation for the association of myopia with formal education (Goldschmidt 1968). Before corrective lenses were widely used, myopes may well have been at a disadvantage in occupations such as hunting, farming, and warfare. Therefore, myopes may have done poorly at surviving, mating, and transmitting their genes to offspring; or they may have gravitated toward urban, sedentary, and literate occupations where their comfort with nearwork tasks may have been an advantage. Were the etiology of myopia largely genetic, predisposing genes would become concentrated in certain social groups, as a result of this pattern of natural selection and occupational choice and the strong tendency of humans to choose mates of similar social and economic backgrounds. Over time, genetic differences between social classes would be perpetuated and increased. In fact, assuming that correlations among relatives are due to polygenic inheritance, a few generations would suffice for such genetic stratification to arise (Spivey 1976). This interesting possibility would be difficult to evaluate, but might be relevant in settled European populations. However, the likely influence of vision activity on refraction is sufficient to account for associations of refractive error with education, regardless of the role of assortative mating. Moreover, the changing prevalence of myopia in native North Americans suggests that vision activity can influence the refraction of growing children directly to cause rapid shifts in population frequency distributions.

□ Emmetropization

Sorsby (reviewed in Sorsby 1980) suggested that refractive state clusters around emmetropia due to the coordinated growth of the eye. This process of emmetropization is largely automatic, large eyes tending to have relatively flat corneas and small eyes relatively curved corneas, with appropriate intermediate combinations occurring such that refractive error tends to be low or moderate. Sorsby presented data indicating correlation of ocular components in persons with low and moderate refractive error and inadequate correlation in higher refractive error. He drew a distinction between low ametropia, which he designated correlation ametropia, and high ametropia, attributable to anomalous values of one or another component of refraction, which he designated component ametropia.

On such a model, variation in both low and high refractive error would be due in part to less-than-perfect correlation between components of refraction, and resemblances between relatives might be greater for components than for refractive error itself. Available data do suggest this (Young and Leary 1972; Sorsby and Benjamin 1973; Alsbirk 1977, Alsbirk 1979, Johnson et al. 1979). Sorsby and Benjamin (1973) measured offspring-parent resemblances in eighteen families in which both parents had axial lengths in the emmetropic range and nineteen families in which one parent had an anomalous axial length. Resemblances in both refraction and component values were relatively small in the second group, consistent with a genetic basis for the distinction between correlation and component ammetropia. Genetic correlations for ocular component values larger than those for refractive error itself are consistent with the suggestion that genetic control of ocular development is very tight, with environmental perturbations determining slight departures from perfect emmetropia. In other words, emmetropization is really only another way of looking at the control of ocular development in evolutionary terms.

□ The Heredity of Ocular Refraction

Resemblances among relatives in refractive error probably do not result from polygenic inheritance only. Rather, they may be due in part or indeed largely to environmental influences, specifically relatives' resemblances in vision activity. The best evidence for such influences is the reduction in measured familial resemblances obtained in the Newfoundland data by statistical adjustment of refraction measurements for vision activity (Bear et al. 1981). If this association were coincidental, or if people adjusted their vision activities to suit their refraction for some reason, this statistical adjustment would not change genetic correlations in a consistent way, as is found. Supporting evidence comes from the finding of Chen et al. (1985) that twin children with similar vision activity were more often similar in refraction than twins with dissimilar vision activity. Conceivably, such findings could be due to vision activity covarying with some other unknown influence on refraction, but it is difficult to imagine what that influence might be. There are indications of a small contribution of dominant genes to population variation at low and moderate values of refractive error. High refractive errors may in some instances be inherited as single gene traits. Evolutionary possibilities, such as tighter genetic control of the components of refraction than of refraction itself, and social stratification of the genes predisposing to myopia, remain interesting suggestions at present.

FUTURE DIRECTIONS

The epidemiology and genetics of refractive error are not as yet well characterized compared to those of other clinically significant quantitative variation, such as serum lipid levels (see, for example, Deeb et al. 1986). Few unqualified conclusions can be drawn about specific genotypic and environmental contributions to refractive error variation in the population, and genotype-environment interactions remain essentially unexplored. An influence of vision activity, shifting refraction toward minus values, seems undeniable. Familial resemblances in refraction may be affected, perhaps to a large extent by relatives' resemblances and differences in vision activity. Factors that account for little of the population variation in refraction can nonetheless shift the population frequency distribution sufficiently to alter greatly the prevalance of refractive errors requiring correction. Improving epidemiological and genetic insight will require longitudinal family studies in which children can be followed for several years, with repeated measurements made of their refraction, ocular components, vision activity, growth and development, and nutrition. The children and their parents should be studied as family units to distinguish genetic effects from those of familial environment.

Specification of the actual genes relevant to the development of refractive error might eventually prove possible. The classical formulation of polygenic inheritance assumes that the individual genes influencing the value of a quantitative trait have small, essentially equal effects. This assumption is reasonable when nothing is known of the physiological mechanisms that underly variation in the trait (Vogel and Motulsky 1979, 150). When the physiology of trait variation is known, however, it is sometimes found that alleles of one or more genes determine large differences in individual values for the trait and have measurable influences on trait variation. For instance, the three different alleles of the gene for apolipoprotein E, a peptide involved in cholesterol transport in the bloodstream, account for a measurable proportion of population variation in serum cholesterol levels (Sing and Davignon 1985).

The physiological mechanisms that influence the development of refractive error are obscure. However, a genetic study that might reveal some of these mechanisms can be proposed. Just as genetically determined variation in the structure of lipid transport proteins might reasonably be expected to influence the efficiency of serum lipid transport, and thus individual values of serum lipid levels and population variation in these attributes, some genes are likely candidates for influencing ocular refraction. For instance, high myopia is often a feature of inherited disorders due to abnormalities of collagen (Maumenee 1982), some of which have been shown to be due to mutations of the structural genes for various of the collagen molecules (Cheah 1985). This suggests that it would be worthwhile, in families in which high myopia was apparently being transmitted as a single gene condition, to follow the transmission of specific alleles at the genes that code for collagen molecules to determine whether any were co-inherited along with the high myopia. This could be accomplished most efficiently by tracing the inheritance of "marker" DNA variation in and near the collagen genes (White et al. 1985). Co-inheritance would indicate that variation in collagen structural genes was relevant to the development of high myopia and would identify gene products (specific collagen molecules) to study in order to understand better how inherited (and environmentally induced) high myopia occurs. Associations could then be sought between relevant collagen genes and low and moderate refractive errors. This strategy could be applied for any gene, assuming its products seemed relevant to ocular development or the responsiveness of ocular development to environmental influences; collagen genes simply provide a good example. Potentially, this approach provides information simultaneously about the inheritance of refraction and the physiology of its variation; conversely, if this approach proved unproductive when comprehensively applied for a large number of potentially relevant genes, this would suggest that, ordinarily, no single gene has a large influence on ocular development, relative to the other genes involved.

REFERENCES

Alsbirk PH. Variation and heritability of ocular dimensions. Acta Ophthalmol 1977;55:443–456.

Alsbirk PH. Refraction in adult West Greenland Eskimos. Acta Ophthalmol 1979;57:84–95.

Alward WM, Bender TR, Demske JA, Hall DB. High prevalence of myopia among young adult Yupik Eskimos. Can J Ophthalmol 1985;20:241–245.

Angle J, Wissman DA. Age, reading and myopia. Am J Optom Physiol Optics 1978;55:302–308.

Angle J, Wissman DA. The epidemiology of myopia. Am J Epidemiol 1980;111:220–228.

Ashton GC. Nearwork, school achievement and myopia. J Biosoc Sci 1985a;17:223–233.

Ashton GC. Segregation analysis of ocular refraction and myopia. Hum Hered 1985b;35:232–239.

Baldwin WR. A review of statistical studies of relations between myopia and ethnic, behavioral and physiological characteristics. Am J Optom Physiol Optics 1981;58:516–527.

Bartsocas CS, Kastrantas AD. X-linked form of myopia. Hum Hered 1981;31:199–200.

Bear JC, Richler A. Ocular refraction and inbreeding: a population study in Newfoundland. J Biosoc Sci 1981;13:391–399.

Bear JC, Richler A, Burke G. Nearwork and familial resemblances in ocular refraction: a population study in Newfoundland. Clin Genet 1981;19:462–472.

Benirschke K, Kim CK. Multiple pregnancy. N Engl J Med 1973;288:1276–1284, 1329–1336.

Boniuk V. Refractive problems in native peoples (the Sioux Lookout Project). Can J Ophthalmol 1973;8:229–233.

Cass E. A decade of northern ophthalmology. Can J Ophthalmol 1973;8:210–217.

Cheah KSE. Collagen genes and inherited connective tissue disease. Biochem J 1985;229:287–303.

Chen C-J, Cohen BH, Diamond EL. Genetic and environmental effects on the development of myopia in Chinese twin children. Ophthalmol Pediat Genet 1985;6:113–119.

Crow JF. Basic Concepts in Population, Quantitative, and Evolutionary Genetics. New York: WH Freeman and Co, 1986.

Deeb S, Failor A, Brown BG, et al. Molecular genetics of apolipoproteins and coronary heart disease. Cold Spring Harbor Symp Quant Biol 1986;51:403–409.

Donders FC. On the Anomalies of Accommodation and Refraction of the Eye. Trans. Moore WD. London: New Sydenham Society, 1864.

Duke-Elder S, Abrams D. System of Ophthalmology, vol V. Ophthalmic Optics and Refraction. St. Louis: CV Mosby Co, 1970.

Dunphy EB, Stoll MR, King SH. Myopia among American male graduate students. Am J Ophthalmol 1968;65:518–521.

Eriksson AW, Lehmann W, Forsius H. Congenital cornea plana in Finland. Clin Genet 1973;4:301–310.

Falconer DS. Introduction to quantitative genetics. London: Longman, 1981, 2nd ed.

Fisher RA. The correlation between relatives on the supposition of mendelian inheritance. Trans R Soc Edinburgh 1918;52:399–433.

Fledelius H. Prematurity and the eye. Acta Ophthalmol 1976;suppl 128.

Fodor JG. Epidemiology of hypertension. Medicine North America 1980;1:1–4.

Gardiner PA. Dietary treatment of myopia in children. Lancet 1958;1:1152–1155.

Gardiner PA, James G. Association between maternal disease during pregnancy and myopia in the child. Br J Ophthalmol 1960;44:172–178.

Garner LF, Kinnear RF, Klinger JD, McKellar MJ. Prevalence of myopia in school children in Vanuatu. Acta Ophthalmol 1985;63:323–326.

Gmelin RT. Myopia at West Point: past and present. Milit Med 1976;141:542–543.

Goldschmidt E. On the etiology of myopia. Acta Ophthalmol 1968;suppl 98.

Goss DA, Erickson P, Cox VD. Prevalence and pattern of adult myopia progression in a general optometric practice population. Am J Optom Physiol Opt 1985;62:470–477.

Goss DA, Erickson P. Meridional corneal components of myopia progression in young adults and children. Am J Optom Physiol Opt 1987;64:475–481.

Grosvenor T. A review and a suggested classification system for myopia on the basis of age-related prevalence and age of onset. Am J Optom Physiol Opt 1987;64:545–554.

Halasa AH, McLaren DS. The refractive state of malnourished children. Arch Ophthalmol 1964;71:827–831.

Harrison GA, Weiner JS, Tanner JM, Barnicot NA. Human biology. Oxford: Oxford University Press, 1977, 2nd ed.

Hegmann JP, Mash JA, Spivey BE. Genetic analysis of human visual parameters in populations with varying incidences of strabismus. Am J Hum Genet 1974;26:549–562.

Hirsch MJ. The relationship between measles and myopia. Am J Optom Arch Am Acad Optom 1957;34:289–297.

Holm S. Les états de la réfraction oculare chez les palénégrides au Gabon Afrique Équatoriale Française. Acta Ophthalmol 1937;suppl 13.

Johnson GJ, Matthews A, Perkins ES. Survey of ophthalmic conditions in a Labrador community. I. Refractive errors. Br J Ophthalmol 1979;63:440–448.

Karlsson JL. Concordance rates for myopia in twins. Clin Genet 1974;6:142–146.

Keller JT. A comparison of the refractive status of myopic children and their parents. Am J Optom 1973;50:206–211.

Lalouel JM, Rao DC, Morton NE, Elston RC. A unified model for complex segregation analysis. Am J Hum Genet 1983;35:816–826.

Lane BC. Calcium, chromium, protein, sugar and accommodation in myopia. Doc Ophthalmol Proc Series 1981a;28:141–148.

Lane BC. Elevation of intraocular pressure with daily sustained closework stimulus to accommodation lowered tissue chromium and dietary deficiency of ascorbic acid (vitamin C). Doc Ophthalmol Proc Series 1981b;28:149–155.

Majima A, Nakajima A, Ichikawa H, Watanabe M. Prevalence of ocular anomalies among school children. Am J Ophthalmol 1960;50:139–146.

Maumenee IH. The eye in connective tissue diseases. In Daentl DL, ed. Clinical, Structural and Biochemical Advances in Hereditary Eye Disorders. New York: Alan R Liss Inc, 1982;53–67.

Maurice DM, Mushin AS. Production of myopia in rabbits by raised body temperature and increased intraocular pressure. Lancet 1966;2:1160–1162.

Mausner JS, Bahn AK. Epidemiology: An Introductory Text. Philadelphia: WB Saunders, 1974.

McLaren DS. Nutrition and eye disease in East Africa: Experience in Lake and Central Provinces, Tanganyika. J Trop Med Hyg 1960;63:101–122.

McLaren DS. Nutritional Ophthalmology. London: Academic Press, 1980.

Miller RW. Distant visual acuity loss among Japanese grammar school children: The roles of heredity and environment. J Chron Dis 1963;16:31–54.

Morgan RW, Munro M. Refractive problems in Northern natives. Can J Ophthalmol 1973; 8:226–228.

Morgan RW, Speakman JS, Grimshaw SE. Inuit myopia: An environmentally induced "epidemic"? Can Med Assoc J 1975;112:575–577.

Neel JV, Schull WJ, Kimura T, et al. The effects of parental consanguinity and inbreeding in Hirado, Japan. III. Vision and hearing. Hum Hered 1970;20:129–155.

Nettleship E. A pedigree of congenital night blindness with myopia. Trans Ophthalmol Soc UK 1912;32:21–45.

Otsuka J. Research in myopia. Acta Soc Ophthalmol Jpn 1967;71.

Pärssinen TO. Relation between refraction, education, occupation and age among 26- and 46-year-old Finns. Am J Optom Physiol Opt 1987;64:136–143.

Peckham CS, Gardiner PA, Goldstein H. Acquired myopia in 11-year-old children. Br Med J 1977;1:542–544.

Post RH. Possible cases of relaxed selection in civilized populations. Humangenetik 1971; 13:253–284.

Propping P, Vogel F. Twin studies in medical genetics. Acta Genet Med Gemellol 1976; 25:249–258.

Richler A, Bear JC. Refraction, nearwork and education. A population study in Newfoundland. Acta Ophthalmol 1980a;58:468–478.

Richler A, Bear JC. The distribution of refraction in three isolated communities in western Newfoundland. Am J Optom Physiol Opt 1980b;57:861–871.

Richler A, Bear JC, Snow AA, et al. The Marystown family study of refractive error: Measuring vision activity. Proceedings of the 1986 Annual Meeting of the American Academy of Optometry. 1986;18p (abstract).

Sato T. The Causes and Prevention of Acquired Myopia. Yokohama: Kanehara Shuppan Co., Ltd., 1957.

Schull WJ, Neel JV. The effects of parental consanguinity and inbreeding in Hirado, Japan. V. Summary and interpretation. Am J Hum Genet 1972;24:425–453.

Shotwell AJ. Plus lens, prism, and bifocal effects on myopia progression in military students, part II. Am J Optom Physiol Opt 1984;61:112–117.

Sing CF, Davignon J. Role of apolipoprotein E polymorphism in determining normal plasma lipid and lipoprotein variation. Am J Hum Genet 1985;37:268–285.

Skeller E. Anthropological and ophthalmological studies on the Angmagssalik Eskimos. Meddelelser om Grønland 1954;107.

Sorsby A. Biology of the eye as an optical system. In: Duane TD, ed. Clinical Ophthalmology, revised ed. Hagarstown, MD: Harper and Row, 1980.

Sorsby A, Sheridan M, Leary, GA. Vision, visual acuity, and ocular refraction of young men: Findings in a sample of 1033 subjects. Br Med J 1960;1:1394–1398.

Sorsby A, Benjamin B. Modes of inheritance of errors of refraction. J Med Genet 1973; 10:161–164.

Sorsby A, Fraser GR. Statistical note on the components of ocular refraction in twins. J Med Genet 1964;1:47–49.

Sorsby A, Sheridan M, Leary GA. Refraction and its components in twins. Medical Research Council special Report Series No. 303. London: HMSO, 1962.

Sorsby A, Leary GA, Fraser GR. Family studies on ocular refraction and its components. J Med Genet 1966;3:269–373.

Sperduto RD, Seigel D, Roberts J, Rowland M. Prevalence of myopia in the United States. Arch Ophthalmol 1983;101:405–407.

Spivey BE. Quantitative genetics and clinical medicine. Trans Am Ophthalmol Soc 1976; 74:661–707.

Taylor HR. Racial variations in vision. Am J Epidemiol 1981;113:62–80.

Tscherning M. Studier over myopiens aetiologi. Copenhagen: København, 1882.

Vogel F, Motulsky AG. Human Genetics: Problems and Approaches. New York: Springer-Verlag, 1979.

Waardenburg PJ. Genetics and Ophthalmology, vol II, Chapter 23. Assen: Koninklijke Van Gorcum & Comp NV, Publishers. 1963.

Weale RA. Ocular anatomy and refraction. Doc Ophthalmol 1983;55:361–374.

White R, Leppert M, Bishop DT, Barker D, Berkowitz J, Brown C, Callahan P, Holm T, Jerominski L. Construction of linkage maps with DNA markers for human chromosomes. Nature 1985;313:101–105.

Woodruff ME. Vision and refractive status among grade 1 children in the Province of New Brunswick. Am J Optom Physiol Opt 1986;63:545–552.

Woodruff ME, Samek MJ. A study of the prevalence of spherical equivalent refractive states and anisometropia in Amerind populations in Ontario. Can J Public Health 1977; 68:414–424.

Young FA. An estimate of the hereditary component of myopia. Am J Optom Arch Am Acad Optom 1958;7:337–345.

Young FA, Leary GA, Baldwin WR, West DC, Box RA, Harris E, Johnson C. The transmission of refractive errors within Eskimo families. Am J Optom Arch Am Acad Optom 1969;46:676–685.

Young FA, Leary GA. The inheritance of ocular components. Am J Optom Arch Am Acad Optom 1972;49:546–555.

Young FA, Leary GA, Zimmerman RR, Strobel DA. Diet and refractive characteristics. Am J Optom Arch Am Acad Optom 1973;50:226–233.

__5__

Childhood Myopia

David A. Goss

□

■

THE FIRST FIVE YEARS OF LIFE

The wide distribution of refraction at birth, as reported by Cook and Glasscock (1951), was noted in Chapter 2. In another study, Goldschmidt (1969) also found a wide distribution of refraction at birth: In both of these studies, refraction was measured by cycloplegic retinoscopy, and in both studies the prevalence of myopia was about 25%. In a study of normal full-term infants conducted in Massachusetts by Mohindra and Held (1981), a wide distribution of refraction was again found, but the prevalence of myopia was approximately 50% — double the percentage reported in the previous studies. In the Mohindra and Held study, refraction was determined not by cycloplegic retinoscopy but by near retinoscopy — a noncycloplegic procedure in which the infant presumably watches the retinoscope light at a distance of 50 cm in an otherwise dark room (Mohindra 1977, Borghi and Rouse 1985).

Studies of refraction in premature (low-birth-weight) infants show a high prevalence of myopia, which decreases during the first several months of life, many myopic infants being emmetropic by 1 year of age (Fletcher and Brandon 1955, Scharf et al. 1975, Yamamoto et al. 1979). It has been shown that the eyes of premature infants have relatively steep corneas. This may be due to the immaturity of the eye.

□ Changes in Refraction

Much of our current knowledge of changes in refraction during the first 5 years of life comes from studies reported by Mohindra and Held (1981) and by Ingram and Barr (1979). In the study described previously, Mohindra and Held (1981) reported on spherical equivalent refractive errors of 400 normal full-term infants and preschool children. Their subjects ranged in age from birth to 5 years and were divided into seven age groups, the youngest group being from birth to 4 weeks and the oldest being from 2.5 to 5 years old.

The mean refractive error found by Mohindra and Held was −0.70 D in the 0- to 4-week group, shifting toward hyperopia with increasing age, to +0.59 D in the 2.5- to 5-year group. As shown in Figure 5.1, the refractive error distribution curve narrowed markedly during the 5-year period, the standard deviation declining from 3.20 D in the 0- to 4-week group to 0.85 D in the 2.5- to 5-year group. Most of the change in mean refractive error and standard deviation occurred during the first year of life. These findings suggested that although a large proportion of children are myopic at birth, almost all of them decrease in myopia or become hyperopic by the end of 1 year; whereas some of the infants born with hyperopia tend to decrease in hyperopia during the same period. The decrease in myopia during the first year of life is consistent with the suggestion by Goldschmidt (1969) that the wide range of refractive error at birth is due to a wide range in the degree of maturity of the eye at birth and that when an infant is born with myopia, the amount of myopia decreases as the eye continues to develop after birth.

In the United Kingdom, Ingram and Barr (1979) reported on refractions of 148 children at 1 year of age and again at 3.5 years. Over this age span they found, as did Mohindra and Held, that the prevalence of both myopia and astigmatism decreased and the prevalence of emmetropia increased. Most children with myopia or emmetropia at 1 year of age shifted toward hyperopia; whereas most children with hyperopia of 1.00 to 2.25 D shifted toward emmetropia. Children having

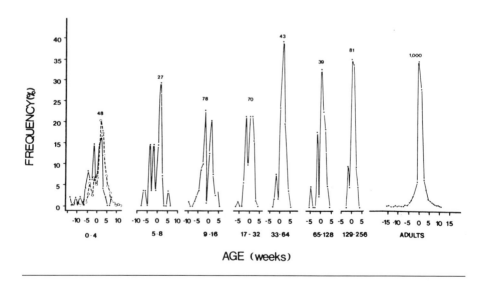

Figure 5.1. Change in the distribution of refraction during the first 5 years of life. (From Mohindra and Held 1981. Reprinted by permission.)

2.50 D of hyperopia or more were approximately equally split between shifts toward more and less hyperopia. Additional studies of refractive changes during the early years of life — in particular, longitudinal studies — are needed.

_____■_____

THE SCHOOL YEARS

Monroe Hirsch conducted a longitudinal study of refraction in Ojai, California, beginning the study in 1954 and continuing it until 1967 (Hirsch 1955, 1961, 1962, 1963, 1964a, 1964b, 1967). One of the few longitudinal studies of refraction using a nonvisually selected population, the Ojai study consisted of data obtained from semiannual vision screenings conducted during the 12-year period. Although 1,200 children were originally enrolled in the study, by the time the study was completed only some 200 children remained. Refractive data consisted of the means of the spherical equivalent refraction for the right and left eyes of each subject, obtained by retinoscopy.

In one of the reports on the Ojai study, Hirsch (1961) used visual inspection of refractive error plots to assess the linearity of the change in refractive error with age, from age 6 to 7 through age 11 to 12. Typical plots are shown in Figure 5.2. A comparison of plots E and F with the other four plots demonstrates the high rate of change in refractive error of the myopic children (that is, high rate of progression) as compared with the rates of change for hyperopic or emmetropic children. In a later report Hirsch (1962) calculated rates of change in refraction in diopters per year, using the least squares method, for those individuals previously determined to have linear (as opposed to curvilinear) changes in refractive error, and found a mean slope of −0.07 D per year. The distribution of rates of change was negatively skewed, due to the greater rates of change of the myopes.

Findings similar to those of the Ojai study were reported in an unpublished thesis by Langer (1966), based on manifest retinoscopic refractions performed at intervals of approximately 2 years on schoolchildren in Leaside, Ontario, a suburb of Toronto. The children were followed from the age of 5 or 6 years to 15 or 16 years. Changes in refraction for 93% of the children were judged to be linear (including all of the children having 0.50 D of myopia or more). The mean slopes (rates of change in refractive error) were found to be −0.21 D per year for girls, and −0.16 D per year for boys. The means were more negative than the medians, due to the negative skew in the distribution produced by the myopes. The rates were more negative in the Langer study than in the Hirsch study because the Langer study had a greater prevalence of myopia.

The results of both the Hirsch study and the Langer study demonstrate that rates of change in refraction during the school years are greater for myopes than for hyperopes. This was previously reported by Hofstetter (1954) and, more re-

Figure 5.2. Typical plots of binocular mean spherical equivalent refractive error vs age. (From Hirsch 1961. © The Am Acad of Optom 1961. Reprinted by permission.) Increasing myopia is downward along the y axis. The majority of subjects had plots such as C and D. Some became more hyperopic such as plot A, and several had little or no change, such as plot B. Plots E and F were typical of the myopes.

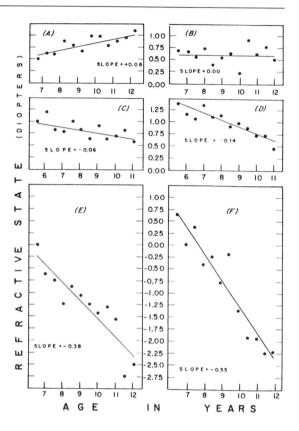

cently, by Mäntyjärvi (1985a). Using records from an optometric practice in Bloomington, Indiana, Hofstetter (1954) presented scatterplots of the rate of change of binocular mean spherical equivalent refractive error vs the refraction at the initial examination, on the basis of three age categories beginning with age group 10 to 20 years. For almost all of the myopes, changes were in the direction of increased myopia; but for the hyperopes, the refractive changes were almost normally distributed, the mean and mode both being at or near zero. On the basis of these results, Hofstetter suggested that when an adolescent shifts into myopia, a sudden increase in the rate of refraction occurs.

Mäntyjärvi (1985a) presented data from an ophthalmologic clinic in a community health center in Kuopio, Finland. For forty-six hyperopic children followed for 5 to 8 years, the mean change in refraction was -0.12 D (± 0.14 D) per year, whereas for 133 myopes the mean change was -0.55 D (± 0.27 D) per year. However, for thirty children who were hyperopic at the beginning of the period of observation and then became myopic, the mean change was -0.21 D (± 0.21 D) per year while hyperopic but -0.60 D (± 0.45 D) after they became myopic. Three examples from this group of thirty children are presented in Figure 5.3;

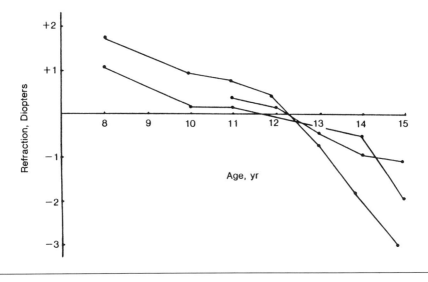

Figure 5.3. Examples of the spherical equivalent refractive error (right eye) obtained under cycloplegia in three children who shifted from hyperopia to myopia before the age of 15. (From Mäntyjärvi 1985a.)

these examples confirm Hofstetter's statement that when an adolescent shifts into myopia, a sudden increase in the rate of change of refraction occurs.

An important advantage of a longitudinal study of refraction is that it enables one to predict the changes in refraction that will occur for an individual child or for a group of children. When the refraction of the Ojai children had been followed for a period of 8 years, Hirsch (1963b) reported on the predictability of refractive error at age 13 to 14, based on refractive error at age 5 to 6. The predictions were based on data for 766 eyes of 383 children who remained in the study for the 8-year period. At 13 to 14 years of age, there were ninety-two eyes with 0.50 D of myopia or more, sixty-nine eyes with 1.00 D of hyperopia or more, and 605 eyes having refractions between -0.50 and $+1.00$ D, which Hirsch called the emmetropic category. For the analysis of data he randomly selected 100 of the 605 emmetropic eyes. The results of this analysis are shown in Table 5.1. As shown in this table, one may make the following predictions: (1) Those children entering school with hyperopia of 1.50 D or more will still be hyperopic by age 13 to 14; (2) those children entering school with a refraction between $+0.50$ D and $+1.24$ D will be emmetropic at age 13 to 14; (3) those children entering school with a refraction between 0.00 and $+0.49$ D will tend to become myopic by age 13 to 14; and (4) those children who were myopic on entering school are likely to become more myopic by age 13 to 14. Hirsch also found that proportionally more children with against-the-rule astigmatism upon entering school developed myopia than those with no astigmatism or with-the-rule astigmatism.

Table 5.1. Number of Individuals in the Ojai Study at Various Refractive Error Levels at age 13 to 14 years Compared to Refractive Error at Age 5 to 6 Years

Spherical equivalent refraction at age 5–6	Spherical equivalent refraction at age 13–14		
	Myopia ($\geq$0.50 D)	Emmetropia (-0.49 to $+0.99$ D)	Hyperopia ($\geq$1.00 D)
Over -0.26 D	4	0	0
-0.25 to -0.01 D	6	0	0
0.00 to $+0.24$ D	7	6	0
$+0.25$ to $+0.49$ D	37	4	0
$+0.50$ to $+0.74$ D	21	33	5
$+0.75$ to $+0.99$ D	15	41	10
$+1.00$ to $+1.24$ D	2	15	14
$+1.25$ to $+1.49$ D	0	1	7
Over $+1.50$ D	0	0	33
Totals	92	100	69

From Hirsch, 1964b.

PREVALENCE OF MYOPIA AS RELATED TO AGE

Myopia not only progresses in amount during the school years, but the prevalence of myopia increases throughout this period, as illustrated by vision screenings performed in elementary schools in the Los Angeles area by Hirsch (1952) and in Pullman, Washington by Young et al. (1954). The Hirsch and Young data may be compared to data from Langer's thesis (1966), which was a longitudinal study. Data from these studies are summarized in Table 5.2. For girls, the largest increases in prevalence occurred at age 10 to 11 in the Hirsch study, at age 8 to 9 in the Young et al. study and at age 12 to 13 in the Langer study. For boys, the largest increases in prevalence occurred at age 12 to 13 in the Hirsch and Langer studies and at age 10 to 11 in the Young et al. study. In the Hirsch and Young et al. studies, the most common age of onset of myopia in girls appears to precede that of boys by approximately 2 years. However, interpretation of these studies is subject to the limitations and nature of cross-sectional studies and the age spans by which the data were grouped.

Results of several studies have shown that the earlier the age of onset of myopia, the greater the amount that is eventually developed. François and Goes (1975)

Table 5.2. Prevalences of Myopia in Studies in the Los Angeles Area, in Pullman, Washington, and in Leaside, Ontario*

| | Prevalence of myopia greater than 1.00 D | | | | | |
| | Hirsch | | Young et al. | | Langer | |
Age	Girls	Boys	Girls	Boys	Girls	Boys
5–6 yrs	0.45	0.67	4.17	0.00	0.00	0.00
7–8 yrs	0.98	0.90	2.60	5.62	0.00	1.54
9–10 yrs	2.01	1.82	19.44	9.68	6.71	5.11
11–12 yrs	5.77	3.08	20.00	27.27	10.26	5.71
13–14 yrs	5.78	5.08	25.71	28.57	19.58	15.01

*From Hirsch 1952, Young et al. 1954, and Langer 1966, respectively.

Table 5.3. Comparison of Amount of Myopia at Age 15 to 16 Years to Age of Onset of Myopia

Age of onset	No	Mean spherical equivalent refraction at age 15–16 ($\pm$ SD)
7–10 yrs	40	-4.46 (± 1.63) D
11–13 yrs	122	-2.87 (± 1.15) D
14–15 yrs	52	-1.66 (± 1.00) D

From Mäntyjärvi 1985b.

reported that of forty eyes in which myopia was discovered before the age of 10 years, eleven developed more than 7.00 D of myopia; whereas of twenty-six eyes in which myopia was found after 10 years of age, none progressed to more than 4.00 D. Septon (1984) polled optometry students at Pacific University in Oregon and found a correlation coefficient of -0.57 for the age at which the students reported first wearing corrective lenses and the amount of myopia in the first year of optometry school (age range for these students was 20.7 to 37.5 years).

In a longitudinal study of 214 myopic children (136 girls and 78 boys) in Kuopio, Finland, Mäntyjärvi (1985b) compared the age at which myopia was first discovered to the amount of myopia at 15 or 16 years of age. As shown in Table 5.3, the earlier the onset of myopia, the greater the amount at the age of 15 to 16 years.

Rosenberg and Goldschmidt (1981) analyzed the progression of myopia in patients examined in a Danish ophthalmology practice. For thirty girls whose myopia was first discovered at 9 or 10 years of age, the mean annual refractive change was −0.47 D (±0.28 D) per year, whereas for girls whose myopia was found at 11 or 12 years it was −0.37 D (±0.42 D) per year.

PATTERNS OF MYOPIA PROGRESSION

A useful method to grasp the general characteristics of myopia progression is to inspect graphs of refractive error vs age for several individuals. Bücklers (1953) plotted the refractive error in a single principal meridian for 110 eyes of patients who had been followed for two or three decades in his ophthalmology practice. As shown in Figure 5.4, the earlier the onset of myopia, the greater its rate of progression; in addition, the curves tend to flatten toward the end of the progression period. Mandell (1959) collected data from an optometric practice in southern California. Although he intended to evaluate the effect of bifocal correction on myopia progression, his plots (Figure 5.5) also serve to illustrate the general rule

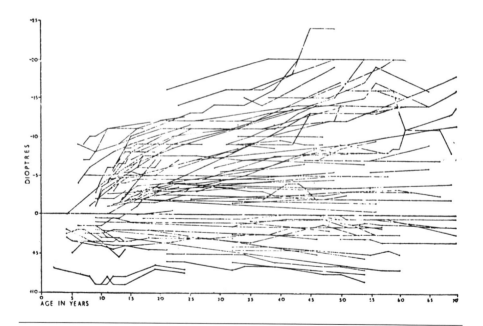

Figure 5.4. Composite graph of changes in refraction in 110 eyes. (From Bücklers 1952. Reprinted by permission.) Refractive error is plotted along the y axis with increasing myopia going upward on the graph, and age in years is along the x axis. Note that change in refraction is most common among myopes before about 15 or 16 years of age.

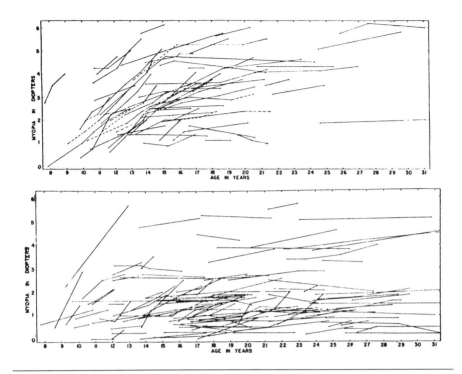

Figure 5.5. Plots of amount of myopia (D) vs age. (From Mandell 1959. © The Am Acad of Optom 1959. Reprinted by permission.) Each individual line represents change for one person's refractive error. The top panel shows refractive changes for wearers of bifocal lenses (except for periods indicated by dashed lines), and the bottom panel shows refractive changes for wearers of single vision lenses. Note that both graphs are flatter after about 15 years of age, and that there is noticeable individual variability in the slopes before that age.

that myopia tends to progress up to about 15 or 16 years of age, after which it may show lesser progression or stability.

My colleagues and I collected longitudinal records of 559 patients from five optometric practices. Records were selected on the basis of the following criteria: (1) four or more examinations between the ages of 6 and 24 years, (2) myopia of at least 0.50 D at one or more of the examinations, (3) no more than 2.50 D of astigmatism, (4) no strabismus or amblyopia, (5) no contact lenses, (6) no ocular pathology, and (7) no systemic pathology which might affect ocular findings. The practices from which the data were taken were located in northwestern Iowa (n = 74), southern Indiana (n = 141), northern Illinois (n = 190), and northeastern Oklahoma (two practices, n = 154). The refractive data consisted of subjective refraction findings recorded in the optometrist's clinical files; in most analyses, the principal meridian nearest horizontal for the right eye was used. Typical

Figure 5.6. Graphs that are typical representations of our sample. (From Goss and Winkler 1983. © The Am Acad of Optom 1983. Reprinted by permission.) Upper panel, graphs for five male subjects; lower panel, graphs for five female subjects.

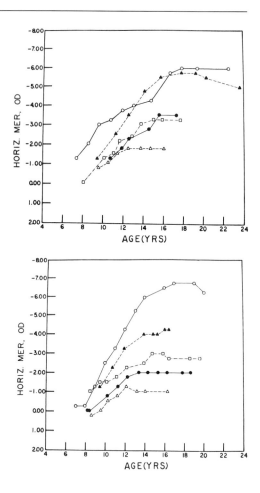

plots of refractive error as a function of age are shown for five males and five females, in Figure 5.6.

☐ Age of Onset

On the basis of the data plotted for each of the 559 patients, we derived the individual ages of onset and the rates of progression, using observations at or before 15 years of age for those subjects for whom four or more refractions were recorded during that age span (Goss and Cox 1985). For 158 boys, the mean rate of childhood myopia progression was −0.40 D (±0.24 D) per year; for 145 females, the mean was −0.43 D (±0.25 D) per year. The differences between the mean rates for boys and girls was not statistically significant at the 0.05 level.

We calculated an index of onset age for each subject by extrapolating the regression line for points at or before 15 years of age to zero refractive error. We then calculated the coefficient of correlation between onset age and the mean of the refractive measurements taken after 17 years of age. The coefficients of correlation were $+0.42$ for males (n = 49) and $+0.61$ for females (n = 31). Thus, the earlier myopia appears, the more likely it will progress to a higher amount, a finding that is consistent with the studies discussed earlier.

□ Age at Cessation of Progression

We defined the age of cessation of myopia progression for a given individual as the age at which the regression line of refractive error vs age intersects a horizontal representing the mean amount of myopia beyond the age of 17 years (Goss and Winkler 1983). The data pool for this analysis was the first 299 patient records we collected. We found a statistically significant difference in mean cessation ages for males and females ($P < .0001$). For those subjects on whom sufficient data were available for the analysis, mean cessation age was 16.66 (± 2.10) years for sixty-six males, and 15.21 (± 1.74) years for females. Considerable individual variation was noted. Cumulative frequency distributions for cessation age are given in Figure 5.7. The cessation age, as defined above, is an index of the age of cessation of childhood

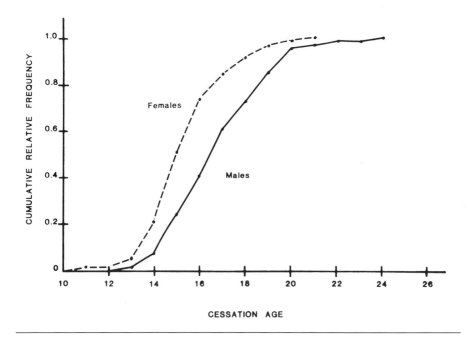

Figure 5.7. Cumulative distributions of childhood myopia progression cessation ages for males (n = 66) and females (n = 57). (From Goss and Winkler 1983. © The Am Acad of Optom 1983. Reprinted by permission.)

Table 5.4.   Average Amount of Myopia from Goss and Cox (1985) and 50th Percentile of Height from Lowrey (1978)*

Age (yrs)	Mean amount of myopia (diopters)		Median height (cm)	
	Males	Females	Males	Females
8	−0.87(64)	−0.93(58)	130.0	128.0
8.5	−1.01(81)	−1.12(73)	132.8	130.5
9	−1.32(102)	−1.37(94)	135.5	132.9
9.5	−1.47(119)	−1.57(112)	137.9	135.8
10	−1.64(135)	−1.71(129)	140.3	138.6
10.5	−1.75(152)	−1.86(151)	142.3	141.7
11	−1.91(168)	−1.93(162)	144.2	144.7
11.5	−2.04(180)	−2.11(171)	146.9	148.1
12	−2.12(192)	−2.26(189)	148.6	151.9
12.5	−2.19(195)	−2.40(196)	152.3	154.3
13	−2.29(200)	−2.52(205)	155.0	157.1
13.5	−2.40(207)	−2.59(204)	158.9	158.4
14	−2.50(205)	−2.65(194)	162.7	159.6
14.5	−2.55(203)	−2.73(191)	165.3	160.4
15	−2.62(201)	−2.74(185)	167.8	161.1
15.5	−2.67(204)	−2.71(177)	169.7	161.7
16	−2.72(200)	−2.71(167)	171.6	162.2
16.5	−2.78(193)	−2.71(158)	172.7	162.4
17	−2.77(184)	−2.75(144)	173.7	162.5
17.5	−2.77(175)	−2.77(134)	174.1	162.5
18	−2.82(158)	−2.90(121)	174.5	162.5

*For the myopia data the number of subjects from which the average was determined is given in parentheses.

myopia progression and does not infer that further progression is not possible during the young adult years (Goss 1987a).

It was hypothesized that the earlier cessation of childhood myopia progression for females could be related to the cessation of general body growth (Goss and Winkler 1983). We did not have height data for our sample, but we did compare our average myopia to American growth norms (Table 5.4). On the basis of this table, it may be noted that the age after which median height shows relatively little change corresponds closely to the age after which the progression of myopia is relatively small.

□ Corneal Power Changes

Changes in corneal refracting power as determined by keratometry were compared to rates of myopia progression for those subjects on whom three or more keratometer findings before the age of 15 were available. Mean rates of corneal power change were found to be not significantly different from zero, even though mean rates of myopia progression were about 0.50 D per year; consequently, correlations between rates of corneal power change and rates of myopia progression were not statistically significant. Thus it appears that corneal power changes play a negligible role in childhood myopia progression.

USE OF BIFOCAL LENSES

Many practitioners have introduced clinical interventions to try to slow or stop myopia progression. These techniques, which are discussed in Chapter 20, have not been universally or consistently effective. One common method is the prescription of bifocal lenses (Grosvenor 1980, Goss 1982, Young et al. 1985, Grosvenor et al. 1987). In three of the five practices from which our data were drawn, bifocal lenses were used almost as often as single-vision lenses for young myopes. Rates of myopia progression, derived as described earlier, were used to assess the effect of bifocal lenses on myopia progression (Goss 1986a). Fifty-two subjects wore single vision lenses for the entire period for which myopia progression was determined, and sixty wore bifocals for the same period. The mean rates of progression were found to be -0.44 (± 0.26) D per year for the single-vision group and -0.37 (± 0.24) D per year for the bifocal group. This difference was not statistically significant. However, when the groups were further categorized in terms of median nearpoint phoria and median nearpoint binocular cross cylinder net, the bifocal group was found to have lower rates of progression than the single-vision group for patients with nearpoint esophoria and higher nearpoint binocular cross cylinder findings. This result suggests that bifocals can reduce the rate of myopia progression in some cases, specifically those in which a bifocal may help to relieve asthenopia (Goss 1986b). These findings are consistent with the report of Roberts and Banford (1967) and a re-analysis of the Houston myopia control study (Goss and Grosvenor 1990), and they could partially explain the wide disparity of results that have been reported for the use of bifocal lenses in myopia.

YOUNG-ADULT MYOPIA

This sample of patients (from the five optometric practices) was also used to study trends of myopia progression in young adults (Goss, Erickson, and Cox 1985; Goss and Erickson 1987). Although the young adult period is considered to be a time of relatively stable refraction, some individuals do experience increases in myopia (National Academy of Sciences Working Group 58, 1989). We performed three analyses to characterize young-adult myopia: (1) a subjective categorization of patterns based on plots of refractive error vs age, (2) a determination of rates of progression based on linear regression slopes, and (3) an analysis of changes in corneal refracting power. Most of the available data points used for analysis were for subjects between the ages 20 and 25 years.

□ Patterns of Progression

A sufficient number of data points were available for sixty-three males and fifty-three females. We identified three patterns of progression: (1) adult stabilization, (2) adult continuation, and (3) adult acceleration. Adult stabilization, the most common pattern (87% of females and 68% of males), consists of rapid progression during childhood and early adolescence, followed by slight or no progression in adulthood. In adult continuation (25% of males and 13% of females), myopia progresses in the young adult years, but at a slower rate than in childhood. In adult acceleration (6% of males and no females), myopia progression accelerates during young adulthood.

□ Rates of Progression

Rates of myopia progression for those young adults with three or more data points at or beyond 18 years of age ranged from +0.09 D to −0.36 D per year for males (n = 60) and from +0.19 D to −0.25 D per year for females (n = 48). Means were −0.07 (±0.09) D per year for males, and −0.03 (±0.09) D per year for females; the difference was statistically significant at the 0.05 level (Goss, Erickson, and Cox 1985). It is of interest that not only are these rates of myopia progression lower than those for childhood myopia, but they show that for some young adults the amount of myopia decreases with age.

□ Corneal Power Changes

To determine whether the cornea plays a significant role in the progression of myopia in young adults, we compared changes in corneal refracting power to rates of myopia progression for those subjects whose myopia progressed during the early adult years. For this analysis, we used only those subjects for whom three keratometer findings were available after the age of 18 years (twenty-two men and fifteen women) (Goss and Erickson 1987). Rates of corneal power change for the two principal meridians were calculated by linear regression and were compared to rates of myopia progression. As shown in Table 5.5, statistically significant cor-

Table 5.5. Coefficients of Correlation (r) and Linear Regression Equations of Rate of Young Adulthood Myopia Progression (y) on Rate of Keratometer Power Change (X)*

	N	r	Linear regression equation
Principal Meridian Nearest Horizontal			
Males	22	$+0.34\ (P < .2)$	$Y = (+0.24)X - 0.06$
Females	15	$+0.58\ (P < .05)$	$Y = (+0.66)X - 0.002$
Total	37	$+0.38\ (P < .05)$	$Y = (+0.33)X - 0.04$
Principal Meridian Nearest Vertical			
Males	22	$+0.68\ (P < .001)$	$Y = (+0.78)X - 0.09$
Females	15	$+0.69\ (P < .005)$	$Y = (+0.70)X - 0.01$
Total	37	$+0.54\ (P < .001)$	$Y = (+0.51)X - 0.05$

*Corneal steepening was given a negative sign to make the sign the same as the myopia progression rate it would produce (increase in myopia). Statistical significance of the correlation coefficients is given in parentheses.

relations were found for both principal meridians for females, but only for the principal meridian nearest vertical for males. Regressions of rates of myopia progression on rates of corneal power change yielded slopes of about 0.60, which compare well to the 0.68 slope found by Erickson and Thorn (1977) for refractive changes in orthokeratology. Unfortunately, data on the other components of refraction were not available for these subjects; however, on the basis of our data, it appears that the cornea plays a significant role in the progression of adult myopia.

OCULAR COMPONENT CHANGES IN MYOPIA

□ Childhood Myopia

Most of the available evidence indicates that axial elongation is responsible for the development and progression of childhood myopia. On the basis of his longitudinal studies, Sorsby (1980) noted that the greatest changes in refractive error in children occurred when anomalous axial elongation was not adequately compensated by a reduction in the refracting power of the eye, the latter being mostly the result of a reduction of the power of the crystalline lens.

Table 5.6. Mean ($\pm$ SD) Changes in Refractive Error and Ocular
Components in 1 Year in Myopes

Age span (yrs)	No. eyes	Change in refractive error (D)	Change in corneal power (D)	Change in lens power (D)	Change in axial length (mm)
7–10	18	−0.602 ($\pm$0.266)	−0.064 ($\pm$0.084)	−0.357 ($\pm$0.309)	+0.318 ($\pm$0.105)
11–15	15	−0.699 ($\pm$0.382)	−0.029 ($\pm$0.076)	−0.233 ($\pm$0.151)	+0.321 ($\pm$0.164)
16–22	9	−0.132 ($\pm$0.153)	−0.016 ($\pm$0.162)	−0.047 ($\pm$0.187)	+0.028 ($\pm$0.040)

*From Tokoro and Kabe (1964).

   Studies by Tokoro and his colleagues in Japan and by Fledelius in Denmark also show that the optical component change most important in childhood myopia is axial elongation. Tokoro and Kabe (1964) published data about changes in refractive error, corneal power, lens power, and axial length for forty-two eyes of myopes between the ages of 7 and 22 years. The mean changes shown in Table 5.6 show that for the 7- to 10-year and 11- to 15-year age categories myopia increases, axial length increases, lens power decreases, and corneal power decreases slightly. However, after the age of 16, which is close to the mean age at which myopia ceases to progress, changes in the components are much smaller: Note particularly that the mean axial length change after age 16 is negligible. In another paper, Tokoro and Suzuki (1969) presented plots of refractive error and axial length changes as a function of age. These plots show the familiar sequence of large increases in myopia up to about 15 or 16 years of age, after which the curve flattens; their patterns of axial length increases are strikingly similar. A cross-sectional study (Goss et al. 1990) suggests that the axial elongation of the eye responsible for childhood myopia progression slows at about the same age as does general body growth.
   In a study designed primarily to look at the effects of low birth weight on refraction during childhood, Fledelius (1976, 1980, 1981a, 1981b, 1982a, 1982b) performed two follow-up examinations at age 10 and age 18 on children born in a Copenhagen hospital. Data for seventy low-birth-weight subjects and sixty-seven full-term subjects are summarized in Table 5.7. As shown in this table, mean changes in anterior corneal radius, anterior chamber depth and lens thickness between 10 and 18 years of age are not significantly different from zero; however, mean changes in axial length are large, varying from 0.48 to 0.90 mm, and compare very closely to changes in vitreous length. Changes in axial length and vitreous length were found to be significantly correlated with changes in myopia.

Table 5.7. Changes in Refractive Error and the Ocular Components from 10 to 18 Years of Age

Group	N	Mean change refractive error	Mean change anterior corneal radius (mm)	Mean change anterior chamber depth (mm)	Mean change lens thickness (mm)	Mean change vitreous length (mm)	Mean change axial length (mm)
LBW Males	36	−1.75 (±1.66)	−0.004 (±0.071)	+0.08 (±0.16)	+0.03 (±0.18)	+0.77 (±0.76)	+0.90 (±0.77)
LBW Females	34	−1.29 (±0.03)	−0.005 (±0.055)	+0.08 (±0.11)	−0.01 (±0.17)	+0.58 (±0.48)	+0.64 (±0.52)
FT Males	36	−1.26 (±1.23)	+0.020 (±0.061)	+0.17 (±0.18)	−0.02 (±0.12)	+0.58 (±0.53)	+0.73 (±0.60)
FT Females	31	−1.07 (±0.91)	+0.003 (±0.055)	+0.09 (±0.11)	−0.02 (±0.12)	+0.41 (±0.52)	+0.48 (±0.52)

*From Fledelius 1981a, 1982a, 1982b.
LBW = low birthweight
FT = full term

Although the eyes of the low-birth-weight myopes were found to be smaller than those of the full-term myopes, for both groups the mechanism for the progression of myopia appeared to be axial elongation (Fledelius 1981b).

□ Young-Adult Myopia

The conclusions reached by studies of ocular component changes in young adult myopia are not consistent. The existence of a relationship between corneal steepening and the progression of young-adult myopia, described earlier in this chapter (Goss and Erickson 1987), appears to be supported by data published by Baldwin (1962). His graphic display appeared to show decreases in corneal power in childhood myopia progression and increases in corneal power in young-adult myopia progression. Data published by Kent (1963) also support the idea that the cornea steepens during myopia progression: For one subject, he found that shifts in myopia of 0.94 and 0.75 D, for the right and left eyes, were associated with increases in corneal refracting power of 0.58 and 0.64 D. On the other hand, Adams (1987) found a minimal corneal power change and a greater than average axial length measurement for a subject (himself) in whom myopia progressed considerably during the young adult years. The role of axial length was supported in a study by McBrien and Millodot (1987) who found that mean axial length was greater in myopes with onset after 15 years of age than in emmetropes of the same age.

MYOPIA PROGRESSION: SUMMARY AND RECOMMENDATIONS

On the basis of the results summarized in this chapter, two mechanisms are suggested for the progression of myopia: one for childhood myopia and one for myopia during the young adult years. The former exhibits more rapid progression than the latter, and is mainly due to axial elongation; the latter is related, in some cases, to an increase in corneal refracting power. The earlier myopia appears in childhood, the greater the amount at the cessation of childhood myopia progression. Females tend to have earlier onset of myopia and earlier cessation of childhood myopia progression, and less likelihood of progression during the young adult years.

The earlier cessation of myopia progression in females can be likened to the earlier cessation of bodily growth in females. The cessation age of childhood myopia progression appears to correspond to a cessation of axial elongation, which in turn may occur because the hormonal influences leading to the termination of bone and general body growth might also lead to the cessation of the growth of the sclera. These possible interrelationships should be investigated.

Possible neurohumoral or biochemical growth factor influences on axial elongation, suggested by Raviola and Wiesel (1985), Wickham (1986) and Wallman et al. (1987), should also be studied. They might explain, for instance, the axial elongation that occurs as a result of visual deprivation in animals and humans. It has also been hypothesized that decrease in retinal image quality accompanying accommodative disorders could play a role in axial elongation and myopia (Goss 1988).

Although clinical interventions to slow or stop the progression of myopia have been largely unsuccessful, the results reported here (Goss 1986a) together with those of Roberts and Banford (1987) suggest that bifocals reduce the rate of progression for myopes who have esophoria at nearpoint and for those who have high nearpoint binocular cross cylinder nets. Future research should attempt to replicate these results with carefully designed prospective studies and should investigate possible mechanisms for these results. One possible explanation is that the lag of accommodation implied by a high nearpoint binocular cross cylinder finding could be similar to visual deprivation in eliciting ocular growth (Goss 1988). Correction of this problem with bifocal lenses would restore clear retinal imagery. Such a mechanism would have physiologic significance: Without a bifocal correction, retinal image clarity could be attained by axial elongation. It is conceivable that such a mechanism could be mediated by secretion of growth factors from retinal amacrine or ganglion cells, which are responsive to border information (Cohen 1987).

CLINICAL ISSUES

Procedures for the management of myopia have been discussed by Goss and Eskridge (1987) and are presented in chapters in this volume by Grosvenor, Jensen and Goldschmidt, and Waring.

Parents of myopic children, as well as the children themselves, are often concerned about expected future changes in the myopia. The generalized trend of childhood myopia progression is a rapid increase in myopia after onset, continuing to the mid to late teens. However, there are considerable variations in age of onset, rate of progression, age of cessation, likelihood of progression during the young adult years, and other factors. Therefore, when discussing myopia progression with patients or their parents, predictions should be made only in the most general terms.

In clinical trials of interventions, such as the use of bifocal lenses, experimental and control subjects should be matched with respect to parameters such as age, sex, amount of myopia, and nearpoint phoria status. Additional characteristics of a well-designed clinical trial include masking of examiners, adherence to appropriate measurement protocols, and appropriate statistical treatment (Ederer 1975,

Goss 1982, Young et al. 1985). Most of the studies discussed in this chapter did not require sophisticated equipment and, with proper planning, could be performed in the practitioner's office, using routine patients as subjects. Practitioners should be encouraged to undertake such studies.

——— ■ ———————————————————————————

REFERENCES

Adams AJ. Axial elongation, not corneal curvature, as a basis of adult onset myopia. Am J Optom Physiol Opt 1987;64:150–152.

Baldwin WR. Corneal curvature changes in high myopia vs. corneal curvature changes in low myopia. Am J Optom Arch Am Acad Optom 1962;39:349–355.

Baldwin WR. Some relationships between ocular, anthropometric, and refractive variables in myopia. Ph.D. Thesis. Indiana University, Bloomington, 1964.

Borghi RA, Rouse MW. Comparison of refraction obtained by "near retinoscopy" and retinoscopy under cycloplegia. Am J Optom Physiol Opt 1985;62:169–172.

Bücklers M. Changes in refraction during life. Br J Ophthalmol 1953;37:587–592.

Cohen AI. The retina. In: Moses RA, Hart WM Jr., eds. Adler's Physiology of the Eye, 8th ed. St Louis: CV Mosby Co, 1987;458–490.

Cook RC, Glasscock RE. Refractive and ocular findings in the newborn. Am J Ophthalmol 1951;34:1407–1413.

Criswell MH, Goss DA. Myopia development in nonhuman primates — a literature review. Am J Optom Physiol Opt 1983;60:250–268.

Curtin BJ. The Myopias — Basic Science and Clinical Management. Philadelphia: Harper & Row, 1985;177–234.

Ederer F, ed. The randomized controlled clinical trial — National Eye Institute workshop for ophthalmologists. Am J Ophthalmol 1975;79:752–789.

Erickson P, Thorn F. Does refractive error change twice as fast as corneal power in orthokeratology? Am J Optom Physiol Opt 1977;54:581–587.

Fledelius H. Prematurity and the eye — ophthalmic 10-year follow-up of children of low and normal birth weight. Acta Ophthalmol 1976;54 (Suppl 128):1–245.

Fledelius HC. Ophthalmic changes from age of 10 to 18 — a longitudinal study of sequels to low birth weight. I. Refraction. Acta Ophthalmol 1980;58:889–898.

Fledelius HC. The growth of the eye from age of 10 to 18 years — a longitudinal study including ultrasound oculometry. Doc Ophthalmol Proc 1981a;29:211–215.

Fledelius HC. Myopia of prematurity — changes during adolescence — a longitudinal study including ultrasound oculometry. Doc Ophthalmol Proc 1981b;29:217–223.

Fledelius HC. Ophthalmic changes from age of 10 to 18 years — a longitudinal study of sequels to low birth weight. III. Ultrasound oculometry and keratometry of anterior eye segment. Acta Ophthalmol 1982a;60:393–402.

Fledelius IIC. Ophthalmic changes from age of 10 to 18 years — a longitudinal study of sequels to low birth weight. IV. Ultrasound oculometry of vitreous and axial length. Acta Ophthalmol 1982b;60:403–411.

Fletcher MC, Brandon S. Myopia of prematurity. Am J Ophthalmol 1955;40:474–481.

François J, Goes F. Oculometry of progressive myopia. Bibl Ophthalmol 1975;83:277–282.

Goldschmidt E. Refraction in the newborn. Acta Ophthalmol 1969;47:570–578.

Goss DA. Attempts to reduce the rate of increase of myopia in young people — a literature review. Am J Optom Physiol Opt 1982;59:828–841.

Goss DA. Refractive status and premature birth. Optom Monthly 1985;76:109–111.

Goss DA. Effect of bifocal lenses on the rate of childhood myopia progression. Am J Optom Physiol Opt 1986a;63:135–141.

Goss DA. Ocular Accommodation, Convergence, and Fixation Disparity: A Manual of Clinical Analysis. New York: Professional Press, 1986b;61–70, 89–99.

Goss DA. Matters arising: Cessation age of childhood myopia progression. Ophthalmol Physiol Opt 1987a;7:195–196.

Goss DA. Linearity of refractive change with age in childhood myopia progression. Am J Optom Physiol Opt 1987b;64:775–780.

Goss DA. Retinal image-mediated ocular growth as a possible etiological factor in juvenile-onset myopia. In: Vision Science Symposium/A Tribute to Gordon Heath. Bloomington: Indiana University, 1988;165–183.

Goss DA, Cox VD. Trends in the change of clinical refractive error in myopes. J Am Optom Assoc 1985;56:608–613.

Goss DA, Cox VD, Herrin-Lawson GA, et al. Refractive error, axial length, and height as a function of age in young myopes. Optom Vis Sci 1990;67:332–338.

Goss DA, Criswell MH. Myopia development in experimental animals — a literature review. Am J Optom Physiol Opt 1981;58:859–869.

Goss DA, Erickson P. Meridional corneal components of myopia progression in young adults and children. Am J Optom Physiol Opt 1987;64:475–481.

Goss DA, Erickson P, Cox VD. Prevalence and pattern of adult myopia progression in a general optometric practice population. Am J Optom Physiol Opt 1985;62:470–477.

Goss DA, Eskridge JB. Myopia. In: Amos JF, ed. Diagnosis and Management in Vision Care. Boston: Butterworths, 1987;121–171.

Goss DA, Grosvenor T. Rates of childhood myopia progression with bifocals as a function of nearpoint phoria: consistency of three studies. Optom Vis Sci 1990;67:(in press).

Goss DA, Winkler RL. Progression of myopia in youth: age of cessation. Am J Optom Physiol Opt 1983;60:651–658.

Greene PR. Mechanical considerations in myopia: relative effects of accommodation, convergence, intraocular pressure, and the extraocular muscles. Am J Optom Physiol Opt 1980;57:902–914.

Greene PR. Myopia and the extraocular muscles. Doc Ophthalmol Proc 1981;28:163–169.

Grosvenor T. Can myopia be controlled? Part 4: The use of bifocals. Optom Monthly 1980; 71:620–622.

Grosvenor TP. Primary Care Optometry: A Clinical Manual. Chicago: Professional Press, 1982.

Grosvenor TP, Perrigin DM, Perrigin J, Maslovitz B. Houston myopia control study: a randomized clinical trial. Part II. Final report by the patient care team. Am J Optom Physiol Opt 1987;64:482–498.

Gwiazda J, Scheiman M, Mohindra I, Held R. Astigmatism in children: changes in axis and amount from birth to six years. Invest Opthalmol Vis Sci 1984;25:88–92.

Hirsch MJ. The changes in refraction between the ages of 5 and 14 — theoretical and practical considerations. Am J Optom Arch Am Acad Optom 1952;29:445–459.

Hirsch MJ. The Ojai longitudinal study of refractive state. Am J Optom Arch Am Acad Optom 1955;32:162–165.

Hirsch MJ. A longitudinal study of refractive state of children during the first six years of school — a preliminary report of the Ojai study. Am J Optom Arch Am Acad Optom 1961;38:564–571.

Hirsch MJ. Relationship between refraction on entering school and rate of change during the first six years of school — an interim report from the Ojai longitudinal study. Am J Optom Arch Am Acad Optom 1962;39:51–59.

Hirsch MJ. Changes in astigmatism during the first eight years of school — an interim report from the Ojai longitudinal study. Am J Optom Arch Am Acad Optom 1963; 40:127–132.

Hirsch MJ. The longitudinal study in refraction. Am J Optom Arch Am Acad Optom 1964a; 41:137–141.

Hirsch MJ. Predictability of refraction at age 14 on the basis of testing at age 6 — Interim report from the Ojai longitudinal study of refraction. Am J Optom Arch Am Acad Optom 1964b;41:567–573.

Hirsch MJ. Anisometropia: a preliminary report of the Ojai longitudinal study. Am J Optom Arch Am Acad Optom 1967;44:581–585.

Hofstetter HW. Some interrelationships of age, refraction, and rate of refractive change. Am J Optom Arch Am Acad Optom 1954;31:161–169.

Howland HC, Atkinson J, Braddick O, French J. Infant astigmatism measured by photo-refraction. Science 1978;202:331–333.

Ingram RM, Barr A. Changes in refraction between the ages of 1 and 3½ years. Br J Ophthalmol 1979;63:339–342.

Kent PR. Acquired myopia of maturity. Am J Optom Arch Am Acad Optom 1963;40:247–256.

Langer MA. Changes in ocular refraction from ages 5–16. Master's Thesis. Indiana University, Bloomington, 1966.

Lowrey CH. Growth and development of children, 7th ed. Chicago: Yearbook Medical Pub., 1978:84–85.

Mandell RB. Myopia control with bifocal correction. Am J Optom Arch Am Acad Optom 1959;36:652–658.

Mäntyjärvi MI. Predicting of myopia progression in school children. J Pediatr Ophthalmol Strabismus 1985a;22:71–75.

Mäntyjärvi MI. Changes of refraction in school children. Arch Ophthalmol 1985b;103:790–791.

McBrien NA, Millodot M. A biometric investigation of late onset myopia eyes. Acta Ophthalmol 1987;65:461–468.

Mohindra I. A non-cycloplegic refraction technique for infants and young children. J Am Optom Assoc 1977;48:518–523.

Mohindra I, Held R. Refraction in humans from birth to five years. Doc Ophthalmol Proc 1981;28:19–27.

National Academy of Sciences Working Group 58. Myopia: Prevalence and Progression. Washington, DC: National Academy of Sciences, 1989.

Raviola E, Wiesel TN. Effect of dark-rearing on experimental myopia in monkeys. Invest Ophthalmol Vis Sci 1978;17:485–488.

Raviola E, Wiesel TN. An animal model of myopia. N Engl J Med 1985;312:1609–1615.

Roberts WL, Banford RD. Evaluation of bifocal correction technique in juvenile myopia. Optom Weekly 1967;58(38):25–28, 31; 58(39):21–30; 58(40):23–28; 58(41):19–24, 26.

Rosenberg T, Goldschmidt E. The onset and progression of myopia in Danish school children. Doc Ophthalmol Proc 1981;28:33–39.

Saunders H. A longitudinal study of the age-dependence of human ocular refraction-I. Age-dependent changes in the equivalent sphere. Ophthalmol Physiol Opt 1986a;6:39–46.

Saunders H. A longitudinal study of the age-dependence of human ocular refraction. II. Prediction of future trends in medium and high myopia by means of cluster analysis. Ophthalmol Physiol Opt 1986b;6:177–186.

Saunders H. Author's reply. Ophthalmol Physiol Opt 1987;7:196–197.

Scharf J, Zonis S, Zeltzer M. Refraction in Israeli premature babies. J Pediatr Ophthalmol 1975;12:193–196.

Septon RD. Myopia among optometry students. Am J Optom Physiol Opt 1984;61:745–751.

Sorsby A. Biology of the eye as an optical system. In: Safir A, ed. Refraction and Clinical Optics. Hagerstown, MD: Harper & Row, 1980;133–149.

Thorn F, Held R, Li-Luo F. Orthogonal astigmatic axes in Chinese and Caucasian infants. Invest Ophthalmol Vis Sci 1987;28:191–194.

Tokoro T, Kabe S. Relation between changes in the ocular refraction and refractive components and development of the myopia. Acta Societatis Ophthalmologicae Japonicae 1964;68:1240–1253.

Tokoro T, Suzuki K. Changes in ocular refractive components and development of myopia during seven years. Jpn J Ophthalmol 1969;13:27–34.

Wallman J, Gottlieb MD, Rajaram V, Fugate-Wentzek LA. Local retinal regions control local eye growth and myopia. Science 1987;237:73–77.

Wickham MG. Growth as a factor in the etiology of juvenile-onset myopia. In: Goss DA, Edmondson LL, Bezan DJ, eds. Proceedings of the 1986 Northeastern State University Symposium on Theoretical and Clinical Optometry. Tahlequah, Okla: Northeastern State University, 1986;117–137.

Wiesel TN, Raviola E. Myopia and eye enlargement after neonatal lid fusion in monkeys. Nature 1977;266:66–68.

Wiesel TN, Raviola E. Increase in axial length of the macaque monkey eye after corneal opacification. Invest Ophthalmol Vis Sci 1979;18:1232–1236.

Yamamoto M, Tatsugami H, Bun J. A follow-up study of refractive error in premature infants. Jpn J Ophthalmol 1979;23:435–443.

Yinon U. Myopia induction in animals following alteration of the visual input during development: a review. Curr Eye Res 1984;3:677–690.

Young FA, Beattie RJ, Newby FJ, Swindal MT. The Pullman study — a visual survey of Pullman school children. Part II. Am J Optom Arch Am Acad Optom 1954;31:192–203.

Young FA, Leary GA, Grosvenor T, Maslovitz B, Perrigin DM, Perrigin J, Quintero S. Houston myopia control study: a randomized clinical trial. Part I. Background and design of the study. Am J Optom Physiol Opt 1985;62:605–613.

—6

Young-adult Myopia

William R. Baldwin,
Anthony J. Adams, and
Pamela Flattau

☐

The U.S. Air Force has been concerned about the high percentage of Academy cadets who are emmetropic at admittance but develop myopia during the 4-year training program. As a result, the Air Force requested that the National Research Council's Committee on Vision determine whether there have been significant changes, over the years, in the prevalence of myopia among adults who are eligible for Academy training, and to identify the variables that might predict refractive error changes in young adults.*

The impact of both juvenile and young-adult myopia on the recruitment and retention of Air Force Academy students is substantial and has enormous economic and social consequences. Qualifications for military pilots currently specify no refractive error greater than 0.25 D of myopia in any meridian, although waivers may be granted for myopia up to 1.25 D. A high prevalence of myopia in the applicant pool necessarily places constraints on recruitment. Students who are either qualified at entry or have a waiver run the risk of losing their waivers for pilot qualification should they develop myopia greater than 1.25 D by the time they complete 4 years of study. This poses a real problem for the U.S. Air Force, not to mention for students' career plans.

Since 1878, reports have been published concerning groups of young men be-

---

*To accomplish its task, the Committee on Vision formed a Working Group on Myopia Prevalence and Progression, consisting of the following members: Anthony Adams, chair (University of California), William Baldwin (University of Houston), Irving Biederman (University of Minnesota), Brian Curtin (Manhattan Eye and Ear Clinic), Sheldon Ebenholtz (State University of New York), David Goss (Northeastern State University), George Hutchison (Harvard University), Johanna Seddon (Massachusetts Eye and Ear Infirmary), and Joshua Wallman (City University of New York). This Working Group reviewed more than 500 articles on myopia. The present chapter is based on their report, which has recently been published through the National Research Council's Committee on Vision (Myopia: Prevalence and Progression, Washington, DC: National Academy Press, 1989).

Table 6.1.   U.S. Naval Academy Entrants Who Became Myopic, 1956

Spherical equivalent refraction at entrance (Homatr 0.4%)	17–18 yrs		19 yrs		20 yrs		21 yrs	
	N	%	N	%	N	%	N	%
+1.00 D and above	119	1.5	61	1.5	32	2	64	3
+0.62 D to +1.00D	156	11	54	8	50	4	65	2
+0.50 D or less	169	77	110	44	94	39	153	15

From Hynes 1956.

tween the ages of 17 and 21 years who have been examined to determine uncorrected visual acuity or refractive status before admission to college or military officer training, and then again after a period of time. Studies of those 17 to 21 years of age at entrance generally report that subjects are unlikely to become myopic if they have hyperopia greater than 0.75 D in the least plus meridian (perhaps as much as 1.25 D if refraction is determined under cycloplegia), even in those environments in which hyperopes of low degree often become myopic and in which myopes show progression. Shifts toward myopia occur approximately twice as often in myopes as in low hyperopes, and the mean magnitude of the change is somewhat greater. More recently, young men from 17 years to the mid to late thirties have been evaluated before beginning and after exposure to extensive nearwork in nonacademic settings.

Some studies show that subjects who are low hyperopes at 17 years of age are more likely to show changes than those low hyperopes who are older, as shown in Table 6.1. Movement from low hyperopia into low myopia, as well as progression of existing myopia, appear to be more common among younger adults than has traditionally been assumed.

MYOPIA IN COLLEGE STUDENTS

College students represent the most accessible group within the age range of interest. The first author to report the prevalence of myopia among college students was Ware (1813), who found that 25.2% were myopic. His and other prevalence figures for college students are given in Table 6.2.

Studies of prevalence of myopia among college students in the United States and Europe provide evidence that prevalence is similar in both areas over time. Among those prevalence rates listed in Table 6.3 are several figures for students

Table 6.2. Studies of Myopia Prevalence Among College Students in the United States and Other Countries, 1871–1985

Investigator	Year	Prevalence %	Location
College Students in the United States			
Derby	1877b	35.0	Harvard
Derby	1880	35.0	Amherst (lower division)
Derby	1882	47.2	Amherst (upper division)
Randall	1885	52.5	Composite of 6 European and 2 U.S. studies (2,436 subjects)
Agnew	1887	28.5	Brooklyn Polytechnic
Agnew	1887	40.0	New York College
Burnett	1911	15.0	University of California
Hall	1935	35.0	Washington
Dunphy	1968	44.0	Harvard (Business and Law Schools)
Septon	1984	75.0	Optometry students
Schell et al.	1985	81.0	Optometry students
College Students in Other Countries			
Erismann	1871	43.0	Germany
Pfluger	1875	40.0	Germany
Seggel	1879	81.0	Germany
Cohn	1881	53.0	Germany
Collard	1881	30.0	Germany
Durr	1883	35.0	Germany
Van Anrooy	1884	31	Germany
Fleischer	1907	50.0	Germany
Ware	1813	25.2	England
Kotelmann*	1877	49.0	England
Smith	1880	20.0	England
Clarke	1924	20.0	England
Parnell	1951	32.0	England
Emmert[a]	1876	76.0	Switzerland
Francesschetti	1935	24.0	Switzerland
Vogt		24.0	Switzerland
Tscherning	1882	32.4	Denmark
Tamura	1932	12.0	Japan
Banerjee	1933	35.0	India
Li and Rush	1920	55.0	China

*Cited by Randall (1885).

Table 6.3. Studies of Myopia Prevalence Among Young Adults By Age and Other Variables, 1848–1953

Investigator	Year reported	% Myopic		Sample and criteria
		Group A	Group B	
Szokalsky*	1848	13.0 (1st yr. college)	17.0 (upper division)	France
Loring	1877	26.0 (U.S.)	63.0 (German)	College students
Loring	1877	26.0 (U.S.)	44.0 (Soviet)	College students
Agnew	1877	29.0 (precollege)	37.0 (seniors)	College students
Derby	1880	35.4 (at entrance)	47.2 (at graduation)	College students
Collard†	1880	23.0 (scientific and professional)	42.0 (humanities)	College students
Collard†	1881	30.0 (ages 17–22)	27.0 (ages 24–27)	Military recruits
Tscherning	1882	2.4 (farmers and fishermen)	32.4 (advanced students)	Military conscriptees (Germany)
Seggel	1884	2.4 (farm workers)	56.7 (compositors and writers)	
Jackson	1932	25.7 (ages 15–20)	19.6 (ages 20–30)	Clinic sample
Tassman	1932	24.7 (ages 15–20)	22.0 (ages 20–30)	Clinic sample
Boynton	1936	18.2 (at entrance)	23.9 (at graduation)	visual acuity 20/50 or worse −1.50 or above
Nakamura	1954	20.0 (White)	30.0 (Nisei)	Military recruits
Sutton and Ditmars	1970	45.0 (at entrance)	60.0 (at graduation)	West Point cadets
Gmelin	1976	51.0 (at entrance)	67.0 (at graduation)	West Point cadets
Roberts and Rowland	1978	29.9 (age 12)	33.2 (age 17)	General
Sperduto	1983	23.9 (ages 12–17)	27.7 (ages 18–26)	General
Fiedelius	1983	32.6 (−0.25D or above)	10.3 (−1.75D or above)	Clinic sample

*Cohn (1867).
†Collard (1881).

aged 17 to 22 years. Schuster (1911) reported that 18% of Oxford undergraduates "have distinctly bad eyesight." He gave no explanation about the derivation of this figure, which corresponds closely with Parnell's (1951) prevalence data of Oxford undergraduate males with visual acuity of 6/60 (20/200) or worse. Employing 6/9 (20/30) as a criterion for myopia, Parnell found a 49.9% prevalence of myopia among a group of male students representing all undergraduate levels at the same university. It can be expected that almost all who exhibit this visual acuity at that age would be myopes of greater than 0.25 D spherical equivalent (Peters 1961).

Several studies in Germany provide prevalence data for college students (Cohn 1881, Durr 1883, Erismann 1871, Fleischer 1907, Pfluger 1875, Van Anrooy 1884). The highest prevalence (58%) reported was by Seggel (1884), and the lowest (30%) was reported by Collard (1881). Seggel's sample was made up of older students, and it may be presumed that they had spent more years in university study. Although several studies have reported a slight decrease in the prevalence of myopia after age 20, this may be due to the addition of nonstudents to samples at older ages and, in clinical samples, to the failure of adults whose myopia is stable to seek care. Longitudinal studies seldom report significant decreases in myopia prevalence before age 40.

Reports from a large number of investigations in the United States and in various European countries were examined by Randall (1885). The data permitted comparison of prevalence of myopia among more than 40,000 secondary school and college students. About 28% of the total group met Randall's criterion for myopia (-0.25 D or greater). Of college groups that provided sufficient data, 52.5% had myopia of 0.25 D or more. Table 6.3 presents prevalence figures from studies of college students in the United States and other countries when various study criteria could be assessed.

Unquestionably, many young adults who enter college level educational programs or who assume roles that involve extensive nearwork become less hyperopic or more myopic. For very low hyperopes, the change may be great enough to produce a low degree of myopia. Even a greater number of myopes become more myopic. The former group represents a unique concern to those organizations that require unaided visual acuity of 6/6 (20/20) or better at the end of training periods as well as at the beginning. Presently U.S. Air Force and U.S. Navy academies enforce these requirements for those who would become pilots or Naval line officers.

U.S. military cadets have backgrounds similar in most respects to those who matriculate in U.S. colleges and universities (Houston 1972). However, most cadets are in the top 10% of their high school classes, whereas few colleges or universities surveyed were this selective. The prevalence of myopia among cadets in the West Point studies (Brown 1986, Gmelin 1976) was not significantly different from that reported for first year students in other colleges.

As already noted, Parnell (1951) classified 32% of first-year Oxford students as myopic. He then computed distance visual acuity loss after 1 year for 150 male and 107 female students and found similar rates of acuity loss for both sexes. Thirteen percent of those whom he originally classified as myopic showed a reduction of visual acuity within 1 year; there was no significant visual acuity loss among hyperopes. Boynton (1936) found that 18.2% of college students had unaided visual acuity of 6/15 (20/50) or poorer during the first year of study, rising to 23.9% at graduation. He noted that those with poorer acuity at entrance tended to change the most and that better students tended to have poorer visual acuity.

Luckeish and Moss (1940) reported a decrease in visual acuity for 21% of a class of U.S. college students during one academic year, although unaided visual acuity improved for many during summer vacation. In addition, they found a small decrease in myopia among many grade school children during summer vacation (Luckeish and Moss 1939). A similar result was found by Owens (1985) and by Owens and Harris (1986) who reported data on 160 college freshmen. After measuring myopic shifts during the academic year, individual refractive states changed toward the entrance refractive error at the end of the summer vacation period. These studies suggest pseudomyopia (that is, myopia that may be reversible) as the basis for some of the visual acuity loss.

Most studies that report an increase in the prevalence of myopia among students during the first years of college are cross-sectional, and do not reflect selective withdrawal of students from the sample. The increased prevalence among graduate level students (Table 6.3) may reflect this selection factor, as well as that of myopic onset during the college years.

Three studies of graduate level students provide longitudinal data. Zadnick and Mutti (1987) found that 47% of a sample of eighty-seven myopic law students seeking care at the university clinic showed a myopic shift of -0.50 D or more between cycloplegic examinations conducted at various intervals during a 3-year period. Riffenburgh (1965) selected three subjects from a population of graduate students and six others who began occupations that involved intensive nearwork who were not myopic at age 20 but who developed myopia. The mean change was estimated to be from -0.75 to -1.50 D per year over a period of 2 to 5 years. Riffenburgh reports having seen several patients in whom "mild nearsightedness that had not progressed after the age of 15 years suddenly began to increase again in the twenties, associated at this time with demanding near work." Schell et al. (1986) reported a myopic shift of -0.50 D or greater in 30% of two successive classes of optometry students. Seventy-eight percent of this group of 109 subjects, having a mean age of 25 years, were myopic at entrance.

------ ■ --

MYOPIA IN MILITARY PERSONNEL

One of the first authors to comment on myopia in military personnel was Ware (1813) who reported that "among officers of the Queen's Guard many were myopic, while of 10,000 footguards less than half a dozen were myopic." Parnell (1951) compared unaided visual acuity of 279 male undergraduates at Oxford University to prevalence figures for over 90,000 18-year-old men from England and Wales who took National Service Board examinations in 1939. Oxford students had a higher prevalence of low visual acuity at all age levels (6/9 (20/30) or less, 49.9% vs 11.4%; 6/6 (20/20) or better, 16.8% vs 26%). Tscherning (1882) examined records of 38,900 Danish recruits and found a prevalence of myopia (1.50 D or greater) of 8.3% of the total group. This ranged from 2.4% for farmers and fishermen to 32.28% for advanced students. Seggel (1884) compared prevalence of myopia of the same magnitude among German conscripts and reported 2.4% for farm workers and 56.7% for compositors and writers.

In a later study of Danish draftees, designed to compare results with those of Tscherning, Goldschmidt (1968) reported a myopia prevalence of 9.2% with a similar occupational stratification. After correcting his data for differences in representation of occupational groups, Goldschmidt reported that the difference in prevalence (8.3% for Tscherning vs 9.2% for Goldschmidt) virtually disappeared. Many of the factors affecting prevalence were similar, fortuitously or by design, in the three studies (those of Parnell, Tscherning, and Goldschmidt) including a mean age of approximately 20 years. Stromberg (1936) found myopia of 1.00 D or greater in 4.8% of 20-year-old men who were entering the Swedish army.

Using the same classification criterion for myopia, Steiger (1913) in Germany and Sorsby et al. (1960) in England found myopia prevalences of 13.1 and 11.6%, respectively. Steiger's sample was made up of men 20 to 30 years of age from a clinic population, and Sorsby's sample consisted of young men called up for national service.

Comparing prevalences of myopia of −0.50 D or greater among white and Nisei (Japanese living in the United States) military recruits, Nakamura (1954) reported prevalences of 20% and 30%, respectively. The difference between these two groups was probably real, reflecting an ethnic difference in prevalence.

□ Changes in Myopia during Military Service

The first author to report acuity changes in military academy personnel during their training years was Hayden (1941). He noted that between the years 1934 and 1940, unaided visual acuity dropped below 6/6 (20/20) for 21% of all graduates during the 4-year training period. Based on Peters' (1961) evaluation of visual acuity and myopia, it can be assumed that virtually all of these visual acuity changes were due to refractive shifts into myopia. Hayden compared cycloplegic refraction at entrance to that 4 years later and found that 65% of 127 subjects who were myopic on graduation had been hyperopic when admitted. Furthermore, he reported that the vast majority of candidates whose entrance refraction was plano to +0.25 or even +0.50 D were found to be myopic within 1 or 2 years after admission to the Academy.

In a study of the 1949 and 1950 U.S. Naval Academy graduating classes, Hynes (1956) found that 18% who had met unaided visual acuity requirements at entrance failed the visual acuity test at graduation, virtually all of the acuity loss being due to myopia. In addition, he reported that older candidates are less likely to become myopic. He concluded that if the entering cycloplegic refraction reveals hyperopia above 0.50 D, the attrition rate due to myopia would be less than 10%.

Studying visual acuity of U.S. Naval Academy students, Shotwell (1981) found that those students who spent more time reading than in outdoor activities were more likely to show myopia onset and progression. However, he was unable to demonstrate any preventive effect in a study of the influence of plus lenses for reading (Shotwell 1984).

In a comparison of noncycloplegic refraction results of 418 randomly selected West Point cadets, determined before admission and again at the beginning of the senior year, Brown (1986) found a mean myopic change of 0.66 D. An unpublished study on the U.S. Air Force Academy graduating class of 1980 (Goodson 1983) and a recently published technical report on the U.S. Air Force class of 1985 (O'Neal and Connon 1987) provide refractive error data that permit some comparisons: Both classes showed similar percentages of entering myopes, with about 60% showing a myopic change of 0.50 D or more and 25% showing a change of 1.00 D or more after 2 or 3 years. For the 1985 group, the percentage of entering hyperopes, emmetropes, and myopes who exhibited no shift or with a hyperopic or myopic shift of 0.25 D or more is shown in Figure 6.1.

Mean refractive error changes over the 2.5-year period in the O'Neal and Connon (1987) study are given in Table 6.4 for various levels of entering refractive error. This table also shows the percentage of eyes at each refractive error level that showed a myopic change of 0.25 D or more, 0.50 D or more, or 0.75 D or more. Figure 6.2 shows that larger percentages of myopic eyes shifted toward greater myopia, at all initial levels of myopia, than did low hyperopes. This figure also shows that the greater the initial myopia, the greater the myopic change tended to be. The mean myopic shift by level of entering refractive error is shown, for the O'Neal and Connon (1987) data, in Figure 6.3. The mean myopic shift was similar (about 0.50 D) for hyperopes, emmetropes, and low myopes but was about double that amount (0.80 to 1.00 D) for myopes of 1.00 D and above.

U.S. Naval Academy studies have shown that those who initially exhibit 6/6 (20/20) visual acuity but develop myopia of low degree after entrance into the Academy have two characteristics in common: (1) They are more likely to be at the lower end of the age spectrum at entrance, and (2) refraction is likely to be between +0.50 and −0.50 D in one or both principal meridians. These studies also indicate that the myopia that develops is of low degree, and that many cadets having more than 0.50 D of hyperopia lose some of their hyperopia during the student years.

Refractive changes of naval submarine crew members were compared with those of National Guardsmen (both groups 22 to 29 years old) over a 3- to 5-year period (Kinney et al. 1980). Fifty-one percent of the submariners showed unaided

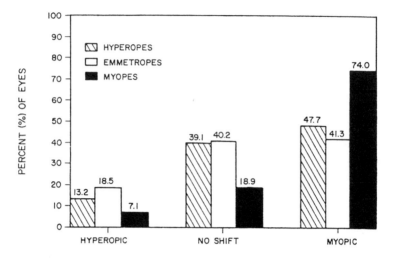

Figure 6.1. Percentage of eyes in each spherical equivalent (SPEQ) refractive error category showing no shift in refraction or a shift of 0.25 D or more in the hyperopic or myopic direction, during the 2.5-year period between entrance exams and third academic year exams, for 994 eyes from the U.S. Air Force Academy class of 1985. (From O'Neal and Connon 1987. © The Am Acad of Optom 1987. Reprinted by permission.)

Table 6.4. Myopic Shift After 2.5 Years in the U.S. Air Force Academy Class of 1985

Spherical equivalent refraction at entrance	Total number (eyes)	Mean change	Standard deviation	Percentage shifting −0.25 or more	Percentage shifting −0.50 or more	Percentage shifting −0.75 or more
+1.00 and above	35	−0.37	±0.51	65.7	37.1	20.0
+.25 to +.87	336	−0.16	±0.34	45.8	19.6	7.3
+.12 to −.12	184	−0.21	±0.45	41.3	25.0	14.7
−.25 to −.87	192	−0.38	±0.48	68.2	43.8	22.6
−1.00 and above	247	−0.70	±0.70	77.8	64.0	48.4

Calculated from O'Neal and Connon 1987.

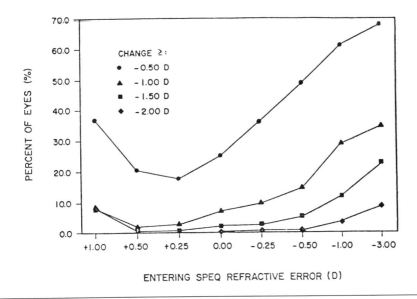

Figure 6.2. Percentages of eyes in selected spherical equivalent (SPEQ) refraction ranges with a myopic shift equal to or greater than the amount shown, during the 2.5-year period between entrance exams and the third academic year exams, for 994 eyes from the U.S. Air Force Academy class of 1985. Note that the refractive error scale has unequal intervals. (From O'Neal and Connon 1987. © The Am Acad of Optom 1987. Reprinted by permission.)

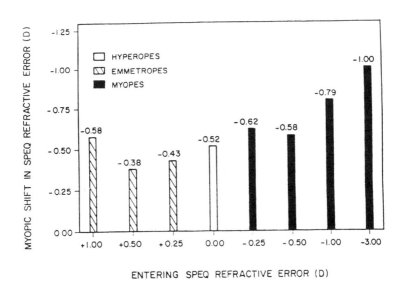

Figure 6.3. Mean myopic shift in spherical equivalent (SPEQ) refraction during the 2.5-year period between entrance exams and the third academic year exams, for 664 eyes showing any amount of myopic shift (−0.12 D or more) from the U.S. Air Force Academy class of 1985. (From O'Neal and Connon 1987. © The Am Acad of Optom 1987. Reprinted by permission.)

visual acuity loss, as compared to 20% of the National Guardsmen. Greene (1970) found that servicemen (all of whom were college graduates) tended to become myopic or to progress in myopia when confined within ICBM sites, the mean change for those showing a myopic shift over a 4-year period being approximately −0.65 D.

Myopic changes of U.S. Air Force pilots were compared to those of navigators

Table 6.5.   U.S. Air Force Pilots and Navigators Who Became Myopic by More than 0.25 D, 1983

Elapsed time (years)	Pilots (percentage)	Navigators (percentage)
1–5	2.4	7.8
6–10	7.4	10.4
11–15	10.4	22.6
16–20	17.6	24.7
Total	7.8	13.6

From Provines et al. 1983.

Table 6.6.   Pilots and Navigators Who Developed More Than 0.25 D of Myopia by Various Initial Refractive Error Levels

Initial spherical equivalent refractive error	N	Did not become myopic (more than −0.25 D)	Did become myopic (more than −0.25 D) (%)
Pilots			
−0.25 to plano	248	205	43 (17.3)
+0.12 to +0.37	251	231	20 (8.0)
+0.50 to +0.75	193	191	2 (1.0)
> +.87	100	100	0 (0.0)
Total	792	727	65 (8.2)
Navigators			
−0.25 to plano	153	109	44 (28.8)
+0.12 to +0.37	142	132	10 (7.0)
+0.50 to +0.75	119	112	7 (5.9)
+0.87 to +1.12	31	29	2 (6.5)
> +1.25	16	16	0 (0.0)
Total	461	398	63 (13.7)

From Provines et al. 1983.

by Provines et al. (1983). Both groups of subjects were 20 to 25 years old when initial refractive data were collected, and refractive data were obtained again after periods ranging from 1 to 20 years. As shown in Table 6.5, a higher percentage of navigators became myopic at all time intervals after the initial examination. Table 6.6 permits comparison of the Provines et al. data with those of the two U.S. Air Force Academy classes reported by Goodson (1983) and O'Neal and Connon (1987). Virtually none of those exhibiting hyperopia of 1.00 D or greater at first encounter became myopic, although a high percentage shifted in a myopic direction. A significant number of those near emmetropia became myopic by 0.50 D or more. Data extracted from the Provines et al. study indicate that the prevalence of myopia continues to increase throughout the prepresbyopic years among both pilots and navigators.

Other authors have reported myopia developing and progressing among individuals in this age range. Diamond (1957) found that sixteen of sixty-seven pilots (24%) became myopic (from 0.25 to 1.25 D) after the age of 21. All who became myopic were emmetropes or very low hyperopes between the ages of 21 and 31 years. Kent (1963) found similar changes in a small sample of naval officers.

□ Effects of Changing Refractive and Acuity Criteria

On the basis of his findings regarding visual acuity loss of emmetropes and low hyperopes during academy training, Hayden (1941) recommended that at least 1.00 D of hyperopia be required for admission into the Naval Academy.

The prevalence of hyperopia in men of military age is so small that if the Navy were to follow Hayden's suggestion, the applicant pool would be greatly diminished. For example, Bennett and Rabbetts (1984) found that only 20% of patients receiving free eye care services in England had refractive states between +1.12 and +2.00 D, and many of those wearing prescriptions greater than +2.00 D would have been disqualified for admission to the academy on the basis of visual acuity or refractive criteria. In a study by Brown and Kronfeld (1929) in which refraction was performed under atropine cycloplegia, only 10% of a group of subjects had hyperopia of 1.25 D or above. In other reports, Brown (1986) reported that less than 1% of 836 West Point cadets had hyperopia of 1.00 D or more; Gmelin (1976) reported that only 0.05% of cadets in the 1970 entering class had 1.00 D of hyperopia or more; Biederman (1986) estimated that the percentage of 18-year-old academy-eligible men having hyperopia of 1.00 D or more may be as low as 1%.

Beginning in 1960, the U.S. Military Academy at West Point instituted liberal admission policies concerning refractive errors, with the result that between 1964 and 1968, 45% to 51% of entering students were myopic (Sutton and Ditmars 1970). In addition, these authors reported that at graduation, the prevalence of myopia among those who were not myopic at entrance increased by an average of 15% for the four classes. As a point of reference, Rengstorff (1972) reported at about the same time that 33% of the total U.S. Army active duty personnel wore corrective lenses to achieve 6/6 (20/20) visual acuity. It was also noted by Sutton and Ditmars (1970) that more than half of the admittees ranked in the top 10% of their high school classes, and 80% had won varsity letters in one or more sports.

Unfortunately, many military academy studies are subject to biases that make interpretation of progression data difficult. Before entry into military academies, candidates receive refractive examinations from family practitioners (optometrists and ophthalmologists) who might be expected to empathize with applicants and underestimate myopia. Also, candidates with hyperopia are more likely to be identified as emmetropic since cycloplegic refractions are not routine before entry into the academies. To the extent that this is true, myopic shifts would be underestimated in hyperopia and overestimated in myopia.

CHANGES IN THE OPTICAL COMPONENTS OF THE EYE

The mechanisms that produce myopic onset or progression in young adults are unclear. Goss and Erickson (1987) and Kent (1963) examined longitudinal data and found that corneal steepening accompanied progression of myopia in some young adults. On the other hand, Adams (1987) found that axial length increase accounted for all of his own adult-onset myopia. Schell et al. (1986) reported that most adult myopic shifts found in a group of optometry students were accounted for by axial elongation. McBrien and Millodot (1987) found that axial elongation accounted for myopic changes in their young adult sample.

Change in accommodative tonus, that is, comparing the accommodative state of the light-adapted eye fixating a distant target to the accommodative state in total darkness (also called dark focus or resting level of accommodation) has been implicated as the cause of late-onset myopia by some investigators. Owens and Harris (1986) reported that significant myopic shifts were found when noncycloplegic refractions were performed at the beginning and the end of each of the freshman semesters, and that myopic shifts were also found when accommodative focus was measured in darkness (dark focus). Marked individual and trial-to-trial differences in susceptibility to accommodative hysteresis effects have been reported (Ebenholtz 1985). McBrien and Millodot (1988) found that after sustained nearwork, dark focus increased among low hyperopes, emmetropes, and myopes, but decreased among higher hyperopes. Ebenholtz (1983) raised the interesting thought that those individuals with consistent accommodative hysteresis effects might have a higher risk for myopia and proposed that this hypothesis be studied.

■

CONCLUSIONS

An exhaustive review of the relevant literature uncovered no experiment specifically designed to answer the questions within the charge of the Working Group. Consequently, most of the conclusions drawn are necessarily tentative and were inferred from considering multiple studies. Very few of the cited reports resulted from investigations undertaken to test hypotheses. What appears to be needed is considerably more research targeted to answer specific questions, designed so that results of different investigators can be compared, and so that relatively small numbers of cohorts can be studied over an extended time.

The traditional view is that myopia rarely has its onset in young adults and that progression of myopia rarely occurs among this age group. It is now clear that progression among adult myopes who enter an academic environment occurs with significant frequency, although less in degree than among juvenile myopes. Although the progression of some young adult myopia may be due to the fact that stabilization of juvenile myopia occurs at a later age, the frequency of progression among college students and military cadets is much greater than predicted by studies of the age at which juvenile myopia stabilizes (Goss and Winkler 1983, Saunders 1984 and 1986).

Studies of uncorrected visual acuity loss indicate that at least 20% of nonmyopes become myopic during the 4-year period after entrance into college or military academy. It appears that there is a distinct form of myopia, or myopic shift, for which young adults who enter academic environments are at risk.

Virtually all students bound for military academies with noncycloplegic refractive errors at entrance of $+1.00$ D or more in any principal meridian retain uncorrected visual acuity of 6/6 (20/20) or better in each eye at the end of 4 years of study. However, if this criterion were to be used as a pass-fail basis for selecting military academy applicants, it would provide an unrealistic constraint on the eligible pool.

■

REFERENCES

Adams AJ. Adult onset myopia: evidence for axial length elongation not corneal curvature increases the basis. Am J Optom Physiol Opt 1987;64:150–152.

Agnew C, Williams A. Near sightedness in the public schools. New York Medical Record 1877;12:34–36.

Bennett AG, Rabbetts RB. Clinical Visual Optics. London: Butterworths, 1984;434–441.

Biederman I. Unpublished communication to working group on myopia prevalence and progression, 1986.

Boynton RE. Variations in visual acuity among college students. Sight Saving Rev 1936; 6:263.

Brown M. Unpublished study of refractive error in U.S. Military Academy Cadets. West Point: U.S. Military Academy, 1986.

Brown EVL, Kronfeld P. The refraction curve in the U.S. with special reference to the first two decades. Proceeding of the 13th International Congress, of Ophthalmology 1929; 13:87–98.

Cohn H. Die Augen der Medicinstudierenden. Winer Med Jahresbucher Vienna 1881; 1:21.

Collard AC. De oogen studenten aau te rijks-universitat te utrecht. Utrecht: Inaug. Diss., 1881.

Derby H. Near sight in the young. Boston Med Surg J 1880;102(b):620–621.

Diamond KS. Acquired myopia in airline pilots. J Aviation Med 1957;28:559–568.

Durr. Die refraction von 414 Schulern nach anwendung von Homatropin. Arch fur Ophthalmol 1883;29:103.

Ebenholtz SM. Accommodative hysteresis: a precursor for induced myopia. Invest Ophthalmol Vis Sci 1983;24:513–515.

Ebenholtz SM. Hysteresis magnitude and decay rate as a function of fixation-target distance from the dark focus. Invest Ophthalmol Vis Sci 1985;26:269.

Erismann G. En beitrage sur Entwicklungsgescheichte der Myopie, gestutzt die Untersuchung der Augen von 4358 Schulern. Arch Ophthalmol 1981;17:1–79.

Fledelius HC. Is myopia getting more frequent? A cross-sectional study of 1,416 Danes aged 16 years +. Acta Ophthalmol 1983;61(4):545–559.

Fleischer B. Uber verebung von Kurzschtigkeit. Berl Ophthalmol Ges 1907;34:238–247.

Gmelin RT. Myopia at West Point: past and present. Mil Med 1976;141:542–543.

Goldschmidt E. On the etiology of myopia. Acta Ophthalmol (Suppl 98). Copenhagen: Munksgaard, 1968.

Goodson RA. Refractive error changes in Air Force Academy cadets. Unpublished study, USAF School of Aerospace Medicine, Radiation Sciences Division, Brooks Air Force Base, Texas, 1983.

Goss DA, Erickson PM. Meridional corneal components of myopia progression in young adults and children. Am J Optom Physiol Opt 1987;64:475–481.

Goss DA, Winkler RL. Progression of myopia in youth: age of cessation. Am J Optom Physiol Opt 1983;60(8):651–658.

Greene MR. Submarine myopia in the minutemen. J Am Optom Assoc 1970;41:1012–1016.

Hayden R. Development and prevention of myopia at the United States Naval Academy. Arch Ophthalmol 1941;25:539–541.

Houston JW. A Comparison of New Cadets at U.S. Military Academy with Entering Freshmen at other Colleges — Class of 1975. Ib4.03-372-030. Off Institutial Res, West Point, NY: U.S. Military Academy, 1972.

Hynes EA. Refractive changes in normal young men. Arch Ophthalmol 1956;56:761–767.

Jackson E. Norms of refraction. JAMA 1932;98(2):132–137.

Kent PR. Acquired myopia of maturity. Am J Optom Arch Am Acad Optom 1963;40:247–256.

Kinney JA, Luria SM, Ryan AP, et al. The vision of submariners and National Guardsman: a longitudinal study. Am J Optom Physiol Opt 1980;57:469–478.

Loring EG. Is the human eye changing its form under the influence of modern education? Transactions of the International Medical Congress. 1876. Printed for the Congress, 1877.

Luckeish M, Moss F. Ocular changes in school children during the fifth and sixth grades. Am J Optom Arch Am Acad Optom 1939;16:443–449.

Luckeish M, Moss F. Functional adaptation to near vision. J Exp Psychol 1940;26:352–356.

McBrien NA, Millodot M. Differences in adaptation of tonic accommodation with refractive states. Invest Ophthal Vis Sci 1988;29:460–468.

McBrien NA, Millodot M. A biometric investigation of late onset myopic eyes. Acta Ophthalmol 1987;65:461–468.

National Research Council Committee on Vision. Myopia: Prevalence and Progression. Washington, DC: National Academy Press, 1988.

Nakamura Y. Postwar ophthalmology in Japan. Am J Ophthalmol 1954;38:413.

O'Neal MR, Connon TR. Refractive error change at the United States Air Force Academy — class of 1985. Am J Optom Physiol Opt 1987;62:344–354.

Owens DA. Near work and myopia: a longitudinal study of accommodative tonus and refractive error. Am J Optom Physiol Opt 1985;62:64.

Owens DA, Harris D. Oculaomnotor adaptation and the development of myopia. ARVO Abstracts, 1986.

Parnell RW. Sight of undergraduates. Br J Ophthalmol 1951;35:467–472.

Peters HB. The relationship between refractive error and visual acuity at 3 age levels. Am J Optom Arch Am Acad Optom 1961.

Pfluger. Untersuchung der Augen von 529 Lehrnen. Klin Monatsbl Augenheilkd und fuer Augenartzliche Fortbildung 1875;13:324.

Provines WF, Woessner WM, Rahe AJ, Tredici TJ. The incidence of refractive anomalies in the USAF rated population. Aviat Space Environ Med 1983;54:622–627.

Randall BE. The refraction of the human eye. Am J Med Sci 1885b;90:123.

Rengstorff RH. Spectacles and contact lenses: a survey of military trainees. Mil Med 1972; 137:13–14.

Riffenburgh RS. Onset of myopia in the adult. Am J Ophthalmol 1965;59:925–926.

Roberts J, Rowland M. Refraction status and motility defects of persons 4–74, United States, 1971–1972. Vital Health Statistics 1978;11(206):1–124. Publication No. (PHS) 78–1654. Washington, DC: U.S. Department of Health, Education and Welfare.

Saunders H. Age-dependence of human refractive errors. Ophthalmic Physiol Opt 1984; 4:281.

Saunders H. A longitudinal study of the age dependence of human ocular refraction — II. Prediction of future trends in medium and high myopia by means of cluster analysis. Ophthalmic Physiol Opt 1986;6(2):177–186.

Schell K, Sewell L, Huey S, et al. Ocular components contributing to myopia and myopia progression in adults. Am J Opt Physiol Opt 1986;63:63P.

Seggel S. Uber normal Sehscharfe und die besiehung der Sehscharfe sur Refraction. Von Graefe's Arch Ophthalmol 1884;30:69–140.

Shotwell AJ. Plus lenses, prisms and bifocal effects on myopia progression in military students. Am J Optom Physiol Opt 1981;58:349–354.

Shotwell AJ. Plus lenses, prisms and bifocal effects on myopia progression in military students. Part II. Am J Optom Physiol Opt 1984;61:112–117.

Shuster E. First results from the Oxford Anthropometric Laboratory. Biometrica 1911;8:40–51.

Sorsby A, Sheridan M, Leary GA, Benjamin B. Vision, visual acuity and ocular refraction of young men. Br Med J 1960;1:1394–1398.

Sperduto RD, Seigel D, Roberts J, Rowland M. Prevalence of myopia in the United States. Arch Ophthalmol 1983;101(3):405–407.

Steiger A. Die Entstchung der Spharicshen Refraktionen des Menschlichen Auges. Berlin: S. Karger, 1913.

Stromberg E. Uber Refraktion and Aschsenldnge des Menschlichen Auges. Acta Ophthalmol 1936;14:281–291.

Sutton MR, Ditmars DL. Vision problems at West Point. J Am Optom Assoc 1970;41:263–265.

Szokalsk, Prager Vierteljahrschr, 1848;165 (Cited by Cohn 1881).

Tassmann IS. Frequency of the various kinds of refractive errors. Am J Ophthalmol 1932; 15:1044–1053.

Tscherning M. Studier over Myopiens Aetiologi. Copenhagen: C. Myhre, 1882.

Van Anrooy. De Oogen der Studenten aan te Rijks-SUnibversiteit te Leiden. Leiden: Inaug. Diss., 1884.

Ware J. Observations relative to the near and distant sight of different persons. Philos Trans R Soc London 1813;1:31.

Zadnik KS, Mutti DO. Refractive error changes in law students. Am J Optom Physiol Opt 1987;(in press).

__7__

Hyperopia

Jerome Rosner

☐

Almost two decades ago, Grosvenor (1971, p. 376) observed: "In the literature concerning the refractive state of the eye, myopia has routinely received most of the attention, hyperopia being pretty well ignored."

He illustrated this by reporting about a 4 to 1 prevalence of published papers devoted to myopia as compared to hyperopia, and went on to point out that:

> Many methods have been devised with the aim of preventing the onset of myopia and of controlling its progression, but little effort, if any, has been directed towards the prevention or control of hyperopia. Much attention has been given to the formulation of theories to account for the etiology of myopia, but little attention has been given to theories concerning hyperopia . . . perhaps the time has come for us to stop worrying about myopes, and to pay a little more attention to the problems that hyperopes may have. (P. 377)

The balance of his paper documented some of these problems: differences between myopes and hyperopes in intelligence test scores, reading ability, and academic placement, with the former group consistently outperforming the latter.

Grosvenor's remarks continue to be germane. If anything, the imbalance between the resources allocated to the study of myopia versus those concerned with hyperopia is even greater than it was 20 years ago. A remarkable amount of effort has been expended in investigating myopia during these two decades; symposia have been conducted (for example, see Fledelius et al. 1980); numerous books and papers have been written (for example, see Curtin 1985 and its extensive list of citations). Relatively little effort has been dedicated to hyperopia and, to a great extent, much of what has been written about it during these past two decades derives serendipitously from studies designed to investigate myopia, in which hyperopia provided the basis for comparison. It is not difficult to rationalize this bias. Myopia is often a progressive condition and, as this occurs, the myopic eye becomes more at risk to a variety of seriously debilitating secondary conditions. Hyperopia, in contrast, rarely progresses significantly and the hyperopic eye is not at risk to anything but whatever effects the hyperopia itself generates. Acknowledging this, but also recognizing that Grosvenor's observation continues to be pertinent, the primary goals of this chapter are to summarize what has been learned about the etiology of hyperopia, to identify certain characteristics of hyperopia, and to discuss their clinical implications.

ETIOLOGICAL FACTORS

Until recently, exceptionally little attention was given to the etiology of hyperopia. Conventional wisdom and the existing empirical evidence linked the condition to congenital and, perhaps, inherited factors (Sorsby et al. 1957); virtually no one proposed that hyperopia was in any way influenced by postnatal environmental factors.

Thinking has changed somewhat of late, in large part as a spin-off of the research devoted to identifying the etiological factors of myopia. There is now evidence that, in humans, ocular pathological conditions that involve foveal vision and that occur before age 3 years are typically accompanied by hyperopia (for example, optic nerve hypoplasia, toxoplasmosis, optic atrophy; Nathan et al. 1985). This new information suggests that disruption of central vision early in life prematurely halts the natural emmetropization process, leaving the individual hyperopic.

Animal studies also seem to substantiate this reasoning. Specifically, it has been shown that raising an animal (for example, monkey, cat, chicken) from birth in a light-free environment — regardless of whether its eyelids are sutured — is apt to lead to hyperopia, whereas raising the animal in a lighted environment with the eyelids sutured, or with sight blurred by some optical device, is more likely to cause the onset and/or progression of myopia (Raviola and Wiesel 1978, 1985; Regal et al. 1976; Yinon and Koslowe 1984; Yinon et al. 1984; Gottlieb et al. 1987).

CHARACTERISTICS OF HYPEROPIA

Hyperopia, unlike myopia, is not acquired (except in ocular conditions where central vision impairment occurs before the age of 3 years; see previous discussion). Nor does hyperopia normally worsen significantly over time. Although there is some evidence that hyperopia increases moderately in some children between the ages of 3 and 7 (Kempf et al. 1928, Brown 1938, Slataper 1950), it is not enough to be of clinical importance. Hyperopia does become more prevalent in the adult years, perhaps attributable to a tendency for latent hyperopia to become more overt with age, perhaps because the axial length of the eye tends to become smaller with age (Grosvenor 1987). In any event, the relatively small amount of change and the age at which this occurs dampens its importance as a clinical question.

Hyperopia has a high prevalence in young children. Most neonates are 1.00 D or more hyperopic, with the mean refractive error being about +2.00 D (Cook and Glasscock 1951, Goldschmidt 1969). An exception to this finding is the report of Mohindra and Held (1981) of a mean spherical refraction of neonates of −0.70 D; however, these authors acknowledged that they did not carry out cycloplegic refractions, as did Cook and Glasscock and Goldschmidt. The process of emmetropization reduces the prevalence of hyperopia somewhat during the school years, with the result that only about 26% of the adolescent population are hyperopic (Hirsch 1964). The trend reverses again as presbyopia ensues; by age 75, about half the population is hyperopic (Hirsch 1958).

Hyperopia is a significant factor in esotropia, even among those cases that appear to be congenital in origin. Almost 90% of congenital (infantile) esotropes are hyperopic, although in most cases it is less than 3.00 D (Robb and Rodier 1986, Hiles et al. 1980, Nelson et al. 1987). The percentage is even more skewed, of course, in accommodative esotropia; well over 90% are hyperopic, most in excess of 3.00 D (Mazow et al. 1984, Raab 1984).

Hyperopia is an important factor in children's school performance. A substantial amount of evidence in regard to this appears in the Grosvenor paper, cited earlier (see, for example, Eames 1948, Young 1963, Grosvenor 1970). A more recent example is provided in a study that compared the visual characteristics of children who were and children who were not making satisfactory progress in school (Rosner and Rosner 1987). Nineteen percent of the group who had school learning difficulties (total n = 123) were myopic (> −0.25 D), 54% were hyperopic (>+0.75 D). The opposite (and remarkably symmetrical) trend was displayed by the group of children who did not have school learning difficulties (n = 453). Fifty-four percent of that group were myopic and only 16% were hyperopic (chi square $P < .001$). (It should be noted that the subjects in this study were all patients of an eye clinic. Hence, they are not necessarily representative of a normal population. Rather, they probably represent two subgroups: (1) children who were referred to the clinic because they are not doing as well in school as their apparent cognitive abilities would predict, and (2) children who were referred because they manifested acuity deficits and/or ocular discomfort.)

Also reported in this study was a significant difference ($P < .001$) between the adequate and inadequate school achievers in the incidence of visual perceptual skills dysfunction. (Visual perceptual skills, in this context, refers to one's ability to analyze spatially organized patterns systematically in terms of such concrete features as the quantity, magnitude, and interrelationships of its constituent parts [Rosner 1979].) Seventy-eight percent of the inadequate achievers displayed visual perceptual skills dysfunction in contrast to 25% of the children designated as adequate achievers. This is particularly relevant because hyperopia, in addition to being related to school achievement, has been shown to be a significant factor in the rate at which children develop visual perceptual skills (Rosner and Gruber

1985). In a study involving 710 elementary schoolchildren (6 to 12 years old; all eye-clinic patients), they reported that substandard visual analysis skills were observed in 82% of the hyperopes ($> +0.75$ D), 38% of the emmetropes, and only 14% of the myopes (> -0.25 D) ($P < .001$).

Hyperopes tend to manifest higher dioptric levels of dark focus — tonic accommodation (TA) — than do emmetropes and myopes. This has been shown with adults, TA being assessed under laboratory conditions with an optometer (Maddock et al. 1981, McBrien and Millodot 1987), and with children, ages 6 to 14 years (Rosner and Rosner 1988a), using a clinical measurement method described by Tsuetaki and Schor (1987).

CLINICAL RELEVANCE AND IMPLICATIONS OF THESE CHARACTERISTICS

In respect to the prevalence of hyperopia in young children, the clinical management of hyperopia varies greatly among practitioners. Although most would agree about whether to prescribe compensatory lenses for a 1-year-old who manifests 1.00 D of hyperopia, consensus disintegrates for greater amounts. Some practitioners are inclined to discourage use of compensatory lenses as long as strabismus is not present, even with refractive errors approximating $+7.00$ D (Raab 1982). They reason that benign neglect at this very young age will not be detrimental; the child's amplitude of accommodation is far in excess of what is required to cope with the hyperopia and, besides, children of this age do not engage in much near-point activity. Other clinicians take a different position, especially when the hyperopia exceeds 3.00 D; this in recognition of the fact that such children, left untreated, are more prone to binocular difficulties — amblyopia and/or strabismus — by age 3½ (Ingram et al. 1986).

The *clinical implication* is that it may be that the conventional wisdom of previous decades — that convex lenses should not be prescribed until the child demonstrates a "need" for them — is not as correct as once believed. Relatively moderate amounts of hyperopia may be significant in some young children. The clinician should weigh the clinical evidence carefully and with an open mind when considering how to manage a young child with moderate hyperopia.

It may also turn out to be true that partial, rather than full lens correction, is not as desirable as some believe. A bifocal lens will serve better because it can provide full compensatory power for near fixation until the patient's accommodation has relaxed to the point where full-correction, single-vision lenses do not blur distance vision.

With respect to hyperopia among esotropes, there is less disagreement among practitioners about lens application when the patient is strabismic, but even in those instances some apply lenses more enthusiastically than do others. For example, Rethy and Gal (1968), in describing their experiences with 1,040 young esotropes, of whom 1,006 were hyperopic, proposed the following regimen: (1) prescribe slightly more plus than indicated by atropine refraction, (2) never allow the patient to have both eyes open at the same time as long as they are strabismic, and (3) reassess refractive status regularly, increasing convex power as much as the patient will tolerate. They report a remarkable 90% cure rate.

The *clinical implication* is that latent hyperopia may be more prevalent than currently believed, especially among esotropes. Contrary to popular practice, perhaps surgical treatment for what appears to be congenital esotropia should be deferred until innervational factors have been completely ruled out by repeated cycloplegic refraction, even if that means a delay until well past the child's eighth birthday. The Rethy and Gal report certainly suggests this regimen. So too, to some extent, does the documented high incidence of accommodative strabismus that manifests for the first time after strabismus surgery (Hiles et al. 1980).

With respect to the relationship between hyperopia and inexplicable school learning difficulties, we noted earlier that hyperopia tends to have a negative effect on the development of visual perceptual skills and that visual perceptual skills, in turn, have a strong influence on how well a child learns the basic skills of the primary grades. It has also been shown that elementary school-aged, hyperopic ($> +2.25$ D) children who obtained their first lenses before the age of 4 years are much less apt to lag in visual perceptual skills development than are those who obtained their first glasses after their fourth birthday (Rosner and Rosner 1986).

Buckminster Fuller, the eminent inventor and global planner, provides an interesting insight about the link between hyperopia and school-related performance with the following anecdote. He states,

> I was born cross-eyed. Not until I was four years old was it discovered that this was caused by my being abnormally farsighted. My vision was thereafter fully corrected with lenses. Until four, I could see only large patterns, houses, trees, outlines of people with blurred coloring. While I saw two dark areas on human faces, I did not see a human eye or a teardrop or a human hair until I was four. Despite my new ability to apprehend details, my childhood's spontaneous dependence only upon big pattern clues has persisted. (Fuller, 1967, P. 14)

Fuller, born in 1895, did not fare well in the organized educational system but sustained nevertheless and lived long enough to gain world acclaim for such inventions as the geodesic dome, dymaxion house, and the floating tetrahedronal city. During the 1960s, his writing and designing, which stressed a "do more with less" philosophy, made him a very popular figure not only in industry and design, but also among the college students of that decade — a decade when eroding natural environments became a concern to more than a few. Fuller closes his introspection,

> There is luck in everything. My luck is that I was born cross-eyed, was ejected so frequently from the establishment that I was finally forced either to perish or to employ some of those faculties with which we are all endowed — the use of which circumstances had previously so frustrated as to have put them in the deep freezer, whence only hellishly hot situations could provide enough heat to melt them back into usability. (P. 18)

The *clinical implication* is that hyperopia in preschool children, if not recognized and managed effectively, is likely to contribute to school learning difficulties, even in children whose cognitive abilities are average or above. The degree of hyperopia, the critical threshold below which the hyperopia may be safely ignored, remains to be determined. Perhaps in the interim, clinicians should consider taking the risk of prescribing lenses that they previously believed to "make no difference."

In respect to the relationship between tonic accommodation and hyperopia, as noted earlier, hyperopes tend to display higher TA than do emmetropes and myopes. Although this phenomenon has not yet been studied enough to justify conclusive statements, it hints at having clinical relevance for a number of reasons. One that has been speculated for a while is the link between the personality characteristics of hyperopes as compared to myopes (Gawron 1981, 1983). In essence, the construct proposes that hyperopes tend to be global-thinking extroverts; myopes, detail-oriented introverts. (Recall Buckminster Fuller's story, earlier.) One explanation for this theory is that myopes are more strongly innervated by the sympathetic nervous system (SNS), hyperopes by parasympathetic nervous system (PNS). Both systems contribute to accommodation and their respective influences are revealed by the individual's TA level (Garner 1983).

Coming closer to the scope of the vision care profession, it has been suggested that the human eye engages in two types of accommodation: positive and negative. The hypothesis is that the eye's state of rest is not at optical infinity, as once believed, but rather at the dark focus or resting point of accommodation, described above as TA (Charman 1982). When something beyond that point is to be seen clearly, the eye has to exercise negative accommodation; for objects closer than the dark focus, positive accommodation is required. The former is driven primarily by the SNS; the latter by the PNS. Inasmuch as the TA of hyperopes tends to be high, they appear to be more strongly controlled by PNS; myopes, with lower TA, are controlled by SNS. Incorporating the notion that the emmetropization process is, at least in part, influenced by TA (Van Alphen 1961), it could be speculated that the reason the refractive status of the average hyperope does not change as much over time as does the refractive status of the myope (Mäntyjärvi 1985) is that his elevated TA prematurely halts the emmetropization process.

Recent evidence indicates that although TA is highly correlated with refractive status, within-refractive-group differences in TA appears to be highly correlated with the adequacy of visual perceptual skills development (Rosner and Rosner 1988b). Specifically, although hyperopic ($>$ $+0.75$ D) 6- to 12-year-old children tend to display higher TA than do emmetropic children who, in turn, tend to display higher TA than do myopic ($>$ -0.25 D) children (P < .05), those within each of the refractive groups who display relatively high TA also tend to display substandard visual perceptual skills development; those within each of the refractive groups who display relatively low TA also tend to display at least adequate visual perceptual skills development (P < .01). Stated simply, children with low TA may be much more likely to have age-appropriate visual perceptual skills than are children with high TA.

The clinical implication is that tonic accommodation may provide an index of one aspect of basic cognitive development in children, although the reason for this is unclear. Perhaps it is because of some critical interaction between the PNS and SNS; perhaps it is because of some imbalance (deficit/overabundance) of one of the PNS and/or SNS neurotransmitter substances that mediate CNS biochemical functions, not only in the eye but elsewhere in the brain as well. Clearly, all of this is speculation, but it does have some tentative basis in fact.

CONCLUSIONS

Hyperopia among humans is a very prevalent phenomenon. It has not drawn much special attention from researchers or clinicians, probably because it is perceived to be an innocuous condition, a deficiency in optical focusing power that can be overcome by eyes that have adequate amplitude of accommodation, and can be compensated for with convex lenses if it causes signs or symptoms that the patient (or parent) cannot ignore. It does not progress, at least not to the extent that it causes concern. It does not appear to generate significant secondary disorders. Although some children with high degrees of hyperopia may develop amblyopia if lens application is delayed too long, this does not involve very many children and, besides, most of them seem to have other, presumably unrelated, problems that also make them different; and these often take precedence over their vision problems. (Recall, again, Buckminster Fuller's story.)

The central theme of this chapter is that even a moderate degree of hyperopia, if left unattended, may have a significant and detrimental influence on various aspects of a young child's behavior, such as how readily the child develops the capacity to view spatially organized information in an analytical manner and how well and easily the child gets started in school. If that turns out to be the case, then the key question is threshold: How much hyperopia is enough to justify lens application and at what age? That question, at present, is moot; but if it is important, then it is bound to be answered in time. Surely, it will not be a single number at a specific age, analogous to 6/6 (20/20) criterion in visual acuity. It is much more likely to require interpretation as part of an interaction between the amount of hyperopia, the tonic levels of accommodation and vergence, the adaptability of those processes, and other unknown factors. (For a discussion of these exquisitely interrelated visual functions, see Schor 1988.) Whatever the answer turns out to be, it is time to think more about the question.

REFERENCES

Brown EVL. Net average yearly change in refraction of atropinized eyes from birth to beyond middle age. Arch Ophthalmol 1938;19:719–734.

Charman WN. Accommodation and the autonomic nervous system. Ophthalmic Optn 1982;22:469–473.

Cook RC, Glasscock RE. Refractive and ocular findings in the newborn. Am J Ophthalmol 1951;34:1407–1413.

Curtin BJ. The Myopias: Basic Science and Clinical Management. Philadelphia: Harper & Row, 1985.

Eames TH. Comparison of eye conditions among 1000 reading failures, 500 ophthalmic patients, and 150 unselected children. Am J Optom Physiol Opt 1948;31:713–717.

Fledelius HC, Alsbirk PH, Goldschmidt E. Third International Conference on Myopia. Doc Ophthalmol Proceedings Series 28. Copenhagen: Dr W. Junk Publications, 1980.

Fuller B. Man with a chronofile. Saturday Review 1967;1:14–18.

Garner LF. Mechanisms of accommodation and refractive error. Ophthalmic Physiol Opt 1983;3:287–293.

Gawron VJ. Differences among myopes, emmetropes, and hyperopes. Am J Optom Physiol Opt 1981;58:753–760.

Gawron VJ. Ocular accommodation, personality, and autonomic balance. Am J Optom Physiol Opt 1983;60:630–639.

Goldschmidt E. Refraction in the newborn. Acta Ophthalmol 1969;47:570–578.

Gottlieb MD, Fugate-Wentzek LA, Wallman J. Different visual deprivations produce different ametropias and different eye shapes. Invest Ophthalmol Vis Sci 1987;28:1225–1235.

Grosvenor T. Refractive state, intelligence test scores, and academic ability. Am J Optom Physiol Opt 1970;47:355–361.

Grosvenor T. The neglected hyperope. Am J Optom Physiol Opt 1971;48:376–382.

Grosvenor T. Reduction in axial length with age: an emmetropizing mechanism for the adult eye? Am J Optom Physiol Opt 1987;64:657–663.

Hiles DA, Watson A, Biglan AWW. Characteristics of infantile esotropia following early bimedial rectus recession. Arch Ophthalmol 1980;98:697–703.

Hirsch M. Changes in refractive state after the age of 45. Am J Optom Arch Am Acad Optom 1958;35:229–237.

Hirsch M. Predictability of refraction at age 14 on the basis of testing at age six — interim report from the Ojai longitudinal study of refraction. Am J Optom Physiol Opt 1964; 41:567–573.

Ingram RM, Walker C, Wilson JM, et al. Prediction of amblyopia and squint by means of refraction at age 1 year. Br J Ophthalmol 1986;70:12–15.

Kempf GA, Collins SD, Jarman BL. Refractive errors in the eyes of children as determined by retinoscopic examination with a cycloplegic. Public Health Bulletin No. 182. Washington, DC: Government Printing Office, 1928.

Mäntyjärvi MI. Changes of refraction in schoolchildren. Arch Ophthalmol 1985;103:790–792.

Maddock RJ, Millodot M, Leat S, Johnson CA. Accommodation responses and refractive error. Invest Ophthalmol Vis Sci 1981;22:387–391.

Mazow ML, Kaldis LC, Prager TC, Jenkins PF. Accommodative esotropia. Am Orthop J 1984;34:77–82.

McBrien NA, Millodot M. The relationship between tonic accommodation and refractive error. Invest Ophthalmol Vis Sci 1987;28:987–1004.

Mohindra I, Held R. Refraction in humans from birth to five years. In: Fledelius HC, Alsbirk PH, Goldschmidt E, eds: Doc Ophthal Proc Series, vol. 28. The Hague: Dr W. Junk Publishers, 1981.

Nathan J, Kiely PM, Crewther SG, Crewther DP. Disease-associated visual image degradation and spherical refractive errors in children. Am J Optom Physiol Opt 1985;62:680–698.

Nelson LB, Wagner RS, Simon JW, Harley RD. Congenital esotropia. Surv Ophthalmol 1987;31:363–383.

Raab EL. Etiologic factors in accommodative esotropia. Trans Am Ophthalmol Soc 1982; 80:657–694.

Raab EL. Hypermetropia in accommodative esodeviations. J Pediatr Ophthalmol Strabismus 1984;21:194–198.

Raviola E, Wiesel TN. Effect of dark-rearing on experimental myopia in monkeys. Invest Ophthalmol Vis Sci 1978;17:485–488.

Raviola E, Wiesel TN. An animal model of myopia. N Engl J Med 1985;312:1609–1615.

Regal DM, Boothe R, Teller DY, Sackett GP. Visual acuity and visual responsiveness in dark-reared monkeys. Vis Res 1976;10:523–530.

Rethy I, Gal Z. Results and principles of a new method of optical correction of hypermetropia in cases of esotropia. Acta Ophthalmol 1968;46:757–766.

Robb RM, Rodier DW. The broad clinical spectrum of early infantile esotropia. Trans Am Ophthalmol Soc 1986;84:103–116.

Rosner J. Helping Children Overcome Learning Difficulties. NY: Walker Publishing Co. Inc, 1979.

Rosner J, Gruber J. Differences in the perceptual skills development of young myopes and hyperopes. Am J Optom Physiol Opt 1985;62:501–504.

Rosner J, Rosner J. Some observations of the relationship between the visual perceptual skills development of young hyperopes and age of first lens correction. Clin Exp Optom 1986;69:166–168.

Rosner J, Rosner J. Comparison of visual characteristics in children with and without learning difficulties. Am J Optom Physiol Opt 1987;64:531–533.

Rosner J, Rosner J. The relationship between clinically measured tonic accommodation and refractive status in 6–14 year old children. Optom Vis Sci 1989;66:436–439.

Rosner J, Rosner J. The relationship between tonic accommodation and visual perceptual skills development in 6 to 12 year old children. Optom Vis Sci 1989;66:526–529.

Schor C. Influence of accommodative and vergence adaptation on binocular motor disorders. Am J Optom Physiol Opt 1988;65:464–475.

Slataper FJ. Age norms of refraction and vision. Arch Ophthalmol 1950;43:466–481.

Sorsby A, Benjamin B, Davey JB, et al. Emmetropia and its aberrations. Medical Research Council Special Report Series, No. 293, 1957.

Tsuetaki T, Schor CM. Clinical method for measuring adaptation of tonic accommodation and vergence accommodation. Am J Optom Physiol Opt 1987;64:437–449.

Van Alphen WGHM. On Emmetropia and Ametropia. Ophthalmology (suppl) 1961;1–92.

Yinon U, Koslowe KC, Rassin MI. The optical effects of eyelid closure on the eyes of kittens reared in light and dark. Curr Eye Res 1984;3:431–439.

Yinon U, Koslowe KC. Eyelid closure effects on the refractive error of the eye in dark- and in light-reared kittens. Am J Optom Physiol Opt 1984;61:271–273.

Young FA. Reading, measures of intelligence and refractive errors. Am J Optom Physiol Opt 1963;40:257–264.

__8

Changes in Spherical Refraction during the Adult Years

Theodore Grosvenor

☐

■
BACKGROUND

The effect of age on refractive state was well known during the time of Aristotle (384–321 B.C.) who remarked that some people could see nearby objects clearly, but not distant objects; while older people had the opposite problem. Levene (1977) quoted Aristotle, in his *Problematica*, as saying:

> Why is it, that though both a short-sighted and an old man are affected by a weakness of the eyes, the former places an object if he wishes to see it, near the eye, while the latter holds it at a distance? Is it because they are afflicted with different forms of the same weakness? For the old man cannot see the object; he therefore removes the object at which he is looking to a point at which the vision of the two eyes meet. . . . The short-sighted man, on the other hand, can see the object but cannot proceed to distinguish which parts of the thing at which he is looking are concave and which are convex . . . but near at hand the incidence of light can more easily be perceived. (pp. 35–36).

There is no reason to believe, however, that Aristotle understood the nature of refraction and its anomalies. An understanding of myopia and presbyopia and their correction with lenses was evident during the renaissance years (Kepler, 1571–1630; Scheiner, 1575–1650), but it remained for Donders (1864) to insist that some young people needed convex lenses, for distance vision as well as near vision, and to point out that myopia and hyperopia, rather than myopia and presbyopia, were "opposites."

Most of the information in the vision-care literature concerning the prevalence of refractive anomalies on the basis of age as well as the literature concerning *changes* in refraction with age deals strictly with myopia. This emphasis on myopia and the apparent lack of concern for hyperopia can be accounted for as follows:

(1) Although clinically significant hyperopia is present in about 4 percent of children when entering school, hyperopia does not increase in prevalence during the school year nor does it tend to progress in amount with the passage of time. This points to a *genetic* origin, minimizing the probability that environmental influences are involved. (2) Although clinically significant myopia is present in no more than about 2 percent of children when entering school, its prevalence increases markedly during the school years, and once a child becomes myopic the condition tends to progress rapidly for a period of several years. The fact that myopia usually develops only after several years of schooling suggests the possibility of an *environmental* influence.

■
CHANGES DURING INFANCY AND CHILDHOOD

Changes in refraction during infancy and childhood have been discussed in Chapters 2 and 5, and will be only briefly summarized here.

□ Premature Infants

Premature (low birthweight) infants are known to have a high prevalence of myopia, with both the prevalence and the amount of myopia decreasing during the first several months of life (Fletcher and Brandon 1955). These myopic eyes have been shown not to be axially elongated but to be short, incompletely developed eyes having relatively steep corneas and relatively small, steeply curved lenses.

□ Refraction at Birth

Studies making use of cycloplegic retinoscopy for refraction of the newborn have shown a wide distribution of refraction at birth. Cook and Glasscock (1951) and Goldschmidt (1969) show that approximately 25 percent of newborn infants are myopic. Goldschmidt stated that a considerable amount of development of the eyes occurs during the last few months of pregnancy and the first few months of life, with the result that the developmental age of an infant may have an effect on the refraction at birth. He noted also that in the majority of cases this congenital myopia decreases early in life and may disappear altogether.

□ The Preschool Years

Using near retinoscopy, a noncycloplegic procedure in which the child watches the retinoscope light source in an otherwise dark room, Mohindra and Held (1981) reported that the refractive error distribution narrows markedly during the first 5 years of life (see Figure 5.1, Chapter 5). In an earlier study, Kempf et al. (1928) reported a very narrow distribution of refraction for children from 6 to 8 years old, having a mean of +0.75 D. In Chapter 3 (Figure 3.1) Hirsch and Weymouth have illustrated the marked change in the refractive error distribution curve from birth (Cook and Glasscock 1951 data) to age 6 to 8 (Kempf et al. 1928 data). Reporting on noncycloplegic retinoscopy findings for a group of children 2 to 71 months old, Woodruff (1969) noted that the dispersion of refractive error was much reduced by the end of the second year, and seemed to show stability from that time until the end of the fifth year.

□ The School Years

In his longitudinal study of refraction, Hirsch (1961) found that those children who remain within the hyperopic or emmetropic ranges during the school years tend to change, in the direction of less hyperopia, by no more than 0.25 to 0.50 D during the first six years of school, while those children who become myopic during the school years show a progression on the order of 0.25 to 0.50 D per year (see Figure 5.2, Chapter 5). Further, he reported (1964) that the prevalence of myopia (0.50 D or more) increased from less than 2 percent at age 5–6 years to 12 percent at age 13–14, whereas the prevalence of hyperopia (+1.50 D or more) was relatively unchanged during this period.

CHANGES DURING THE EARLY ADULT YEARS

As noted by Hofstetter (1948), changes in refraction occur more slowly during the young-adult years than during any other period of life. This has led to the observation that if it were not for fashion frames and the necessity for contact lens replacements, young adults would be responsible for only a small portion of the practitioner's income!

In one of the few studies involving this age group, Morgan (1958) reported on a nonvisually selected group of subjects who were examined at age 13 and again at age 33. Subjects for the study were 51 women and 44 men, and data were reported separately for the two sexes. Mean changes in refraction during the 20-year period were found to be very small: mean spherical equivalent refraction changed from +0.09 D at age 13 to −0.13 D at age 33 for females, and from +0.39 D at age 13 to +0.35 D at age 33 for males.

A questionnaire was published in *Optometric Weekly* (Grosvenor 1977a) requesting readers to report their own refractive corrections in 5-year intervals between the ages of 15 and 45 years. Of the 191 questionnaires that were returned, 111 contained complete data for ages 20 through 40 years. Refraction in the most plus meridian of the right eye was tabulated for each of these 111 subjects at ages 20, 25, 30, 35, and 40 years (Grosvenor 1977b). As shown in Figure 8.1, mean refraction decreased from −0.08 to −0.18 D during the 20-year period, while the standard deviation increased from 1.47 D at age 20 to 1.92 D at age 40. Refractive error distribution curves for ages 20 and 40 are shown in Figure 8.2. Comparison of these distribution curves indicates very little change in the number of hyperopes (refraction +1.50 D or greater), a decrease in the number of emmetropes (refraction from −0.25 to +1.25 D), and an increase in the number of myopes (−0.50 D or greater) between the ages of 20 and 40 years. It should be noted that the subjects who were emmetropic at age 20 but myopic at age 40 were *late-onset* (or *early-adult-onset*) myopes, as discussed in Chapter 6.

To analyze the data in terms of the refractive changes for individual subjects the data were plotted in the form of a scatterplot (Figure 8.3) (Grosvenor 1977c). Each subject's refraction at age 20 was plotted along the x-axis and refraction at age 40 along the y-axis. If no changes in refraction had occurred during the 20-year period, all data points would have fallen on the broken line, indicating a perfect correlation between refraction at ages 20 and 40. The correlation coefficient for the subjects' data was found to be 0.955, and the regression line (the solid line) was found to have a slope of 1.22 and a y-intercept of −0.03. The relationship

Figure 8.1. Mean refraction and standard deviations, from age 20 to age 40 years. (From Grosvenor 1977b.)

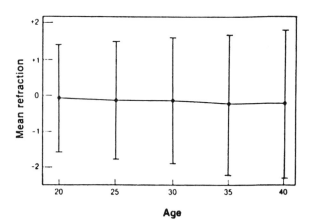

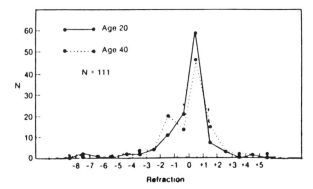

Figure 8.2. Refractive error distribution curves, ages 20 and 40. (From Grosvenor 1977b.)

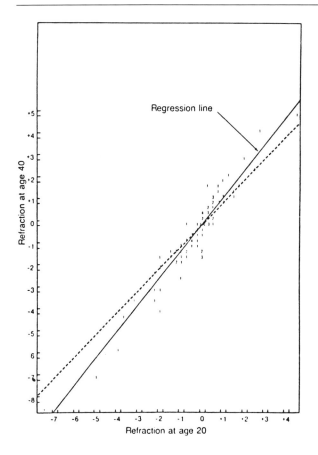

Figure 8.3. Scatterplot of refractive data, comparing refraction at ages 20 and 40 years. (From Grosvenor 1977c.)

between the regression line and the line necessary for a perfect correlation (the broken line) can be interpreted as follows:

1. The small amount of scatter in the *emmetropic* region of the graph, together with the y-intercept value close to zero, indicates that a subject who was emmetropic at age 20 had a good chance of being emmetropic or near-emmetropic at age 40.
2. In the *myopic* region of the graph, the fact that the regression line diverges from the broken line toward increasing myopia indicates that the more myopic a subject was at age 20, the greater the increase in myopia by age 40.
3. In the *hyperopic* region, the divergence of the regression line from the broken line indicates that the more hyperopic a subject was at age 20, the greater the increase in hyperopia by age 40.

To account for these changes, Grosvenor (1977c) suggested that the tendency for myopic eyes to increase in myopia was very likely due to continued axial elongation of an already stretched eye, while the tendency for hyperopic eyes to increase in hyperopia may have been due to a relaxation of accommodation, allowing latent hyperopia to become manifest.

_____ ■ _____

CHANGES DURING THE LATER ADULT YEARS

As with young adults, unselected subjects during their later adult years are not often assembled in large groups that are easily available for vision screening. However, Hirsch (1958) made the point that since almost everyone reaching the age of 45 years will require some professional help, either for distance vision or for near vision, clinical data on patients of this age and beyond can be considered as the equivalent of unselected data.

Hirsch (1958) presented refractive data for 820 patients over the age of 45 years, who were examined in his optometric practice. Of the 820 patients, 460 were women and 360 were men. Hirsch found that the median refractive state increased from $+0.18$ D at age 45–49 years to $+1.02$ D over the age of 75. More importantly, the *dispersion* in refractive state was found to increase markedly with age. Table 8.1 shows that the prevalence of hyperopia ($+1.13$ D or more) increased from 16 percent at ages 45 to 49 to 48 percent at age 75 and over, while the prevalence of myopia (-1.13 D or more) increased from 7 percent at ages 45–49 to 15 percent at age 75 and over. It may be assumed, however, that if Hirsch had used a criterion for myopia of -0.50 D or more, the prevalence of myopia at any age would have been approximately twice the amount he reported for the -1.13 D or more criterion.

Table 8.1.   Spherical Ametropia as a Function of Age*

Age (in years)	Incidence of Ametropia		
	Hyperopia	Emmetropia	Myopia
45–49	16.3%	77.2%	6.7%
50–54	23.5	70.4	6.2
55–59	35.4	59.3	5.0
60–64	40.1	52.3	7.4
65–69	43.9	43.9	12.3
70–74	47.7	43.8	8.8
75 and over	47.9	36.9	15.3

*From Hirsch 1958.

Hirsch noted that the increase in the prevalence of myopia in the older subjects was due to nuclear lens changes affecting approximately 10 percent of this group; and he warned that in view of the increased prevalence of both hyperopia and myopia beyond the age when a +2.00 or +2.25 D addition is required, practitioners should not tell their older patients that a particular lens change is the last that will have to be made.

AGE-RELATED CHANGES IN THE PREVALENCE OF MYOPIA

On the basis of the available data on the prevalence of myopia as a function of age, Grosvenor (1987a) has suggested a classification of myopia based on age-related prevalence and age of onset. As shown in Figure 8.4, *congenital myopia* (i.e., myopia present at birth and of sufficient amount to remain throughout the life span) has a prevalence of approximately 2 percent at all ages; *youth-onset myopia*, having its onset during the school years, has a prevalence that increases in a relatively linear manner, bringing the prevalence of myopia to about 20 percent by age 20; *early adult-onset myopia*, bringing the prevalence of myopia to about 30 percent by the age of 30; and *late-adult-onset myopia*, occurring due to nuclear lens changes as pointed out by Hirsch (1958), accounting for cases of myopia occurring beyond the age of about 55 years.

An obvious characteristic of Figure 8.4 is that the prevalence of both youth-onset myopia and early adult-onset myopia *decreases* markedly with age. As vision-care practitioners routinely observe, those patients having small or moderate amounts of myopia as young adults tend to lose all or a part of their myopia with

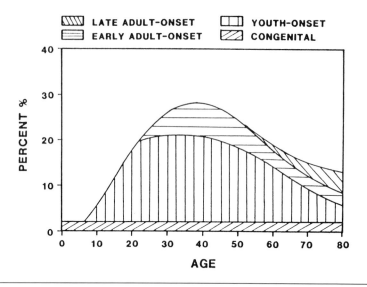

Figure 8.4. Graphical representation of the prevalence of myopia with age, classified as congenital, youth-onset, early adult-onset, and late adult-onset (criterion for myopia is −0.50 D or greater). (From Grosvenor 1987a.)

increasing age. This would seem to be inconsistent with the conclusion (Grosvenor 1977b) that myopes tend to become *more* myopic between the ages of 20 and 40 years; however, consideration of a case history demonstrates that a decrease in myopia may occur somewhat later than the age of 40. The author of this chapter had a spherical equivalent refractive error of −4.75 D at age 21, which gradually increased to −6.50 D at age 45, after which it gradually decreased to −3.50 D at about age 60. A survey of practitioners' records would undoubtedly show that many myopic patients become less myopic, or even emmetropic, with increasing age.

AGE-RELATED HYPEROPIA

Meredith Morgan, a well-known optometric practitioner, educator, and researcher (and the writer of the Foreword for this volume) has suggested the term *age-related hyperopia* to identify the hyperopic shift experienced by many myopes in their later years. In a symposium held at an annual meeting of the American Academy of Optometry, Morgan (1988) presented a paper entitled "My Aging Eyes," in which he made the point that one of the consequences of aging, in his case, was the unfortunate loss of his myopia. He reported that at age 36 his refractive error was

R −2.25 −1.50 × 12.5

L −0.75 −1.25 × 2.5

whereas 37 years later it was

R −0.75 −0.75 × 29

L +0.50 −0.50 × 47.

In a recent letter to the editors of this volume, he described the loss of his myopia in the following manner:

> As you know I was slightly myopic most of my adult life and I enjoyed it. The ability to shave and read without specs was a real advantage which I now miss, being essentially emmetropic. You know today many people live a long time after becoming absolute presbyopes. Along with increasing age comes a decreasing ability to adapt. I think there are going to be a number of very unhappy senior citizens who had successful refractive surgery when young adults.

When reflecting on Dr. Morgan's description of the loss of his myopia, one can only speculate why age-related hyperopia was not identified long ago as a clinical entity! In a report of the refractive status of a "probability sample" of subjects, the U.S. Department of Health, Education and Welfare (1978) published a bar graph (Figure 8.5) showing the percentages of individuals wearing minus as opposed to plus lenses as a function of age. As shown in this graph, at ages 12 to 17 years the percentage of minus vs plus lenses is on the order of 90% vs 10%, while at ages 65 to 74 years the percentages almost completely reverse to about 20% vs 80%.

The clinical implications of this loss of myopia during the later years of life are, in the opinion of this author, of great importance. Young adults who inquire about the possibility of refractive corneal surgery, particularly those having myopia no greater than about 3.00 D — for whom refractive surgery is most likely to be successful — should understand that they will not know how advantageous it was to have been myopic (as noted by Morgan) until they have "lost" their myopia!

□ Prevalence of Age-Related Hyperopia

On the basis of prevalence information available in the literature, it is possible to construct a graph illustrating the prevalence of myopia, hyperopia, and emmetro-

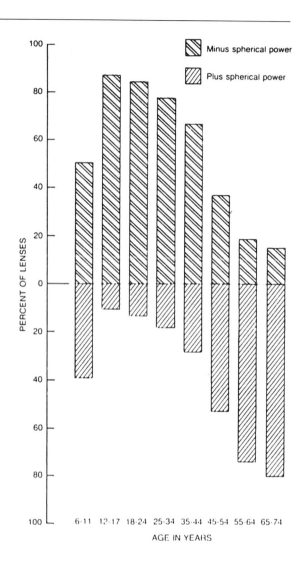

Figure 8.5.
Percentage of
individuals wearing
minus as opposed to
plus lenses. (From
U.S. Dept of Health,
Education and Welfare
1978.)

pia on the basis of age, as shown in Figure 8.6. If we arbitrarily classify any hy-peropia that becomes manifest before the age of 40 as congenital hyperopia — reaching a prevalence of about 10 percent by age 40 — the prevalence of age-related hyperopia increases to about 10 percent by age 50, to 25 percent by age 60, and to about 40 percent by age 70. Those former myopes who have lost their myopia but remain emmetropic beyond age 40 are represented by the lower shaded area on the graph, having a prevalence of about 10 percent by the age of 70.

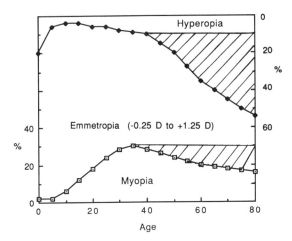

Figure 8.6. Prevalence of myopia (left-hand scale), hyperopia (right-hand scale), and emmetropia on the basis of age. The shaded areas represent the estimated prevalence of age-related hyperopia (upper right) and former myopes who have become emmetropic (lower right).

ARE THERE EMMETROPIZING MECHANISMS IN THE ADULT EYE?

Relatively little attention has been given to the changes occurring in the components of refraction with increasing age. Donders (1864) was aware of the decrease in anterior chamber depth occurring with age, which changes the refraction of the eye in the direction of decreasing hyperopia. He suggested that the crystalline lens develops in such a way as to become flatter with age, causing a decrease in lens power and changing the refraction in the direction of increasing hyperopia, therefore counteracting the effect of the decrease in anterior chamber depth. However, Brown (1974) reported that the crystalline lens becomes *more highly curved* with age, apparently *increasing* in refractive power and therefore adding to the effect of decreased anterior chamber depth, changing the refraction even further in the direction of less hyperopia. This being the case, all eyes would be expected to become relatively myopic with increasing age unless some other refractive component changed, thus driving the refraction in the opposite direction.

□ Reduction in Axial Length with Age?

In two of their studies of refraction and its components, Sorsby et al. (1957, 1962) published data concerning ocular refraction and its components for a large number of subjects of all ages. (In these studies, the axial length of the eye was determined by calculation, based on the results of keratometry and phakometry.) Proposing the existence of one or more *emmetropizing mechanisms* for the adult eye, Grosvenor (1987b) tabulated the Sorsby et al. data, using only data for subjects whose vertical ocular refraction was between plano and +2.00 D. It was possible to tabulate, in 10-year age intervals, right-eye data for 271 subjects ranging from age 4 to 70 years, with roughly equal numbers of males and females in each age group. The results of this tabulation are illustrated in Figure 8.7. In interpreting these graphs, it should be understood that they are based on *cross-sectional* data (consisting of one examination on each of a large number of subjects of various ages) rather than longitudinal data (consisting of repeated examinations on a smaller

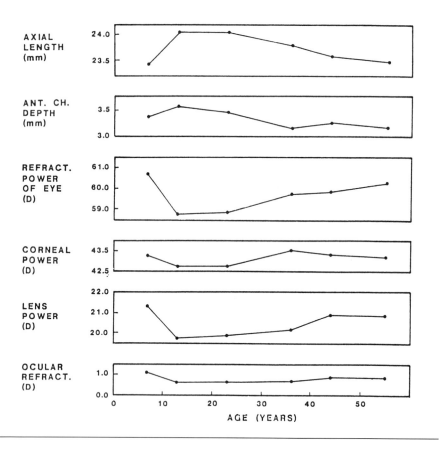

Figure 8.7. Mean values of refraction and its components, by 10-year age intervals, for right eyes of 271 subjects from age 4 to 70 years having a vertical ocular refraction between plano and +2.00 D, based on data published by Sorsby et al. 1957, 1962. (From Grosvenor 1987b.)

number of subjects). With this proviso in mind, the graphs can be interpreted as showing the following tendencies:

1. Mean lens power tends to decrease rapidly during the first two decades of life, from about 21.5 D at age 4 to 9 years to about 19.5 D at age 10 to 19 years, followed by a gradual increase to about 21.0 D beyond the age of 50 years.
2. Mean corneal power tends to decrease from about 43.5 D at age 4 to 9 years to 42.5 D at age 10 to 19 years, gradually increasing to about 43.0 D beyond the age of 50 years.
3. Mean anterior chamber depth tends to increase from about 3.4 mm at age 4 to 9 years to 3.6 mm at age 10 to 19 years, then decrease to 3.2 mm beyond age 50.
4. Mean axial length tends to increase from about 23.5 mm at age 4 to 9 years to 24.0 mm at age 10 to 19 years, then decrease to about 23.5 mm beyond the age of 50 years.

If we consider only those changes occurring beyond the age of 10 to 19 years, the first three (increase in lens power, increase in corneal power, and decrease in anterior chamber depth) all tend to drive the refraction of the eye in the direction of *decreasing hyperopia or increasing myopia;* whereas, only the fourth (decrease in the axial length of the eye) would tend to drive the refraction in the direction of *increasing hyperopia or decreasing myopia.* Based on these results, Grosvenor (1987b) proposed that emmetropization of the adult eye occurs as a result of a decrease in the axial length of the eye with increasing age, which counteracts the combined effects of the increase in lens power, increase in corneal power, and decrease in anterior chamber depth.

The possibility that the eye becomes shorter with age has also been reported by other researchers, including Leighton and Tomlinson (1972), and François and Goes (1971). Using ultrasonography, Leighton and Tomlinson (1972) measured axial lengths of the eyes of 36 "young" subjects (from 19 through 51 years of age) and 36 "old" subjects (from 44 through 92 years of age), and, by plotting a regression line, concluded that mean axial lengths were 23.65 mm at age 20 and 22.97 mm at age 70. Also using axial length data, François and Goes (1971) concluded that the mean axial length was 0.4 mm shorter for subjects older than 50 years than for subjects younger than 50 years. However, both Borish (1986) and Hofstetter (1990) have suggested that the larger eyes of young people may be the result of the larger corporeal size of today's young people as compared to their parents.

Because ultrasound measurement depends on assumed indices of refraction (and, therefore, assumed velocity of ultrasound waves) for the ocular media, an alternative explanation is that age-related changes in refractive indices are responsible for the emmetropization occurring in the adult eye. However, Leighton and Tomlinson (1972) have argued that such changes in indices tend to cancel each other out; an increase in the density of the lens would increase the ultrasound speed, underestimating the lens thickness and also the axial length; whereas, liquefaction of the vitreous would decrease the ultrasound speed, overestimating the vitreous depth and also the axial length of the eye.

Fledelius (1988), after reviewing the available evidence on changes in refraction and its components with age, made the point that there has been a secular trend for people to grow larger in each generation [Recall that this point was also made by Borish (1986) and by Hofstetter (1990).]; and, since larger bodies may have larger eyes, cross-sectional data would tend to show older people as having smaller eyes. Stating that it is biologically difficult to imagine a senile reduction of eye size, Fledelius concluded that the composite oculometric picture "seems to be in favor of eye size stability in old age" (p. 247).

□ Summary

The changes in spherical refraction occurring during the adult years may be summarized as follows:

1. During the early adult years (from ages 20 to 40 years), changes in refraction for most people are relatively small: emmetropes tend to remain emmetropic, while myopes tend to become more myopic and hyperopes tend to become more hyperopic. However, it is interesting to note that, as discussed in Chapters 5 and 6, a significant number of emmetropes become myopic during this period.

2. During the later adult years, there is an increase in dispersion of refractive states; whereas many people who are emmetropic at age 40 remain so, a large group becomes hyperopic in the later years of life while a smaller group becomes myopic, due to nuclear lens changes. On the other hand, many people who are myopic at age 40 gradually begin to lose their myopia, many of whom become emmetropic or even hyperopic (i.e., age-related hyperopes).

3. Since many people remain emmetropic, or nearly emmetropic, during their adult years, we should be able to identify one or more emmetropizing mechanisms. One possible mechanism is a decrease in axial length with increasing age, which drives the refraction of the eye in the direction of increasing hyperopia, thus counteracting the increase in lens power, increase in corneal power, and decrease in anterior chamber depth, all of which tend to drive the refraction in the direction of decreasing hyperopia.

REFERENCES

Borish IM. Personal communication, 1986.
Brown N. The changes in lens curvature with age. Exp Eye Res 1974;19:175–183.
Cook RC, Glasscock RE. Refraction in the newborn. Am J Ophthalmol 1951;34:1407–1413.

Donders FC. On the anomalies of accommodation and refraction of the eye. London: New Sydenham Soc, 1864. Reprinted London: Kreiger, 1979.

Fledelius HC. Refraction and eye size in the elderly. Acta Ophthalmol 1988;66:241–248.

Fletcher MC, Brandon S. Myopia of prematurity. Am J Ophthalmol 1955;40:474–481.

François J, Goes F. Oculometry in emmetropia and ametropia. In: Bock J, Ossoining K, eds. Ultrasonic Medica. Vienna: Verlag der Weiner Med Akad, 1971, 473–515.

Goldschmidt E. Refraction of the newborn. Acta Ophthalmol 1969;47:570–578.

Grosvenor T. Refractive anomalies of the eye, Part II. A survey of adult refractive changes. Optom Weekly January 6, 1977a;68:24–25.

Grosvenor T. A longitudinal study of refractive changes between the ages of 20 and 40: Part 1. Mean changes and distribution curves. Optom Weekly April 14, 1977b;68:386–389.

Grosvenor T. A longitudinal study of refractive changes between the ages of 20 and 40: Part 4. Statistical analysis of data. Optom Weekly April 28, 1977c;68:455–457.

Grosvenor T. A review and a suggested classification system for myopia on the basis of age-related prevalence and age of onset. Am J Optom Physiol Opt 1987a;64:545–554.

Grosvenor T. Reduction in axial length with age: an emmetropizing mechanism for the adult eye? Am J Optom Physiol Opt 1987b;64:657–663.

Hirsch MJ. Changes in refractive state after the age of 45. Am J Optom Arch Am Acad Optom 1958;35:229–237.

Hirsch MJ. A longitudinal study of the refractive state of children during the first 6 years of school: a preliminary report on the Ojai study. Am J Optom Arch Am Acad Optom 1961;38:564–571.

Hirsch MJ. Predictability of refraction at age 14 on the basis of testing at age 6: interim report on the Ojai longitudinal study of refraction. Am J Optom Arch Am Acad Optom 1964;41:567–573.

Hofstetter HW. Optometry: Professional, Economic and Legal Aspects. St. Louis: Mosby, 1948.

Hofstetter HW. Personal communication, 1990.

Kempf GA, Collins SD, Jarman BL. Refractive errors in the eyes of children as determined by retinoscopic examination with a cycloplegic. Public Health Bulletin no. 182. Washington, DC: US Government Printing Office, 1928.

Leighton DA, Tomlinson A. Changes in axial length and other dimensions of the eyeball with increasing age. Acta Ophthalmol 1972;50:815–826.

Levene JR. Clinical Refraction and Visual Science. Stoneham, Mass: Butterworths, 1977.

Mohindra I, Held R. Refraction in humans from birth to 5 years. Doc Ophthalmol Proc Series 28, Third International Conference on Myopia. In: HC Fledelius, PH Alsbirk, E Goldschmidt, eds. The Hague: Dr W. Junk Publishers, 1981.

Morgan MW. Changes in refraction over a period of twenty years in a nonvisually selected sample. Am J Optom Arch Am Acad Optom 1958;31:219–229.

Morgan MW. Vision through my aging eyes. J Am Optom Assoc 1988;59:278–280.

Sorsby A, Benjamin D, Davey JB, et al. Emmetropia and its Aberrations. London: Her Majesty's Stationery Office, 1957.

Sorsby A, Sheridan M, Leary GA. Refraction and its Components in Twins. London: Her Majesty's Stationery Office, 1962.

U.S. Dept of Health, Education and Welfare. Refractive Status and Motility Defects of Persons 4–74 Years, United States, 1971–1972. HEW Publ. No. (PHS) 78-1654. Hyattsville, Md, 1978.

Woodruff ME. Ocular refractive trends in the human eye up to six years of age. Bloomington, In: Unpublished Ph.D. dissertation, 1969.

—9————————————————

Astigmatism

William M. Lyle

☐

Astigmatism, a condition in which the optical system of the eye fails to form a point image of a point object, usually results from the toricity of one or more of the eye's refracting surfaces. Other minor causes of astigmatism are the obliquity of the line of sight with respect to the several optical axes of the eye and the eccentricity of the pupil. A nonuniform index of refraction of one or more of the eye's optical components can also contribute to astigmatism. It is also possible that an astigmatism-like effect could be produced by a toroidal retinal surface, or even by an asymmetry of the projection of the retinal image on the visual centers of the brain — a sort of perceptual astigmatism.

A spherical (nonastigmatic) optical system forms a point image of a point object, whereas in *regular* astigmatism the image of an object point consists of two line foci at different distances along the optic axis and at right angles to one another. The meridians containing the two line foci are known as the *principal meridians* of the eye. The separation between these orthogonal focal lines is called the *interval of Sturm,* and its dioptric dimensions provide a measure of the amount of astigmatism (Figure 9.1). In *irregular* astigmatism, a rare form of astigmatism occurring in conditions involving high corneal toricity, such as keratoconus, the two line foci are not at right angles to one another.

The front surface of the cornea provides about two thirds of the refracting power of the eye and most of the eye's astigmatism. The majority of corneas have the greatest refracting power in the vertical meridian or within 30 degrees of that meridian, resulting in a condition known as *with-the-rule,* or *direct* astigmatism. A minority of corneas have *against-the-rule,* or *inverse* astigmatism, the cornea having its greatest refracting power within 30 degrees of the horizontal meridian; and fewer still have *oblique* astigmatism, in which the meridian of greatest refracting power lies between 30 and 60 degrees or between 120 and 150 degrees.

Residual (internal) astigmatism refers to that part of the total astigmatism not attributed to the cornea's front surface. Residual astigmatism is against-the-rule for most eyes (Neumueller 1953). In Carter's (1963) study 87% of his population had against-the-rule, 2.3% had with-the-rule, and 10.7% had oblique residual astigmatism. Most investigators find residual astigmatism averages between 0.50

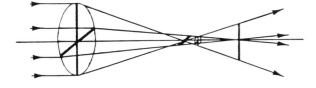

Figure 9.1. The interval of Sturm. If the total refraction of the eye were considered to take place at the plane of the aperture, this would be with-the-rule astigmatism, as the vertical meridian is the meridian of greatest refraction.

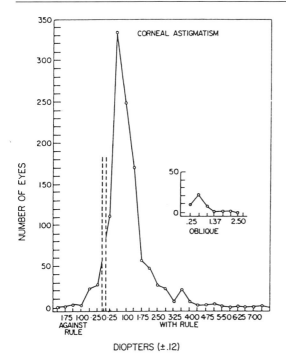

Figure 9.2. Distribution of keratometric astigmatism for 1,208 eyes of patients of various ages. (From Lyle 1971. © The Am Acad of Optom 1971. Reprinted by permission.)

and 0.75 D (Mote and Fry 1939, Kratz and Walton 1949, Loper 1959, Carter 1963, Reading 1972).

A frequency distribution of keratometrically measured astigmatism of 1,208 eyes of patients of various ages was published by Lyle (1971). His distribution curve (Figure 9.2) is leptokurtic, reminiscent of that for spherical ametropia. The modal amount of astigmatism was 0.62 D with-the-rule, and the median was 1.00 D with-the-rule. The corneal astigmatism was with-the-rule for 88% of the patients, against-the-rule for 5%, and oblique for 4%; only 3% had spherical corneas (astigmatism of 0.12 D or less).

The eye's total astigmatism is equal to the anterior corneal (keratometric) astigmatism combined with the residual astigmatism. From Lyle's measures, the majority of eyes have keratometric astigmatism on the order of 1.00 D, with-the-rule and residual astigmatism of about 0.62 D, against-the-rule. The combination of residual astigmatism and keratometric astigmatism results in the human eye commonly having a total astigmatism of about 0.37 D with-the-rule.

SOURCES OF ASTIGMATISM

□ Cornea

Why does the cornea have a toroidal anterior surface? Duke-Elder (1932) proposed that with-the-rule corneal astigmatism was probably related to the fact that the vertical diameter of the eyeball was slightly less than the horizontal diameter; Poos (1950, 1952) suggested that unequal local distribution of blood to the eye might be a cause of astigmatism. Helmholtz (1909) suggested that due to anatomical factors, the eye would be expected to have against-the-rule astigmatism, but this tendency is countered by lid pressure, which tends to cause with-the-rule astigmatism. Marin-Amat (1956) wondered if with-the-rule astigmatism in infants might be due to the frequent constriction of the orbicularis muscle, which is associated with crying.

Duke-Elder (1970) suggested that lid pressure could cause, or could alter, corneal astigmatism; more recently, Grey and Yap (1986) found that tight lids may be a factor in astigmatism. Vihlen and Wilson (1983) found that both with-the-rule astigmatism and the elastic coefficient of the lid declined with age, but they found no evidence that corneal toricity was determined by lid tension; Thorn et al. (1987) concluded that lid pressure differences are not likely to be responsible for the differences in astigmatism between Chinese and Caucasian infants.

For corneas having astigmatism of 1.00 D or more, Wilson et al. (1982) showed that lifting the eyelids reduced the corneal toricity, principally in the horizontal meridian. They concluded that lid pressure produced some with-the-rule astigmatism but generally speaking, lifting the lids had little effect on corneal curvature when the corneal astigmatism was between 1.00 D with-the-rule and 1.00 D against-the-rule. Grey and Yap (1986) found that narrowing the lid aperture in its vertical dimension increased astigmatism by 1.25 to 1.50 D, generally in the with-the-rule direction.

The posterior surface of the cornea acts as a minus lens with a power of 5.00 to 6.00 D. This surface has been reported to produce 0.50 to 0.75 D of against-the-rule astigmatism (Tscherning 1904, Sørensen 1944). However, since the toricity

Table 9.1. Angles between the Visual Axis, the Optic Axis, the Pupillary Axis, and the Line of Sight

Angle	Subtended at	Subtended between
Alpha	Nodal point	The visual axis and the optic axis of the eye
Kappa	Nodal point	The visual axis and the pupillary axis
Lambda	Center of entrance pupil	The pupillary axis and the line of sight

of the front surface of the cornea varies from one cornea to another, it is not surprising that the amount of astigmatism due to the back surface of the cornea varies from 0 to 2.25 D (Bannon and Walsh 1945, LeGrand 1967).

□ Ocular Axes

The eye is not a perfectly centered optical system. The visual axis (the line extending from the object of regard to the center of the fovea, passing through the nodal point) is oblique to the pupillary axis, which is itself somewhat oblique to the optic axis of the lens. In addition, the line of sight (the line extending from the object of regard to the center of the fovea, but passing through the center of the entrance pupil) is not centered with respect to the pupillary axis. The somewhat confusing angles between the visual axis, the optic axis of the eye, the pupillary axis, and the line of sight are summarized in Table 9.1.

Tscherning (1904) considered the value of angle alpha was from 4 to 7 degrees; Sheard (1918) concluded that this angle produced about 0.49 D of against-the-rule astigmatism. Laurence (1926) reported angle kappa to be 5 degrees, and Tscherning (1904) reported it to be from 7 to 9 degrees. According to Banks (1980), angle kappa is twice as large in infants as in adults, a large angle kappa causes increased against-the-rule astigmatism. Loper (1959) found that angle lambda was from 1.1 to 1.6 degrees and concluded that it contributed little to astigmatism. However, angle lambda was reported to be from 2 to 7 degrees by London and Wick (1982), who found it to be larger in infants and in hyperopes, but smaller (about 2 degrees) in myopes. The fovea is eccentrically placed, being 1.25 mm down and temporal from the optic axis (Tscherning 1904).

□ Crystalline Lens

The plane of the lens is slightly oblique to the line of sight. As reported by Tscherning (1904) and by Bannon and Walsh (1945), the lens is normally tilted so that the top is 0 to 3 degrees forward, tending to cause against-the-rule astigmatism. The lens is also tilted about a vertical axis from 0.3 to 7 degrees (Tscherning 1904, Bannon and Walsh 1945), the temporal border being behind the nasal border, resulting in against-the-rule astigmatism. According to Fletcher (1951), the tilt of the lens can result in 0.25 D of against-the-rule astigmatism.

In addition to the obliquity of the lens to the line of sight, its surfaces are considered by some authors to be toroidal. Fletcher (1951) stated that the front surface of the lens is responsible for 0.50 D of with-the-rule astigmatism, whereas the back surface causes more than 0.50 D of against-the-rule astigmatism. According to Sørensen (1944), mean crystalline lens astigmatism in adults is 0.36 D, usually against-the-rule.

□ Other Sources

The possibility that toricity of the retinal surface may be a cause of astigmatism has been noted by Bannon and Walsh (1945) and by LeGrand (1967). Retinal astigmatism has been produced by retinal detachment surgery, particularly by scleral buckling (Burton 1973). Perceptual astigmatism, a visual distortion that may be akin to aniseikonia in that it occurs at higher centers of the brain, has been discussed by Bannon and Walsh (1945).

Measurement uncertainties and errors have been identified as apparent causes of astigmatism (Bannon and Walsh 1946, Brungardt 1969, Roth 1969, Sarver 1969, El-Hage 1971). Off-axis retinoscopy can create an apparent against-the-rule astigmatism, as reported by LeGrand (1967) and London and Wick (1982). An apparent astigmatism of 0.75 to 1.50 D can be produced by off-axis retinoscopy on nonastigmatic eyes.

KERATOMETRIC AND REFRACTIVE ASTIGMATISM COMPARED

During the century that has passed since Javal's development of a clinically useful keratometer, vision practitioners have made use of this instrument to measure the refractive power of the principal meridians of the cornea. The astigmatism indicated by the keratometer differs from refractive astigmatism, or total astigmatism of the eye, as measured by retinoscopy or subjective refraction for several reasons.

1. *Index of refraction for which the keratometer is calibrated.* Helmholtz calibrated the keratometer for an index of refraction of 1.3375, in order to take into

consideration the negative refraction, between 5 and 6 D, at the back surface of the cornea. Since the true index of refraction of the cornea is 1.376, the amount of corneal astigmatism measured by the keratometer is approximately 10% less than the true amount of astigmatism due to refraction at the front surface of the cornea.

2. *Portion of the cornea measured.* The keratometer measures the curvature of a pericentral annulus having an outside diameter of less than 4 mm. The cornea is not a spherical surface (Stone 1962) and flattens toward the periphery (Lotmar and Lotmar 1974, Schultz 1977).

3. *Angle between the corneal apex and the line of sight.* Since the corneal apex does not coincide with the line of sight (Sarver 1969, Mandell 1971) keratometric measurements centered on the line of sight produce results that differ from measurements centered on the normal to the corneal apex (Ludlam and Wittenberg 1966).

4. *Effective power change.* A correcting minus cylinder lens fitted at the spectacle plane (typically, 14 mm from the cornea) has less effective power at the corneal surface than its stated power (Hofstetter 1945, Carter 1980).

5. *Effective power of spherical component of the refractive error.* Due to effectivity consideration, the required correcting cylinder in the spectacle plane differs from that indicated by the keratometer (Hofstetter 1945, Carter 1980), being greater in hyperopes and smaller in myopes than indicated by the keratometer (Neumueller 1953).

6. *Change in effective power with target distance.* The reasons for this slight difference in effective power will be discussed elsewhere in this chapter.

7. *Failure of the principal meridians of the corneal and residual astigmatism to coincide.* When the principal meridians of the corneal and residual astigmatism fail to coincide, the resultant of the two crossed cylinders produces a spherocylindrical effect whose axes and powers differ from those of either of the two crossed cylinders (Long 1976, Carter 1980).

Many rules have been proposed to predict a wearable correcting cylinder at the spectacle plane on the basis of the keratometer finding. The first and most often quoted of these rules is that recommended by Javal; that one should simply multiply the keratometric cylinder by 1.25 and add to this 0.50 D of against-the-rule astigmatism. This and other rules have been only moderately successful in predicting the correcting cylinder (Mote and Fry 1939, Bannon and Walsh 1945, Kratz and Walton 1949). The calculations depend on several approximations, and the result is likely to be identical with the prescribed cylinder only when the principal meridians of the cornea are close to horizontal and vertical. For eyes having with-the-rule or oblique astigmatism, the predicted axis is not likely to be correct unless the cylinder power is over 2.00 D (Carter 1980). A study by Grosvenor et al. (1988) confirms a widely held clinical opinion that a reasonable estimate of the required correcting cylinder can be made by adding 0.50 D of against-the-rule cylinder to the astigmatism shown by the keratometer reading.

■

CHANGES IN ASTIGMATISM WITH AGE

□ Infants and Young Children

A number of recent studies, making use of conventional retinoscopy, near reti-noscopy (a form of retinoscopy performed in the dark, while the infant fixates the retinoscope), and photorefraction, have indicated the presence of considerable astigmatism during the first year of life. In most cases, the astigmatism was found to be against the rule and to decrease during early infancy. The findings of these studies are summarized in Table 9.2; changes in astigmatism during the early years of life are illustrated schematically in Figures 9.3 and 9.4.

The dramatic changes in astigmatism that occur during the first 2 years of life are being studied intensively by several methods. Because keratometry is gener-ally difficult or impossible to perform with infants, the validity of some of the measurements has been questioned, particularly with regard to the effect of mea-surements made off the line of sight (Crewther et al. 1987). However, Howland and Sayles (1984) used photokeratoscopy and concluded that corneal toricity is a major factor in infant astigmatism.

□ Schoolchildren

Mean corneal astigmatism between the ages of 5 and 19 years was found by Sø-rensen (1944) to be 1.08 D, usually with the rule. Phillips (1952) reported that about 75% of patients between the ages of 10 and 20 years had with-the-rule corneal astigmatism, 7% had against-the-rule, and 18% had no corneal astigma-tism. Lyle (1971) found that between 5 and 19 years of age, with-the-rule corneal astigmatism increased at the rate of 0.0033 D per year. In this age group, Sørensen (1944) reported that the mean crystalline lens astigmatism was 0.59 D, usually against-the-rule.

Hirsch (1963) found that 81% of 6-year-olds had less than 0.25 D of astigmatism; by 12 to 14 years of age only 72% had less than 0.25 D of astigmatism. He also noted that at 6½ years of age, 3% had against-the-rule astigmatism, whereas at 12½ years of age, 11.4% had against-the-rule astigmatism and 11% had with-the-rule astigmatism.

□ Young Adults

A large number of investigations have shown that young adults (less than about 40 years of age) have a preponderance of with-the-rule astigmatism; however, studies

Table 9.2. Astigmatism in Infants and Young Children

Investigator(s)	Findings
London and Wick (1982)	83% of a group of premature infants had a-r* astigmatism
Abrahamson et al. (1988)	Nearly 90% of premature infants have a-r astigmatism
Mohindra et al. (1978)	Infants had ten times the prevalence of astigmatism of school-aged children
Howland et al. (1978)	63% of infants had astigmatism of 0.75 D or more
Fulton et al. (1980)	19% of normal infants had astigmatism of 1.00 D or more
Bear and Richler (1983)	Largest amounts of astigmatism found were in infants
Garber (1984)	In Navajo Indians, children had more corneal astigmatism than adults
Atkinson, Braddick, and French (1980); Banks (1980)	Infant astigmatism increases rapidly and reduces to adult levels by 18 months
Howland and Sayles (1987)	Infant astigmatism does not reduce to adult levels until 5 years of age
Nathan et al. (1986)	Astigmatism of 1.00 D or more during first 1 or 2 years, decreasing by age 4 years
Gwiazda, et al. (1984)	Before age 4½ years, most astigmatism was a-r, but w-r† astigmatism tended to develop by school age
Dobson et al. (1984)	Before age 3½ years, a-r astigmatism was more than twice as common as w-r astigmatism
Gwiazda et al. (1985a)	56% of infant astigmatism was a-r, mean amount for the whole group being 2.00 D
Woodruff (1971)	Corneal astigmatism increased between the ages of 2 and 6 years

*Against-the-rule.
†With-the-rule.

of adults beyond the age of 40 years (discussed in the next section) have shown a marked trend for against-the-rule astigmatism to increase.

In a group of patients between the ages of 30 and 40 years, Phillips (1952) found that about 64% had with-the-rule corneal astigmatism, and 18% had against-the-rule corneal astigmatism. In a longitudinal study of a group of subjects examined at age 13 and again at age 33, Morgan (1958) found that with-the-rule astigmatism increased, during this period of time, at a rate which was more rapid in females than in males. Reporting on a study of the refractive errors of 111 optometrists between ages 20 and 40 years, Grosvenor (1977) found that 26% had with-the-rule

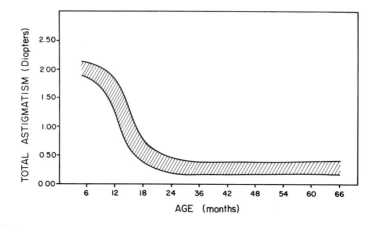

Figure 9.3. Total astigmatism in children up to 5½ years old. The schematic curve represents a trend in amount of astigmatism as reported by various authors. Premature infants are likely to have about 2.00 D of astigmatism, mostly corneal and against the rule.

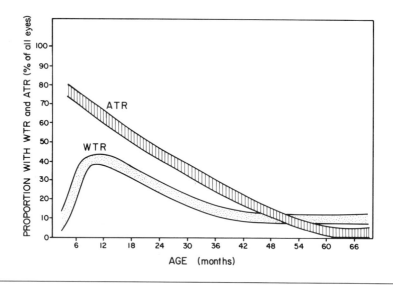

Figure 9.4. Schematic representing relative proportions of against-the-rule and with-the-rule astigmatism up to the age of 5½ years. No data points are shown. The broad curves should emphasize that there is a wide scatter in the results reported by investigators. Problems of definition, criteria, techniques, and interpretation make it difficult to compare results among studies.

and 11% had against-the-rule astigmatism at age 20; and that about 55% showed no significant change in astigmatism between ages 20 and 40 years. On the basis of these results, he concluded that for this subject population, changes in astigmatism between the ages of 20 and 40 years did not occur in any predictable manner.

□ Older Adults

Studies showing a change in the direction of less with-the-rule or more against-the-rule astigmatism in the later adult years have been reported by many authors including Hirsch (1959), Lyle (1971), Anstice (1971), and Baldwin and Mills (1981). The results of these studies are summarized in Table 9.3. In the first of the large-

Table 9.3. Changes in Astigmatism in Older Adults

Investigator(s)	Findings
Stern (1940)	In a large clinical population, astigmatism changed with age in the direction of less w-r* or more a-r†
Hirsch (1959)	For 1,606 eyes of patients over 40 years, astigmatism changed 1.00 D in the a-r direction from age 40 to 80, averaging 0.25 D every 10 years
Lyle (1971)	For 1,208 eyes of patients examined over a 28-year period, prevalence of a-r astigmatism increased from 6% at age 41 to 50 to 27% at age 61 years
Anstice (1971)	621 patients between 5 and 75 years; after age 35 years, both corneal and refractive astigmatism changed in the a-r direction at the rate of 0.20 D every 10 years
Baldwin and Mills (1981)	34 eyes of patients examined at mean age of 51 years and again at mean age of 65 years; refractive astigmatism increased 0.52 D in the a-r direction, and corneal astigmatism increased 0.31 D in the a-r direction
Saunders (1981, 1984)	Proportion of eyes having a-r astigmatism increased rapidly after 40 to 50 years of age
Bear and Richler (1983)	A-r astigmatism was increasingly frequent beyond 45 years of age
Kragha (1986)	W-r astigmatism found in 81% of subjects under age 40, but only in 64% 40 years or older
Satterfield (1989)	In a military population among 1,112 patients examined, 62.9% had measurable astigmatism. Among all with total astigmatism, 70% had 1.00 D or less

*With-the-rule.
†Against-the-rule.

scale studies to be reported, Hirsch (1959) calculated that the average change in astigmatism between the age of 40 and 80 years was 0.25 D each decade, in the direction of increasing against-the-rule astigmatism. Lyle (1971) found no evidence to indicate that the cylinder axis rotated, with time, from a horizontal through an oblique and then to a vertical position; rather, he found that with-the-rule astigmatism gradually decreased in amount with age and against-the-rule astigmatism gradually increased in amount.

Whether this change is primarily a change in corneal astigmatism or in residual astigmatism has been a matter of controversy. However, Stern (1940), Hirsch (1959), Anstice (1971) and Baldwin and Mills (1981) have concluded that the change is primarily in corneal astigmatism (and, this brings about the change in refractive astigmatism). Based on the results of his study in which both keratometric and refractive astigmatism were tabulated, Anstice (1971) noted that if the practitioner has difficulty obtaining accurate retinoscopic or subjective cylindrical data on an older patient, Javal's rule can be used to arrive at a tentative cylindrical correction.

Possible reasons for changes in astigmatism with age are discussed later in this

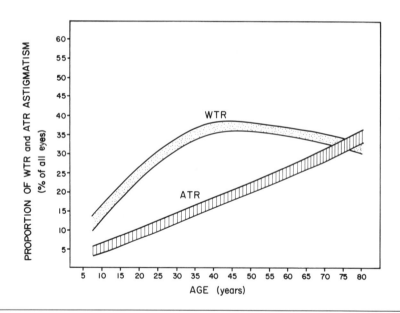

Figure 9.5. These curves are designed to show the trend of changes in the proportion of against-the-rule and with-the-rule astigmatism beyond 6 years of age. No data points are shown. Standard deviations, if calculated, would be very large; the range of values reported is huge. Additional reasons for uncertainty are that some authors report the proportion of against-the-rule astigmatism as a function of all eyes examined. Others report a percentage based on only the eyes with astigmatism. Some report only the astigmatism that exceeds 0.50 D with-the-rule that they consider physiological.

chapter. A schematic representation of changes in astigmatism with age is shown in Figure 9.5.

INFLUENCES ON ASTIGMATISM

□ Genetics

A number of researchers have discussed genetic influences on corneal power and astigmatism. Although some of these reports have indicated that astigmatism is inherited, others have failed to find convincing evidence of inheritance.

Reporting on a study of four generations of one family, Biro (1948) concluded that astigmatism was inherited in an "irregular" autosomal dominant manner. Basing their opinions usually on small pedigrees, the following modes of inheritance have been suggested by various authors: *autosomal dominant* (Gates 1946, Biro 1948, Sorsby 1970, François 1961, Duke-Elder 1962, Waardenburg 1963), *autosomal recessive* (Gates 1946, François 1961), *X-linked recessive* (Sorsby 1970, François 1961), and *polygenic or multifactorial* (Gates 1946, Sorsby 1970, Fatt and Griffin 1983).

On the basis of his study of identical and fraternal twins, Wixson (1958) was convinced that astigmatism was largely inherited. Sorsby (1970) described high astigmatism as an abortive form of keratoconus, which was often inherited in the autosomal recessive manner. Solsona (1975) claimed that over 65% of all astigmatism was congenital, bilateral, and symmetrical and that astigmatism over 0.75 D seemed to be hereditary.

Sorsby et al. (1962) concluded that corneal refracting power is inherited in a multifactorial manner; Grosvenor (1978) suggested that corneal power seems to be inherited. Mash et al. (1975) found that corneal power, but not astigmatism, appeared to be inherited; and Bear and Richler (1983) found that close relatives had similar corneal powers but showed less similarity in their astigmatic errors.

In spite of these reports, a number of authors have reported little or no evidence for the inheritance of astigmatism. For example, on the basis of a study of 2,000 patients, Stern and Rosenberg (1940) reported that corneal astigmatism did not show a clear pattern of genetic transmission; Hofstetter and Rife (1953) concluded that astigmatism was mostly an environmentally determined trait; and on the basis of a study of three or more generations of fifty-one families (1,208 eyes), Lyle (1965) found that no hereditary pattern was discernible for corneal astigmatism under 2.00 D. In the general population, 90% of eyes have less than 2.00 D of astigmatism (Duke-Elder and Abrams 1970), and because amounts of astigmatism under 2.00 D are ubiquitous, a specific mode of inheritance is not readily identifiable. Teikari and O'Donnell (1989), in a comparison of monozygotic and dizygotic twins, found no evidence of the inheritance of astigmatism.

☐ Ethnicity

Certain groups have been identified as having more astigmatism than others. This suggests, but does not prove, that astigmatism is inherited. A number of authors have reported that American Indian children have a greater prevalence of high astigmatism, usually with-the-rule corneal astigmatism, than white children (Lyle et al. 1972, Abraham and Volovick 1972, Wick and Crane 1976, Wong 1976, Hamilton 1976, Heard et al. 1976, Mohindra and Nagary 1977, Garber and Hughes 1983, Adler-Grinberg 1986).

Lyle et al. (1972) studied the prevalence of corneal astigmatism in unselected groups of Amerind children in northern Saskatchewan and in Brantford, Ontario, and in an unselected group of white children in Kitchener, Ontario. They found that mean corneal astigmatism in the northern Saskatchewan Amerind children was significantly higher than that of white children and considerably higher than that of the Brantford Amerind children. Lyle et al. (1972) speculated that the increased prevalence of corneal astigmatism found in Amerind children might depend on ocular rigidity, which itself might relate to diet or heredity. Grosvenor (1977) suggested that corneal rigidity might determine whether the pressure exerted by the tarsal plate in the upper lid induced astigmatism. Relative corneal rigidity may be inherited. As age increases, the coats of the eye become more rigid (McLenachan and Loran 1967, Anstice 1971), thereby altering the influence of lid pressure on the cornea.

☐ Gender

The literature contains a number of reports that females have steeper corneas than males (Woodruff 1971, Mash et al. 1975, Bear and Richler 1983, Fledelius and Stubgaard 1986, Garner et al. 1988). This difference appears to occur because females have smaller eyes than males and has no implications for corneal astigmatism. Although some authors have reported that females have more astigmatism than males (Lyle et al. 1972, Wick and Crane 1976, Bear and Richler 1983), others have found no difference between the sexes (Sørensen 1944, Kragha 1986). Hirsch (1959) found that men are more likely than women to have refractive astigmatism greater than 2.00 D. Theoretical explanations for astigmatic differences between females and males include presumed differences of ocular rigidity and relative lid pressure between the sexes.

☐ Age

It has been suggested that changes in astigmatism with age are due, at least in part, to age changes in pressure exerted on the cornea by the lids. As reported by Gullstrand (1924) and Duke-Elder and Abrams (1970), the suggestion that eyelid pressure can cause astigmatism was made in the nineteenth century by Snellen and Birch-Hirschfield. Masci (1965) found that retracting the eyelids reduced the with-the-rule corneal toricity. As noted earlier, Wilson et al. (1982) performed keratometry on eighteen subjects while the lids were held apart by a speculum and found that, for subjects having with-the-rule corneal astigmatism of 1.00 D or more, retracting the lids reduced the amount of astigmatism. As a result, they concluded that the pressure exerted on the eyeball by the eyelids is a major factor influencing astigmatism.

Because the eyelids become relatively flaccid in the later adult years, due to the loss of tonus of the orbicularis oculi muscle, it is likely that the decreased pressure of the upper lid on the cornea will result in a reduction of with-the-rule corneal astigmatism with increasing age. Reading (1972) and Baldwin and Mills (1981) have proposed that with increasing age, the curvature of the vertical meridian of the cornea remains almost constant, but the steepening which occurs mostly in the horizontal meridian begins in middle age and continues for the rest of the life span, producing against-the-rule astigmatism.

It has also been suggested that pressure or traction of the extraocular muscles, during convergence, may alter corneal curvature by flattening the horizontal meridian (Lopping and Weale 1965, Duke-Elder and Abrams 1970, Bannon 1971, Millodot and Thibault 1985). Because infants generally have against-the-rule corneal astigmatism, it is possible that continued convergence of the eyes, by flattening the horizontal meridian of the cornea, will gradually reduce the amount of against-the-rule astigmatism and could even cause the development of with-the-rule astigmatism.

The well-documented changes in astigmatism with age might be explained on the following basis: For an infant born with against-the-rule astigmatism, convergence of the eyes may be responsible for reducing this astigmatism and for the development, during the preschool years, of with-the-rule astigmatism. During the childhood and young adult years, lid pressure and ocular rigidity tend to remain in balance, with the result that astigmatism changes little during this period. However, in the later years of life, lid pressure decreases due to the relative flaccidity of the orbicularis oculi; and with the concurrent increase in the rigidity of the cornea, with-the-rule corneal astigmatism gradually decreases. When the cornea becomes relatively spherical, the against-the-rule residual astigmatism will manifest as refractive astigmatism.

CLINICAL ISSUES

A variety of methods have been used to measure refractive astigmatism. Most of these are so well known, for example, the fan dial, streak retinoscopy (Francis 1973), the Jackson cross cylinder (Sims and Durham 1986), the Raubitschek test

(Bannon 1958, Eskridge 1958), and will not be discussed here. Readers interested in less well-known methods of measuring astigmatism are referred to studies by Oppenheimer (1924), Haynes (1957), Miller (1961), Gartner (1965), Ludlam and Wittenberg (1966) and Asher (1968).

□ Change in Astigmatism at Near

Although the axis and power of the astigmatic correction are routinely measured for distance fixation only, an occasional patient may require a different cylindrical correction for near vision than for distance vision. A number of mechanisms have been proposed to account for such a difference, including the following:

1. *Effective power change.* Due to the change in effective power, the cylindrical correction required when the eye looks at a near target needs to be greater than that required for distance vision. Percival (1928) and Rabbetts (1973) reported that the cylinder required for near vision is about 9% greater than that needed for distance vision, whereas Bannon (1946) found that nonpresbyopes needed 5 to 10% more cylinder power at near than at distance. However, for astigmatic corrections less than 3.50 D, a change in the cylinder power for near may not be necessary, although an axis change of 5 to 10 degrees can be significant (Rabbetts 1973).

2. *Pressure exerted by the extraocular muscles.* A number of authors including Fairmaid (1959), Löpping and Weale (1965), Bannon (1971) and Millodot and Thibault (1985) have reported that convergence of the eyes is accompanied by a flattening of the horizontal corneal meridian, bringing about a slight increase in with-the-rule astigmatism or a decrease in against-the-rule astigmatism. Löpping and Weale (1965) and Bannon (1971) have estimated that the decrease in power of the horizontal corneal meridian accompanying convergence is from 0.25 to 0.50 D in nonpresbyopic eyes.

3. *Asymmetric contraction of the ciliary muscle.* Whether the ciliary muscle contracts asymmetrically, bringing about an additional source of astigmatism for near fixation, is a matter of controversy. According to Morgan et al. (1943) and Bannon and Walsh (1945), 1.00 D of astigmatic accommodation can be produced in animals by stimulating the cervical sympathetic nerves that supply the eye. In humans, pilocarpine, 10% applied temporally to the cornea on a cotton pledget, produced 1.00 D of with-the-rule accommodation (Halldén and Henricsson 1974). However, Bannon (1946) found little evidence of astigmatic accommodation in humans, Lansche (1966) reported a small change in the astigmatic error when the eyes accommodated, and Denieul (1982) demonstrated on three subjects that the astigmatic error was at a minimum when accommodation was at its resting state (somewhat closer than optical infinity).

4. *Movement of the crystalline lens.* Because the zonular fibers slacken when the eye accommodates, the lens is free to move and may be displaced, decentered, or tilted (Beau-Seigneur 1946, Bannon 1946).

5. *Torsional effects due to convergence.* The eyes extort on near fixation, bringing about a change in cylinder axis (Pascal 1944, Roth 1969). According to Allen and Carter (1967), convergence causes an excyclophoria of about 1.68 degrees. However, Rabbetts (1973) found very little cyclotorsion.

6. *Change in pupil size or position.* It is possible that a different bundle of rays is used for near vision than for distance vision because of changes in pupil size or position (due to eccentricity of the pupil) and the use of a different portion of the cornea (Beau-Seigneur 1946, Bannon 1946, Rabbetts 1973).

7. *Astigmatism due to obliquity of incidence.* When the eye looks through a point other than the center of the correcting spectacle lens, astigmatism due to obliquity of incidence may be present (Bannon 1946, Wang et al. 1983). Normally, this effect is small, but a large effect can be produced by some portions of progressive addition lenses.

8. *Stenopaic effect caused by the eyelids.* When the eyes look downward, the resulting stenopaic effect can alter the apparent astigmatism (Bannon 1946, Grey and Yap 1986).

Fortunately, the difference between the cylindrical correction required at near and at distance is usually too small to be clinically significant. However, for large amounts of astigmatism, the practitioner should measure cylinder axis and power at the nearpoint as well as at distance.

□ Effects of Astigmatism on Acuity

Uncorrected astigmatism can be responsible for a number of adverse effects. The effect of astigmatism on visual acuity depends on the clinical type, as well as the amount, of astigmatism. In simple myopic or compound myopic astigmatism, one or both of the focal lines (for a point object) are located in front of the retina so distance visual acuity will suffer, just as in myopia. In simple hyperopic or compound hyperopic astigmatism, one or both focal lines are located behind the retina, so there is relatively little effect on visual acuity if sufficient accommodation is available. In mixed astigmatism, in which one focal line is located in front of the retina and the other behind, vision may be reasonably good if the circle of least confusion is located near the retina. However, in near vision, for any of the clinical types of astigmatism, the separation of the two focal lines can result in reports of blurring after prolonged nearwork. The axis of the astigmatism greatly influences the ability to read letters (Casanovas 1966, Birnbaum 1978). Vertically oval blur circles may permit reading more readily than horizontally oval blur circles because letters have their orientation mainly in the vertical meridian.

Infants with astigmatism show a preference for gratings at a certain orientation, and grating acuity improves steadily from birth during the first 6 months (Atkinson and French 1979). Gwiazda et al. (1985a) found that in uncorrected infants the focus nearer to the retina tends to be preferred. Kinney (1980) found that placing a +2.00 D cylindrical lens over a person's glasses produced little vision reduction for low-frequency sine waves but large reductions for high-frequency sine waves when the axis of the cylinder was parallel to the orientation of the stripes.

☐ Astigmatic (Meridional) Amblyopia

The visual system can acquire a form of astigmatic amblyopia in which lenses that correct the astigmatism fully and accurately fail to produce normal visual acuity (Martin 1890). Cobb and McDonald (1978) suggested that the critical period for the development of meridional amblyopia occurred before the end of the child's sixth year; others believe the amblyopia develops especially within the first 2 years (Mitchell et al. 1973). According to Mitchell (1979), the critical period for meridional amblyopia is different from and later than the critical period for deprivation amblyopia or strabismic amblyopia.

Meridional amblyopia usually affects both eyes if both have early astigmatism and, in this respect, differs from the amblyopia traditionally associated with high hyperopia or with anisometropia or strabismus. Meridional amblyopia in a child is not detectable much before 3 years of age (Mitchell 1979). Early astigmatism has little effect on visual acuity in the first year of life, even though the mean astigmatism at this age is 2.00 D, being against the rule in about 60% of cases and with the rule in about 40% (Gwiazda et al. 1985b). No evidence for meridional amblyopia was found by Gwiazda et al. (1985a) in the first year of life. Gwiazda et al. (1986) reported that only astigmatism present between the ages of 6 and 24 months correlates with the meridional amblyopia that is detectable later in the child's life. Meridional amblyopia demonstrates a connection between an optical defect and a neural defect: Early visual input affects the neural organization of the visual system.

Experiments by Thibos and Levick (1982) produced astigmatic vision in kittens by fitting them with cylindrical lenses mounted in goggles and found that visual acuity was diminished. Because the eye developed normally in other ways, the defect must have been produced in the brain and not the eye. The reduced resolution, however, was not limited to the orientation, which was blurred during the rearing. Boothe and Teller (1982) were able to produce meridional differences in acuity in monkeys.

The considerable astigmatism present in the first 6 to 36 months of an infant's life diminishes within a few months, but it persists long enough in some children to induce meridional amblyopia, which can be detected later. In the first 2 years of life, the cornea flattens, the keratometer reading decreases by over 7.00 D; the eyeball lengthens by about 6 mm, and the power of the crystalline lens decreases by at least 15.00 D. Based on ultrasound measurements and keratometry, data presented by Gordon and Donzis (1985) revealed smaller amounts and a lower prevalence of astigmatism than data based on photorefraction or near retinoscopy. If most infants at 6 months of age have 2.00 D of astigmatism, it is difficult to explain why only a small proportion of these children develop meridional amblyopia. The precise length of the sensitive period and the minimum amount of astigmatism necessary to produce significant meridional amblyopia are not yet clearly defined.

☐ Rigid Contact Lenses

If a spherical rigid contact lens and the tear film underneath the lens completely neutralize the corneal portion of the eye's astigmatism, the eye's residual astigmatism will be fully revealed. Some confusion has arisen by the use of the term "residual" astigmatism to mean all of the astigmatism manifested by that eye while wearing a contact lens, rather than the residual (internal, physiologic) astigmatism as the term has been used earlier in this chapter. Depending on the lens thickness and the material from which it is made, rigid contact lenses and the associated tear film neutralize all or a part of astigmatism normally measured by the keratometer.

Some practitioners who fit contact lenses tend to overlook uncorrected or undercorrected astigmatism, partly because toric contact lenses introduce further complications and expense and partly because patients express few, if any, complaints when they wear contact lenses that leave some astigmatism uncorrected. For a variety of reasons, many contact lens wearers ignore the effects of up to 0.75 D of uncorrected astigmatism, an amount that most spectacle wearers would not willingly tolerate.

Rigid contact lenses not only neutralize a portion of the corneal astigmatism but often, with the passage of time, cause the cornea to become more toroidal. For example, wearing a flatter-than-normal contact lens in an attempt to reduce myopia (orthokeratology) produces variable effects on corneal toricity, often inducing increased with-the-rule astigmatism (Kerns 1978). The development of with-the-rule corneal astigmatism associated with the wearing of rigid contact lenses has been reported by many authors including Rengstorff (1965, 1971, 1976), Rubin (1967) and Grosvenor (1977). The amount of astigmatism induced by PMMA lenses was reported by Hartstein (1965) to be from 2.50 to 6.00 D; this astigmatism did not always disappear when contact lens wear was discontinued. Grosvenor (1976) has suggested that this astigmatism may result from the pressure exerted by the contact lens, with each blink, on the horizontal meridian of a low-rigidity cornea.

Although rigid contact lenses are often fitted on eyes having keratoconus — and in most cases are the only form of management that provides acceptable visual acuity — Hartstein (1965, 1968) reported that contact lenses may induce keratoconus and with-the-rule astigmatism. Hartstein and Becker (1970) determined ocular rigidity for a group of PMMA contact lens wearers by comparing Shiötz tonometer readings with 5.5 and 10 gram weights, and found that patients who developed with-the-rule astigmatism had lower ocular rigidity than those who did not develop astigmatism; and that those who developed keratoconus while wearing contact lenses had still lower ocular rigidity findings.

Contact lenses usually rotate on the cornea (Harris et al. 1977), and if the lenses contain a cylindrical component, the spherocylindrical refraction will be altered. Tocher (1962) reported that a small tilt of a contact lens can produce from 0.25 to 1.00 D of against-the-rule astigmatism. Oblique astigmatism produced by a contact lens and the associated tear fluid is a random variable that may increase, decrease, or have little effect on the total astigmatism of the system (Sarver 1963).

Rengstorff (1965, 1976, 1977) and Pratt-Johnson and Warner (1965) found that discontinuing PMMA contact lens wear caused an initial increase in with-the-rule astigmatism, but most of the astigmatic change stabilized within about 3 weeks. Rengstorff (1977) suggested that if rigid contact lens wear is to be discontinued, it is preferable to reduce wearing time gradually rather than abruptly.

□ Soft Contact Lenses

Due to their extreme flexibility, spherical soft contact lenses have little or no effect in eliminating corneal toricity; therefore, if significant refractive astigmatism exists, toric soft lenses may be required. Ing (1976) found that soft contact lenses caused little or no change in astigmatism. However, Grosvenor (1978) reported an increase in with-the-rule astigmatism of 0.25 to 0.75 D in wearers of the large, thick soft lenses that were in use at that time. These changes were usually reversed by the use of looser-fitting lenses or by a reduction in lens wearing time.

□ Other Clinical Matters

A common symptom of uncorrected astigmatism is asthenopia, manifested in the form of headaches, tiredness or watering of the eyes. These symptoms are more likely to occur with simple or hyperopic astigmatism that with myopic astigmatism, and are most likely to accompany prolonged near visual tasks. Gullstrand, in his 1924 revision of Helmholtz's Treatise on Physiological Optics, said that 0.50 D of against-the-rule astigmatism produced more symptoms than 1.00 D of with-the-rule astigmatism. Asthenopia also occurs in 65% of those with small amounts of with-the-rule astigmatism.

One school of thought maintains that uncorrected astigmatism in childhood is a frequent cause of myopia (van Alphen 1961). The hyperopic child is believed to accommodate excessively in order to bring each of the line foci in turn onto the retina. According to Birnbaum (1978), against-the-rule astigmatism precedes and predicts the development of myopia. Fulton et al. (1982) suggested that uncorrected astigmatism in a child under 3 years of age can influence the course of myopia. Astigmatism of 1.00 D or more, especially at oblique orientations, has been associated with more myopia. Forcing the eyelids into position to help diminish the optical error associated with astigmatism or myopia may be a supplementary factor.

Astigmatism alters the size and shape of the retinal image because the ametropia is not axial. A 1.00 D difference in cylindrical correction between the two eyes introduces an aniseikonia of about 1.5%, according to Bannon and Walsh (1945). In an eye with astigmatism, the positions of the entrance pupil, exit pupil, and principal planes are different in the two principal meridians (Keating and Carroll 1976).

Partial closure of the lids may alter the astigmatism when a near target is fixated (Bannon 1946). Most eyes show more astigmatism (1.25 to 1.50 D) generally with the rule, when the lids are partly closed (Grey and Yap 1986). Partly closing the lids, therefore, will reduce the effects of against-the-rule astigmatism. If the aperture becomes small enough and the target is bright enough, the increased depth of focus due to the pinhole effect will be helpful, but diffraction provides a limit to the benefit of a smaller aperture.

□ Effects of Ocular Surgery

Both anterior segment and posterior segment ocular surgery can result in astigmatism. Surgical removal of a pterygium usually increases corneal curvature in the horizontal meridian, thus decreasing with-the-rule astigmatism and increasing against-the-rule astigmatism (Bedrossian 1960).

Although refractive surgery is often intended for the correction of spherical refractive errors, many of these procedures (including radial keratotomy, epikeratoplasty, keratophakia, keratomileusis, and epikeratophakia) can alter corneal astigmatism McCartney et al. 1987, Smith 1989). For example, the Ruiz trapezoidal keratotomy procedure is designed to reduce corneal astigmatism in the meridian in which the incisions are placed. In this procedure, cuts in the corneal periphery are placed so as to produce a meridional change of 5.00 to 10.00 D, mostly in the central cornea; but the uncertainty is about 6.00 D (Terry and Rowsey 1986, Deg and Binder 1987). The insertion of a plastic lens into the corneal tissue (keratophakia) can alter corneal astigmatism (Watsky and McCarey 1986). As described by Arons (1987), a surgeon using an excimer laser for refractive keratoplasty can sculpt a new anterior corneal surface in such a way that the desired corneal shape is achieved precisely with minimal damage to the corneal structure.

Cataract surgery has long been known to cause against-the-rule astigmatism, due to a sagging of the cornea (Tscherning 1904). The techniques, materials, and methods used in suturing can greatly influence the amount and the axis of the astigmatism that will be present when the eye heals. According to Singh and Kumar (1976), three sutures produce the least postoperative astigmatism. Modern fine needles and sutures produce much less astigmatism than the older, coarser sutures. The use of the Terry keratometer during surgery can help to reduce the amount of postoperative astigmatism (Swinger 1987). Moore (1980) has reported that the average amount of astigmatism after cataract surgery with the use of an intraocular lens was 2.84 D, compared to 1.50 D when no intraocular lens was used.

Duke-Elder and Abrams (1970) suggest that retinal detachment surgery can produce astigmatism; Burton (1973) noted that episcleral buckling can cause ir-regular astigmatism; and Goel et al. (1983) found that radial buckling procedures caused more than 2.00 D of astigmatism in twenty of thirty-seven eyes. It is of interest that in a recent literature search, nearly one third of the papers on astig-matism were related to the effects of surgery.

REFERENCES

Abraham JE, Volovick JB. Preliminary Navajo optometric study. J Am Optom Assoc 1972; 43:1257–1260.

Abrahamson M, Fabian G, Sjöstrand J. Changes in astigmatism between the ages of 1 and 4 years: a longitudinal study. Br J Ophthalmol 1988;72:145–149.

Adler-Grinberg D. Need for eye and vision care in an undeserved population: refractive errors and other ocular anomalies in the Sioux. Am J Optom Arch Am Acad Optom 1986; 63:553–558.

Allen MJ, Carter JH. The torsion component of the near reflex: a photographic study of the non-moving eye in unilateral convergence. Am J Optom Arch Am Acad Optom 1967; 44:343–349.

Arons IJ. Laser refractive keratoplasty. Optician 1987;193:20, 36.

Amsler M. Pterygium causing corneal astigmatism. Ophthalmologica 1953;126:52–54.

Anstice J. Astigmatism — its components and their changes with age. Am J Optom Arch Am Acad Optom 1971;48:1001–1006.

Asher H. New means for assessment of astigmatism. J Physiol (Lond) 1968;194:72–73.

Atkinson J, Braddick O, French J. Infant astigmatism: its disappearance with age. Vis Res 1980;20:891–893.

Atkinson J, French J. Astigmatism and orientation preference in human infants. Vis Res 1979;19:1315–1317.

Baldwin WR, Mills D. A longitudinal study of corneal astigmatism and total astigmatism. Am J Optom Physiol Opt 1981;58:206–211.

Banks MS. Infant refraction and accommodation. Int Ophthalmol Clin 1980;20(1):205–232.

Bannon RE, Walsh R. On astigmatism. Am J Optom Arch Am Acad Optom 1945;22:101–111, 162–181, 210–219, 263–277.

Bannon RE. A study of astigmatism at the near point with special reference to astigmatic accommodation. Am J Optom Arch Am Acad Optom 1946;23:53–75.

Bannon RE, Walsh R. Reliability of keratometer reading. Am J Ophthalmol 1946;29:76–85.

Bannon RE. Recent developments in techniques for measuring astigmatism. Am J Optom Arch Am Acad Optom 1958;35:352–359.

Bannon RE. Near point binocular problems — astigmatism and cyclophoria. Ophthalmic Optn 1971;11:158–160, 165–168.

Bear JC, Richler A. Cylindrical refractive error: a population study in Western Newfound-land. Am J Optom Physiol Opt 1983;60:39–45.

Beau-Seigneur W. Changes in power and axis of cylindrical errors after convergence. Am J Optom Arch Am Acad Optom 1946;23:111–121.

Bedrossian RH. The effects of pterygium surgery on refraction and corneal curvature. Arch Ophthalmol 1960;64:553–557.

Bennett AG, Rabbetts RB. Refraction in oblique meridians of the astigmatic eye. Br J Physiol Opt 1978;32:59–77.

Birnbaum MH. Functional relationship between myopia, accommodative stress and against-the-rule astigmia: a hypothesis. J Am Optom Assoc 1978;49:911–914.

Biro I. Data concerning the heredity of astigmatism. Ophthalmologica 1948;115:156–166.

Boothe RG, Teller DY. Meridional variations in acuity and CSF's in monkeys (*Macaca nemestrina*) reared with externally applied astigmatism. Vis Res 1982;22:801–810.

Brungardt TF. Reliability of keratometric readings. Am J Optom Arch Am Acad Optom 1969;46:686–691.

Burton TC. Irregular astigmatism following episcleral buckling procedure with use of silicone rubber sponges. Arch Ophthalmol 1973;90:447–448.

Carter JH. Residual astigmatism of the human eye. Optom Weekly 1963;54:1271–1272.

Carter JH. Ophthalmometric prediction of correcting cylinder axis. Am J Optom Physiol Opt 1980;57:15–24.

Casanovas J. The untoward influence of astigmatism on the statement of visual acuity. Am J Ophthalmol 1966;61:1059–1062.

Cobb SR, MacDonald CF. Resolution acuity in astigmats: evidence for a critical period in the human visual system. Br J Physiol Opt 1978;32:38–49.

Crewther DP, McCarthy A, Roper J, Costello K. An analysis of eccentric photorefraction. Clin Exp Optom 1987;70:2–7.

Deg JK, Binder PS. Wound healing after astigmatic keratotomy in human eyes. Ophthalmol 1987;94:1290–1297.

Denieul P. Effects of stimulus vergence on mean accommodation response, microfluctuations of accommodation and optical quality of the human eye. Vis Res 1982;22:561–569.

Dobson V, Fulton AB, Sebris SL. Cycloplegic refractions of infants and young children: the axis of astigmatism. Invest Ophthalmol Vis Sci 1984;25:83–87.

Donders FC. On the Anomalies of Accommodation and Refraction of the Eye. (Translated by Moore WD.) London: New Sydenham Society, 1864:491. Hatton Press edition, 1952.

Dorland G, Dorland D. Oblique cylindrical lenses as a cause of variable vertical prism. Am J Optom Arch Am Acad Optom 1970;47:1006–1010.

Duke-Elder WS. Textbook of Ophthalmology, vol. 1. London: Kimpton, 1932;33.

Duke-Elder S. The Foundations of Ophthalmology, vol. 7. In: System of Ophthalmology, London: Kimpton, 1962;106–113.

Duke-Elder S, Abrams D. Ophthalmic Optics, Refraction, vol. 5. In: System of Ophthalmology, London: Kimpton, 1970;274–295.

El-Hage SG. Suggested new methods for photokeratoscopy. A comparison for their validities. Part 1. Am J Optom Arch Am Acad Optom 1971;48:897–912.

Eskridge JB. The Raubitschek astigmatism test. Am J Optom Arch Am Acad Optom 1958;35:238–247.

Fairmaid JA. The constancy of corneal curvature. An examination of corneal response to changes in accommodation and convergence. Br J Physiol Opt 1959;16:2–23.

Fatt HV, Griffin JR. Genetics for Primary Eye Care Practitioners. Chicago: Professional Press, 1983.

Fledelius HC, Stubgaard M. Changes in refraction and corneal curvature during growth and adult life. A cross-sectional study. Acta Ophthalmol 1986;64:487–491.

Fletcher RJ. Astigmatic accommodation. Br J Physiol Opt 1951;8:73–94, 129–160, 193–224, 1952;9:8–32.

Francis JL. The axis of astigmatism with special reference to streak retinoscopy. Br J Physiol Opt 1973;28:11–22.

François J. Heredity in Ophthalmology. St. Louis: CV Mosby Co, 1961;191–192.

Fulton AB, Hansen RM, Petersen RA. The relation of myopia and astigmatism in developing eyes. Ophthalmology 1982;89:298–302.

Fulton AB, Dobson V, Salem D, et al. Cycloplegic refractions in infants and young children. Am J Ophthalmol 1980;90:239–247.

Garber JM, Hughes J. High corneal astigmatism in the adult Navajo population. J Am Optom Assoc 1983;54:815–818.

Garber JM. Steep corneal curvature: a fetal alcohol syndrome landmark. J Am Optom Assoc 1984;55:595–598.

Garber JM. The relation of astigmatism and hyperopia (more effective plus). J Am Optom Assoc 1985;56:491–493.

Gartner WF. Astigmatism and optometric vectors. Am J Optom Arch Am Acad Optom 1965;42:459–463.

Gates RR. Human Genetics. New York: Macmillan, 1946;156–244.

Goel R, Crewdson J, Chignell AH. Astigmatism following retinal detachment surgery. Br J Ophthalmol 1983;67:327–329.

Gordon RA, Donzis PB. Refractive development of the human eye. Arch Ophthalmol 1985; 103:785–789.

Grey C, Yap M. Influence of lid position on astigmatism. Am J Optom Physiol Opt 1986; 63:966–969.

Grosvenor T. What causes astigmatism? J Am Optom Assoc 1976;47:926–933.

Grosvenor T. A longitudinal study of refractive changes between the ages of 20 and 40. Part 4. Changes in astigmatism. Optom Weekly 1977;68:475–478.

Grosvenor T. Etiology of astigmatism. Am J Optom Physiol Opt 1978;55:214–218.

Grosvenor T, Perrigin DM, Quintero S. Predicting refractive astigmatism: a suggested simplification of Javal's rule. Am J Optom Physiol Opt 1988;65:292–297.

Gullstrand A. The cornea. In: Helmholtz's Treatise on Physiological Optics, 3rd ed. 1909. (Translated by Southall JPC.) The Optical Society of America, 1924. New York: Dover Publications, 1962;317–332.

Gwiazda J, Scheimann M, Mohindra I, Held R. Astigmatism in children: changes in axes and amount from birth to six years. Invest Ophthalmol Vis Sci 1984;25:88–92.

Gwiazda J, Mohindra I, Brill S, Held R. Infant astigmatism and meridional amblyopia. Vis Res 1985a;25:1269–1276.

Gwiazda J, Mohindra I, Brill S, Held R. The development of visual acuity in infant astigmats. Invest Ophthalmol Vis Sci 1985b;26:1717–1723.

Gwiazda J, Bauer J, Thorn F, Held R. Meridional amblyopia *does* result from astigmatism in early childhood. Clin Vis Sci 1986;1:145–152.

Halldén U, Henricsson M. Astigmátism of the lens by asymmetric contraction of the ciliary muscle. Acta Ophthalmol 1974;52:242–245.

Hamilton JE. Vision anomalies of Indian school children: the Lame Deer study. J Am Optom Assoc 1976;47:479–487.

Harris MG, Decker MR, Funnell JW. Rotation of spherical nonprism and prism — ballast hydrogel contact lenses on toric corneas. Am J Optom Physiol Opt 1977;54:149–152.

Hartstein J. Corneal warping due to wearing of corneal contact lenses. A report of 12 cases. Am J Ophthalmol 1965;60:1103–1104.

Hartstein J. Keratoconus that developed in patients wearing corneal contact lenses. Report of four cases. Arch Ophthalmol 1968;82:345–346.

Hartstein J, Becker B. Research into the pathogenesis of keratoconus. Arch Ophthalmol 1970;84:728–729.

Haynes PR. A homokonic cross cylinder for refractive procedures. Am J Optom Arch Am Acad Optom 1957;34:478–485.

Heard T, Reber N, Levi D, Allen D. The refractive status of Zuni Indian children. Am J Optom Physiol Opt 1976;53:120–123.

Helmholtz HLF, von. Helmholtz's treatise on physiological optics, 3rd ed., 1909. Trans. Southall JPC. The Optical Society of America, 1924. New York: Dover Publications, 1962;317–332.

Hirsch MJ. Changes in astigmatism after the age of forty. Am J Optom Arch Am Acad Optom 1959;36:395–405.

Hirsch MJ. Changes in astigmatism during the first eight years of school — an interim report from the Ojai longitudinal study. Am J Optom Arch Am Acad Optom 1963; 40:127–132.

Hofstetter HW. The correction of astigmatism for near work. Am J Optom Arch Am Acad Optom 1945;22:121–134.

Hofstetter HW, Rife DC. Miscellaneous optometric data on twins. Am J Optom Arch Am Acad Optom 1953;30:139–150.

Howland HC, Atkinson J, Braddick D, French J. Infant astigmatism measured by photo-refraction. Science 1978;202:331–333.

Howland HC, Sayles N. Photorefractive measurements of astigmatism in infants and young children. Invest Ophthalmol Vis Sci 1984;25:93–102.

Ing MR. The development of corneal astigmatism in contact lens wearers. Ann Ophthalmol 1976;8:309–314.

Keating MP, Carroll JP. Blurred imagery and the cylinder sine-squared law. Am J Optom Physiol Opt 1976;53:66–69.

Kerns RL. Research in orthokeratology. Part VIII. Results, conclusions and discussion of techniques. J Am Optom Assoc 1978;49:308–314.

Kinney JAS. The effects of astigmatism on sensitivity to sinusoidal and square wave gratings. Am J Optom Physiol Opt 1980;57:372–377.

Kragha IK. Corneal power and astigmatism. Ann Ophthalmol 1986;18:35–37.

Kratz JD, Walton WG. A modification of Javal's rule for the correction of astigmatism. Am J Optom Arch Am Acad Optom 1949;295–306.

Kronfeld PC, Devney C. The frequency of astigmatism. Arch Ophthalmol 1930;4:873–884.

Lansche RK. Asthenopia caused by "against-the-rule" astigmatism. Headache 1966;6:147–151.

Laurance L. Visual Optics and Sight Testing, 3rd ed. London: The School of Optics, 1926; 369–372.

LeGrand Y. Form and Space Vision. Revised ed. Translated by Millodot M, Heath GG. Bloomington: Indiana University, 1967;108, 128.

Lewis HT. Reducing a cylindrical correction. Am J Optom Arch Am Acad Optom 1949; 26:538–542.

Lewis RA. Juvenile hereditary macular dystrophies. In: Newsome RA, ed. Retinal Dystrophies and Degenerations. New York: Raven Press, 1988;115–134.

London R, Wick BC. Changes in angle lambda during growth: theory and clinical implications. Am J Optom Physiol Opt 1982;59:568–572.

Long WF. A matrix formalism for decentration problems. Am J Optom Physiol Opt 1976; 53:27–33.

Loper LR. The relationship between angle lambda and the residual astigmatism of the eye. Am J Optom Arch Am Acad Optom 1959;36:365–377.

Löpping B, Weale RA. Changes in corneal curvature following ocular convergence. Vis Res 1965;5:207–215.

Lotmar W, Lotmar T. Peripheral astigmatism in the human eye: experimental and theoretical model predictions. J Opt Soc Am 1974;64:510–513.

Ludlam WM, Wittenberg S. Measurements of the ocular dioptric elements utilizing photographic methods. Am J Optom Arch Am Acad Optom 1966;43:249–267.

Lyle WM. Changes in corneal astigmatism with age. Am J Optom Arch Am Acad Optom 1971;48:467–478.

Lyle WM, Grosvenor T, Dean KC. Corneal astigmatism in Amerind children. Am J Optom Arch Am Acad Optom 1972;49:517–524.

Lyle WM. The inheritance of corneal astigmatism. Thesis. Indiana University, 1965.

Mandell RB, St. Helen R. Mathematical model of the corneal contour. Br J Physiol Opt 1971;26:183–196.

Marin-Amat M. Les variations physiologiques de la courbe de la cornée pendant la vie. Leur importance et transcendance dans la réfraction oculaire. Bull Soc Belge Ophthalmol 1956;113:251–293.

Martin G. Amblyopie astigmatique. Condition du développement parfait de la vision. Bull Soc Ophthalmol Fr 1890;8:217–224.

Masci E. Sull'astigmatismo oftalmetrico: Modificzioni della curvatura corneale in rapporto alla attivita palpebrale ed alla rigidita sclerale. Bull d'Oculist 1965;44:755–763.

Mash AJ, Hegmann JP, Spivey BE. Genetic analyses of indices of corneal power and corneal astigmatism in human populations with varying incidences of strabismus. Invest Ophthalmol 1975;14:826–832.

McLenachan J, Loran DFC. Angle-closure glaucoma and inverse astigmatism. Br J Ophthalmol 1967;51:441–448.

McCartney DL, Whitney CE, Stark WJ, Wong SK, Bernitsky DA. Refractive keratoplasty for disabling astigmatism after penetrating keratoplasty. Arch Ophthalmol 1987;105:954–957.

Miller RG. A test for astigmatism — a preliminary report. Am J Optom Arch Am Acad Optom 1961;38:681–686.

Millodot M, Thibault C. Variation of astigmatism with accommodation and its relationship with dark focus. Ophthalmic Physiol Opt 1985;5:297–301.

Mitchell DE, Freeman RD. Millodot M, Haegerstrom G. Meridional amblyopia: evidence for modification of the human visual system by early visual experience. Vis Res 1973;13:535–558.

Mitchell DE. Astigmatism and neural development (editorial). Invest Ophthalmol Vis Sci 1979;18:8–10.

Mohindra I, Nagaraj S. Astigmatism in Zuni and Navajo Indians. Am J Optom Physiol Opt 1977;54:121–124.

Mohindra I, Held R, Gwiazda J, Brill S. Astigmatism in infants. Science 1978;202:329–331.

Moore JG. Intraocular implants: the postoperative astigmatism. Br J Ophthalmol 1980;64:318–321.

Morgan MW, Mahoney J, Olmstead HMD. Astigmatic accommodation. Arch Ophthalmol 1943;30:247–249.

Morgan MW. Changes in refraction over a period of twenty years in a nonvisually selected sample. Am J Optom Arch Am Acad Optom 1958;35:281–289.

Mote HG, Fry GA. The significance of Javal's rule. Am J Optom Arch Am Acad Optom 1939;16:362–365.

Nathan J, Kiely PM, Crewther SG, Crewther DP. Astigmatism occurring in association with pediatric eye disease. Am J Optom Physiol Opt 1986;63:497–504.

Neumueller J. Optical, physiological and perceptual factors influencing the ophthalmometric findings. Am J Optom Arch Am Acad Optom 1953;30:281–291.

Oppenheimer EH. Astigmatism in high myopia and a new way of testing it. Am J Ophthalmol 1924;7:530–531.

Pascal JI. Intrinsic variability of astigmatic errors. Arch Ophthalmol 1944;32:123–124.

Percival AS. The Prescribing of Spectacles, 3rd ed. New York: Wright & Sons, 1928;63–64, 184–190.

Phillips RA. Changes in corneal astigmatism. Am J Optom Arch Am Acad Optom 1952;29:379–380.

Poos F. Kausale Genese der sphärischen und asphärischen Refraktionszustände. Graefes Arch Clin Exp Ophthalmol 1950;150:245–278.

Poos F. Der onkotische Blutdruck als Determinationsfaktor bei der Ausbildung der Proportionsnormen in oculo-orbitalen system. Graefes Arch Clin Exp Ophthalmol 1952;152:300–311.

Pratt-Johnson JA, Warner DM. Contact lenses and corneal curvature changes. Am J Ophthalmol 1965;60:852–855.

Rabbetts RB. A comparison of astigmatism and cyclophoria in distance and near vision. Br J Physiol Opt 1973;27:161–190.

Reading VM. Corneal curvatures. The Contact Lens 1972;3(6):23–25.

Rengstorff RH. Corneal curvature and astigmatic changes subsequent to contact lens wear. J Am Optom Assoc 1965;36:996–1000.

Rengstorff RH. Variations in astigmatism overnight and during the day after wearing contact lenses. Am J Optom Arch Am Acad Optom 1971;48:810–813.

Rengstorff RH. Corneal curvature: patterns of change after wearing contact lenses. J Am Optom Assoc 1976;47:357.

Rengstorff RH. Astigmatism after contact lens wear. Am J Optom Physiol Opt 1977;54:787–791.

Roth N. The problem of the undependable cylinder. Surv Ophthalmol 1969;14:112–115.

Rubin ML. The tale of the warped cornea, a real life melodrama. Arch Ophthalmol 1967;77:711–712.

Sarver MD. The effect of contact lens tilt upon residual astigmatism. Am J Optom Arch Am Acad Optom 1963;40:730–744.

Sarver MD. A study of residual astigmatism. Am J Optom Arch Am Acad Optom 1969;46:578–582.

Satterfield DS. Prevalence and variation of astigmatism in a military population. J Am Optom Assoc 1989;60:14–18.

Saunders H. Age dependence of human refractive errors. Ophthalmic Physiol Opt 1981;1:159–174.

Saunders H. The astigmatic modulus and its age-dependence. Ophthalmic Physiol Opt 1984;4:215–222.

Schultz DN. Asymmetry of central and peripheral corneal astigmatism measured by photokeratoscopy. Am J Optom Physiol Opt 1977;54:776–781.

Sheard C. Physiological Optics. Chicago: Cleveland Press, 1918;36–67, 139–146, 236.

Sims CN, Durham DG. The Jackson cross cylinder disproved. Trans Am Ophthalmol Soc 1986;84:355–387.

Singh D, Kumar K. Keratometric changes after cataract extraction. Br J Ophthalmol 1976; 60:638–641.

Smith RS. Refractive surgery. In: Ophthalmology Annual. Reineke RD, ed. New York: Raven Press, 1989;351–361.

Solsona F. Astigmatism as a congenital, bilateral and symmetrical entity. Observations based on the study of 51000 patients. Br J Physiol Opt 1975;32:119–127.

Sørensen SK. L'astigmatisme du christallin, determiné comme la différence entre l'astigmatisme cornéen et l'astigmatism total, illustré par l'examen de ses variations d'après l'âge. Acta Ophthalmol 1944;22:341–385.

Sorsby A, Benjamin B, Davey JB, et al. Emmetropia and its Aberrations; a Study in the Correlation of the Optical Components of the Eye. Medical Research Council Special Report No. 293. London: HM Stationery Office, 1957.

Sorsby A, Sheridan M, Leary GA, Benjamin B. Vision, visual acuity and ocular refraction of young men. Br Med J 1960;1:1394–1398.

Sorsby A, Benjamin B, Sheridan M. Refraction and Its Components During Growth of the Eye from the Age of Three. Medical Research Council Special Report Series No. 301. London: HM Stationery Office, 1961.

Sorsby A, Sheridan M, Leary GA. Refraction and Its Components in Twins. Medical Research Council Special Report, Series No. 303. London: HM Stationery Office, 1962.

Sorsby A. Ophthalmic Genetics, 2nd ed. London: Butterworths, 1970.

Stern CN (with Rosenberg HH). The relative contributions of cornea and lens in the changes of astigmatism with age. Master's Thesis, New York University, 1940.

Stone J. The validity of some existing methods of measuring corneal contour compared with suggested new methods. Br J Physiol Opt 1962;19:205–230.

Swinger CA. Postoperative astigmatism. Surv Ophthalmol 1987;31:219–248.

Teikari JM, O'Donnell JJ. Astigmatism in twin pairs. Cornea 1989;8:263–266.

Terry MA, Roswey JJ. Dynamic shifts in corneal topography during the modified Ruiz procedure for astigmatism. Arch Ophthalmol 1986;104:1611–1616.

Thibos LN, Levick WR. Astigmatic visual and deprivation in cat: behavioral, optical and retinophysiological consequences. Vis Res 1982;22:43–53.

Thorn F, Held R, Fang L-L. Orthogonal astigmatic axes in Chinese and Caucasian infants. Invest Ophthalmol Vis Sci 1987;28:191–194.

Tocher RB. Astigmatism due to the tilt of a contact lens. Am J Optom Arch Am Acad 1962; 39:3–16.

Tscherning M. Optique Physiologique (1898). Translated by Weiland C, 2nd ed. Philadelphia: Keystone Publishing Co., 1904;37, 66, 120–136.

van Alphen GWHM. On emmetropia and ametropia. Ophthalmologica (Suppl) 1961; 142:1–92.

Vihlen FS, Wilson G. The relation between eyelid tension, corneal toricity and age. Invest Ophthalmol Vis Sci 1983;24:1367.

Waardenburg PJ. Genetics and Ophthalmology, vol. II. Oxford: Blackwell, 1963;1201–1285.

Wang G-J, Pomerantzeff O, Pankratov MM. Astigmatism of oblique incidence in the human model eye. Vis Res 1983;23:1079–1085.

Watsky MA, McCarey BE. Alloplastic refractive keratophakia: a comparison of predictive algorithms. CLAO J 1986;12(2):112–117.

Wick B, Crane S. A vision profile of American Indian children. Am J Optom Physiol Opt 1976;53:34–40.

Wilson G, Bell C, Chotai S. The effect of lifting the lids on corneal astigmatism. Am J Optom Physiol Opt 1982;59:670–674.

Wixson RJ. The relative effect of heredity and environment upon the refractive errors of identical twins, fraternal twins, and like-sex siblings. Am J Optom Arch Am Acad Optom 1958;35:346–351.

Wong S. Vision analysis and refractive status of youths in a juvenile detention home population. Am J Optom Physiol Opt 1976;53:112–119.

Woodruff ME. Cross sectional studies of corneal and astigmatic characteristics of children between the twenty-fourth and seventy-second months of life. Am J Optom Arch Am Acad Optom 1971;48:650–659.

__10__

Anisometropia

I. Knox Laird

☐

Interest in anisometropia has been rekindled in recent years by the sometimes unexpected results in several areas of study. Monocular deprivation experiments, designed to induce amblyopia, have in many cases resulted in induced anisomyopia. The increasing use of intraocular lenses after cataract surgery, as well as the manipulation of refractive error by procedures such as radial keratotomy, require careful consideration to minimize the introduction of anisometropic complications.

By definition, anisometropia exists whenever there is a difference between the refractive states of the two eyes. Subcategories of anisometropia are anisomyopia, in which both eyes are myopic; anisohyperopia, in which both eyes are hyperopic; and antimetropia, in which one eye is myopic and the other hyperopic. Anisometropia may be classified as either axial or refractive. In the axial form, the eyes have approximately equal focal powers but differ in overall length; in the refractive form, the eyes have different focal powers as found, for example, in unilateral aphakia. Higher degrees of anisometropia (greater than 2.00 D) are typically, although not exclusively, axial in nature (Sorsby et al. 1962).

Data published by a number of investigators suggest that the prevalence of anisometropia decreases throughout the early childhood period of emmetropization, followed by an increase during and beyond adolescence (Table 10.1). This implies that the preadolescent refractive balance may be fine-tuned by some growth-regulating mechanism that optimizes the development of anisometropia. Evidence for the operation of such a mechanism, in the kitten, has been presented by Hendrickson and Rosenblum (1985) who showed that if anisometropia was induced in newborn kittens by radial keratotomy, their refraction tended to change toward emmetropia and isometropia, but only if accommodation had been left intact.

My thanks to Martin Boase for his assistance in collecting the cross-sectional data, and to Robert Kinnear, Kerry Atkinson, and Graeme Kearney for access to their clinical files.

Table 10.1. Prevalence of Anisometropia Expressed as a Percentage of the Sample Population*

Population age	Investigator(s)	Prevalence
Premature infants	Fulton et al. (1981)[a]	32.0 (N = 146)
Full-term infants	Zonis and Miller (1974)[b]	17.3 (N = 300)
	Fulton et al. (1980)[a]	18.0 (N = 640)
1 to 6 years	Hirsch (1952)[c]	1.0 (N = 1166)
	Ingram (1979)[c]	6.5 (N = 1648)
	Ingram and Barr (1979)[b]	8.5 to 8.8 (N = 148)
	Mayer et al. (1982)[d]	4.0 (N = 291)
5 to 12 years	Flom and Bedell (1985)[b]	3.4 (N = 2762)
5 to 17 years	Blum et al. (1959)[a]	3.5 (N = 1221)
13 to 19 years	Hirsch (1952)[c]	2.4 (N = 1040)
	Hirsch (1967)[b]	6.0 (N = 359)
	Laatikainen and Erkkila (1980)[a]	3.6 (N = 411)
	de Vries (1985)[e]	4.0 (N = 1356)
	Kehoe (1942)[b]†	11.9
	Giles (1950)[c]†	7.4 (N = 2500)
	Lebensohn (1957)[c]†	10.0
	Martinez (1977)[c]	10.7 (N = 2000)
	Fledelius (1984)[a]	9.0 (N = 1200)

*Superscripts indicate criteria for anisometropia.
[a]0.50 D sphere
[b]1.00 D in corresponding meridians
[c]1.00 D sphere
[d]2.00 D cylinder or sphere
[e]not known
†Cited by Borish 1970; 258.

The prevalence of anisometropia depends on the sample studied and the criterion adopted. In a general clinical population, about 10% of patients manifest an interocular difference in spherical equivalent refraction of 1.00 D or more. Data presented in this chapter show that the prevalence reduces to 2.5% if anisometropia is defined as a difference of 2.00 D or more; and that the proportion of anisometropia in each decade increases to age 30 and then declines. Blum et al. (1959), in the Orinda study, demonstrated that the prevalence of anisometropia (1.00 D or more) in children appears to increase slowly with age, from about 2% at age 5 years to about 4% at age 15 years, but the change never reaches statistical significance. Little work appears to have been conducted in the area of genetic transmission of anisometropia, although Sorsby (1972) has cited examples of both dominant and recessive pedigrees.

GROWTH PATTERNS IN ANISOMETROPIA

In the majority of cases, anisometropes are myopic. Schapero (1971) found that anisomyopia was three times more common than anisohyperopia, but that aniso-hyperopes were more likely to develop amblyopia or strabismus, or both. In 200 nonstrabismic anisometropes, Jampolsky et al. (1955) found that anisomyopes were twice as prevalent as anisohyperopes. Analysis of the subjects of the Sorsby et al. study (1962) of the components of anisometropia showed that the number of anisometropic subjects having myopia (in at least one meridian of one or both eyes) was 1.75 times the number of those having hyperopia. For subjects having very high anisometropia (an interocular difference ranging from 5.25 to 15.5 D) Sanfilippo (1978) recorded only one in thirty as having hyperopia in the more ametropic eye.

In a report on the Ojai longitudinal study, Hirsch (1967) reported that although no two anisometropic children followed precisely the same pattern of growth, four general patterns were observed to describe almost all of the children. Three of these four patterns are illustrated in Figure 10.1 (reproduced from Hirsch's report). In this diagram, the heavy lines represent the spherical equivalent refractive state of the two eyes; and the age scale represents a period of 10 to 12 years, from average ages of 6 and 17 years. Hirsch described the following growth patterns:

1. Hyperopia. The three subjects identified in the upper-left graph had no anisometropia when entering school but acquired it at an older age. One subject

Figure 10.1. Three patterns of anisometropia progression. See text for explanation. (From Hirsch 1967. © The Am Acad of Optom 1967. Reprinted with permission.)

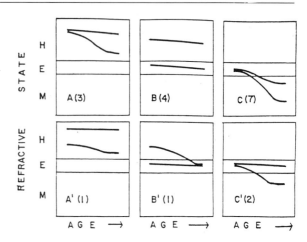

(A', lower left graph) had anisometropia at the initial examination, with the amount increasing during the school years.

2. Hyperopia-emmetropia. At the time of the first examination, five subjects were hyperopic in one eye only, the fellow eye being within the limits of emmetropia (+1.25 to −0.25 D). Four subjects (B) maintained the anisometropia throughout the school years, but one subject (B') became emmetropic in the hyperopic eye.

3. Myopia. The largest group consisted of nine subjects who were emmetropic when entering school but developed myopia in both eyes (C, seven subjects) or one eye (C', two subjects) during the school years.

4. Astigmatism. Three children (not shown in the figure) had anisometropia and marked astigmatism, one or the other meridian differing from the same meridian in the fellow eye by 1.00 D or more.

OCCURRENCE OF AMBLYOPIA

Amblyopia is known to frequently accompany anisometropia. According to von Noorden (1985) amblyopia affects between 2 and 2.5% of the general population. Schapero (1971) noted that 65% of amblyopes are what Phillips (1959) terms "anisometropic amblyopes." Flom and Bedell (1985) found 3.4% of 2,762 schoolchildren (ages 5 to 12) had anisometropia (1.00 D or more difference in power between corresponding meridians of the two eyes). One percent of their sample had amblyopia of 6/12 (20/40) or worse acuity; approximately one third had anisometropia, one third had anisometropia and strabismus, and one third had strabismus. In a study of anisometropes of 2.00 D or more in communities in Thailand and the United States, Tanlamai and Goss (1979) concluded that 50% of those with anisometropia of 4.50 D or more have amblyopia of at least 6/9 (20/30). Flom and Bedell (1985) reported that among their grade school children, the anisometropic amblyopes had an average acuity in the amblyopic eye of 6/18 (20/60); for amblyopes having anisometropia and strabismus the average acuity was 6/28.2 (20/94), and those amblyopes having strabismus only, 6/22.2 (20/74).

INFLUENCE OF BINOCULARITY

In order for the optical image to be in focus on the retina of the eye, the various refractive elements must develop and subsequently grow with a high degree of coordination. One diopter of myopia, causing the world to be blurred beyond 1 meter, could result either from an excessive axial length of about 0.33 mm (an error of approximately 1.5%) or a deficiency in the corneal radius of about .166 mm (an error of approximately 2.2%). This would seem to present nature with sufficient problems without the added constraints of binocular vision, which requires the eyes to cooperate in a unique and highly synchronized manner. The anomalies and adaptations accompanying asymmetric growth in infantile anisometropia suggest that the visual system is quite intolerant of any disharmony during development.

Clinical experience has demonstrated that an interocular difference in refractive error of 1.00 D in humans can lead to a poorly developed quality of binocular vision, with amblyopia in the more ametropic eye (Ingram and Walker 1979). Experiments using anisometropes or artificially induced anisometropia have provided perceptual and electrophysiologic evidence that small levels of monocular defocus can produce significant disruptions in the binocular processes. Using the Howard-Dolman apparatus, Ong (1972) found that the depth error doubled for artificially induced anisometropia of 0.75 D and was worse for myopic focus. Simons (1984) found that degrading the contrast of the image of one eye (lowering contrast to the equivalent of 6/9 (20/30) Snellen acuity) reduced the stereoacuity on the Frisby, Randot and TNO stereotests by twice as much as by simultaneously degrading the contrast for both eyes.

Persson and Wanger (1982) identified a linear relationship between the relative amplitude of the pattern reversal electroretinogram and monocular defocus: 1.00 D of artificially induced anisometropia resulted in a 25% reduction of the electroretinographic amplitude. Interestingly, Fiorentini et al. (1978) demonstrated a correlation between the visually evoked potential and perceptual suppression in anisometropia. They found that an increase in perceptual suppression, resulting from increasing artificial anisometropia, coincided with reduction of the ratio of binocular/monocular evoked potential amplitude. This suggests that the reduced binocular amplitude is due to suppression of the response from the blurred eye. Binocular summation was also shown by Harwerth and Smith (1985) to decline linearly with monocular defocus. They cited an example of a monkey who, when viewing a 12.5 cycle/second grating, reached zero summation as a result of 1.5 D of artificially induced anisometropia. Results such as these illustrate the importance of studying anisometropia because what seem to be small percentage differences in eye parameters have profound effects on the binocular system.

The studies to be reported here were undertaken to supplement the information available on the distribution of refractive error in anisometropia and with the hope of yielding some insight into the etiology and progression of anisomyopia.

A CROSS-SECTIONAL STUDY

□ The Sample

The records of 731 anisometropes were selected from the files of three urban optometric practices (I. K. Laird and M. M. Boase, unpublished data). Records were selected on the basis of the following criteria: at least 2.00 D difference in the vertical meridian of the two eyes, astigmatism less than 3.00 D, ages between 3 and 50 years, and no history of contact lens wear. The sample selected on this basis comprised 390 anisomyopes (53.3%), 255 anisohyperopes (34.9%), and 86 antimetropes (11.8%).

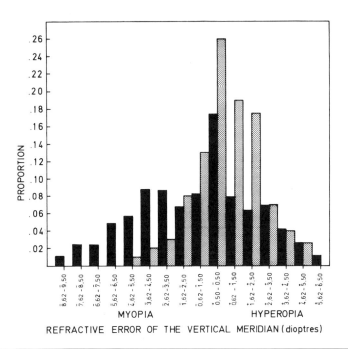

Figure 10.2. Frequency distribution of the vertical meridian refractive error for 731 anisometropes (at least 2.00 D difference in the vertical meridians of the two eyes) denoted by the darker bars, compared with the adult clinical population (N = 4,431) of Brown (cited by Borish 1970) represented by the lighter bars.

☐ Analysis of Data

The distribution of vertical meridian refraction of all eyes (N = 1,462) is shown by the darker bars in Figure 10.2. The tendency toward emmetropization is present, manifesting a significant skew toward moderate myopia. However, the tendency toward emmetropization is less marked than that found for an overall clinical population by Brown (cited by Borish 1970, 9) as shown by the lighter bars in Figure 10.2.

To determine the distribution of the myopic refraction on the basis of age, the refraction data were distributed in 10-year intervals as shown in Figure 10.3. The distribution curves shown in this figure show a very small proportion of aniso-myopes at ages 3 to 10 years, gradually increasing to age 21 to 30 years and then flattening, with an increase in the proportion of anisohyperopes beyond age 30. This increase in the relative prevalence of anisomyopia could be due either to an

Figure 10.3.
Distributions of the vertical meridian refractive error for 731 anisometropes presented in 10-year age groups, as indicated on each graph.

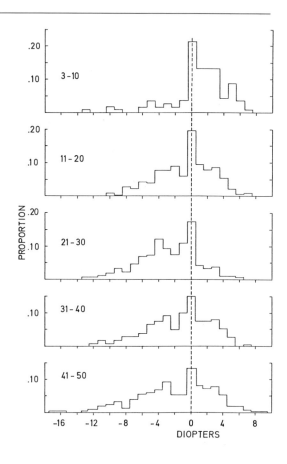

increase in the number of myopes or to an increase in the degree of myopia in existing myopes, or both.

To determine which of these situations exists, the relative proportions of anisomyopes, anisohyperopes, and antimetropes were compared with the mean change in refractive error for each decade of life of the group as a whole. As shown in Figure 10.4, the increased proportion of anisomyopes (open circles) up to the age of 30 years clearly parallels the mean increase in the degree of myopia (shown by the hollow circular symbols) and is directly related to the decrease in the proportion of anisohyperopes (filled circles). Therefore, the increase in the relative prevalence of anisomyopia is due, not to an increase in the number of myopes, but to an increase in the degree of myopia occurring with age.

The cross-sectional data show that higher degrees of anisometropia (4.00 D or more) are associated predominantly with myopia. Of the 130 "high" anisometropes, 96 (or 74%) were either anisomyopes (n = 78) or antimetropes with myopia in the more ametropic eye (n = 18). The fact that 82% of these myopic patients were older than 20 years of age implies that the amount of anisometropia increases with age.

Overall, the results of the cross-sectional study show that both the number of anisomyopes and the amount of their interocular refractive error difference increases with age. On the basis of these conclusions, it was evident that a longitu-

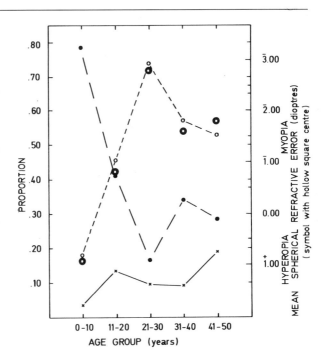

Figure 10.4.
Variations in the proportion of the various anisometropic/antimetropic categories, presented for each 10-year age group. Anisomyopes are depicted by open circles, anisohyperopes by black dots, and antimetropes by crosses. These variations are compared with the mean change in refractive error with age (circular symbol with the hollow center).

dinal study was needed to determine whether individual anisomyopes follow this trend and to discover whether this trend also accounts for the proportional decline of anisohyperopes with increasing age.

------■------

A LONGITUDINAL STUDY OF CLINICAL PATIENTS

□ Previous Relevant Studies

A number of researchers have demonstrated that the amount of anisometropia may either increase or decrease during a person's lifetime. Using a criterion for anisometropia of 1.00 D or more, Hirsch (1967) found that of twenty-one children who were anisometropic at an average age of 17 years, only nine had been anisometropic when first tested at an average age of 6 years; one child who was anisometropic at age 6 "outgrew" the anisometropia by the age of 17 years. Ingram and Barr (1979) found that of twelve anisometropes identified at the age of one year, seven lost their anisometropia during the following 2½ years, and a further eight developed anisometropia during the same period. Friedman et al. (1985) studied the effect of prescribing for marked ametropia in nonstrabismics, prescribing before the age of 3 years and reassessing the results at age 7 years. The sample included six anisometropes (ranging from 3 to 11.00 D) of which three increased and three decreased in amount, during the 4-year period. Lepard (1975) reported that thirty-seven of fifty-five strabismic amblyopes developed anisometropia greater than 1.00 D between the ages of 4 and 14 years.

Seniakina (1979) found that the absence of binocular vision favored the maintenance of anisometropia in children refracted annually between the ages of one and 18 years; whereas in the presence of binocular vision, anisometropia decreased with age.

□ The Sample

To verify the conclusions of the cross-sectional study, a retrospective analysis was made from the clinical files of sixty anisometropes between the ages of 5 and 25 years. None of these had been included in the cross-sectional study. Criteria for inclusion were at least four refractions between the ages of 5 and 25 years, spherical anisometropia of 2.00 D or more (irrespective of the level of astigmatism), no active pathology, and no contact lens wear. The spherical interocular difference of 2.00 D was selected for this study because spherical refraction is presumed to

Figure 10.5. The mean vertical meridian refractive error plotted against age, with the filled circles representing the cross-sectional data (N = 731) and the open circles representing the longitudinal data (N = 60). The cross-sectional data of Sorsby et al. (1962) are analyzed and presented with rescaled coordinates in the inset.

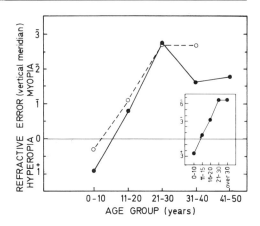

more closely reflect the axial changes associated with growth than cylindrical refraction and because astigmatism shows little change over the time interval sampled. The percentages of subjects in each anisometropic category compared closely with those in the cross-sectional sample: 55% anisomyopes (n = 33); 40% anisohyperopes (n = 24), and 5% antimetropes (n = 3).

The change in mean refractive error with age illustrates the high and significant correlation between the cross-sectional and longitudinal samples (r = 0.95, P < .025), supporting the conclusion that anisometropes, as a group, show a steady increase in the amount of myopia up to age 30 (Figure 10.5). The results of Sorsby et al. (1962) are included on the graph to show their close alignment.

□ Progression of Anisometropia

To explore the patterns of alteration in refractive status of subjects in the longitudinal study, anisomyopes were segregated from anisohyperopes, with antimetropes being included in either category according to the eye with the greater ametropia. Patterns of progression are illustrated in Table 10.2, in terms of the proportions of subjects who maintained anisometropia, who lost anisometropia, or who developed anisometropia (classified as myopes or hyperopes on the basis of the first refraction). These results show that not all subjects increased their level of anisometropia with increasing age.

The longitudinal data revealed two interesting features (not shown in the table). First, half of the patients who were anisometropic at a mean age of 22 years were isometropic before age 10; second, of particular clinical interest are those patients who lost their anisometropia but were left with nonstrabismic amblyopia (four of seven patients) or with strabismic amblyopia (three of seven). The refractive his-

Table 10.2.   Anisometropia Characterized by Its Pattern of Progression with Age, as Found in Study II*

| | Anisometropia category | | | | | |
| | Maintained anisometropia | | Lost anisometropia | | Developed anisometropia | |
	Myopes	Hyperopes	Myopes	Hyperopes	Myopes	Hyperopes
Study II	0.18	0.17	0.05	0.08	0.33	0.18
(N = 68)	(n = 11)	(n = 17)	(n = 3)	(n = 5)	(n = 20)	(n = 11)
Hirsch (1967)	—	0.19	—	0.05	0.43	0.41
Category		B, A'		B'	A	C,C'
Amblyopia	6%	60%	68%	100%	10%	82%
(Study II)	(n = 4)	(n = 10)	(n = 2)	(n = 5)	(n = 2)	(n = 9)

*The proportions (percentages of anisometropes in the sample) in each category are compared with the patterns identified by Hirsch 1967; see Figure 10.1.

Figure 10.6.   Changes in the mean spherical refractive error (D) with age, in anisometropia (data from longitudinal study). The results are categorized according to whether 2.00 D of anisometropia or more was **(a)** maintained, **(b)** lost, or **(c)** developed between the mean ages of 8 and 24 years. Anisomyopes and anisohyperopes are presented separately with the open symbols identifying the mean result of the eye that showed the greater change in refraction over the period recorded. The filled symbols represent the fellow eye.

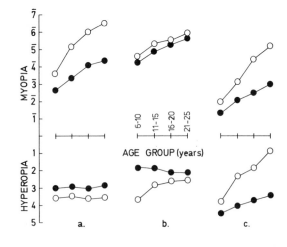

tory of these patients suggests that their anisometropia was a significant factor in the etiology of their amblyopia or strabismus.

An analysis comparing the change in refraction of the eye having the greater overall change in refraction to the eye having the lesser change is shown in Figure 10.6. The patterns of changes in anisometropes identified in this study (Table 10.2 and Figure 10.6) agree well with those presented by Hirsch (1967) and reproduced here in Figure 10.1.

The longitudinal data show that if a child develops anisomyopia during infancy, the anisometropia is more likely to increase than to stabilize or decrease. By comparison, anisohyperopia tends to stabilize or decrease over the same period. This accounts for the observed decrease in the proportion of anisohyperopes in Figure 10.4. These trends are accentuated by the large number of children who develop anisomyopia during adolescence. Unfortunately, if anisometropia of either form occurs during adolescence, it is likely to increase along with a myopic shift in refraction, even up to age 30 years.

■ ASYMMETRICAL OCULAR GROWTH

As Hirsch (1967) has commented, anisomyopia is an enigma for any theory of myopia, particularly if one attempts to account for anisometropia that presents itself during adolescence: The theory must provide an adequate explanation of how the two eyes can grow or stretch asymmetrically. An additional mystery is the large proportion of anisohyperopes (Figure 10.6,c) who show a typically myopic shift while developing their anisometropia; indeed, the progression rates of these patients match those of the anisomyopes (Table 10.3), both during the adolescent and the adult growth phases. These patients are all the more interesting when considered in the light of recent theories of the genesis of refractive error, with the conjectured influence of dark focus (Charman 1982) and possible involvement of accommodative hysteresis (Ebenholtz 1983).

One clue in this puzzle is the evidence just presented that the anisometropia continues to increase with one eye showing a rate of change similar to the 0.115 D per year reported by Goss et al. (1985, Table 10.4) for "adult continuation" myopes. It would be an oversimplification to suggest that the more myopic eye characterizes "adult continuation," whereas the less myopic eye characterizes "adult stabilization," although the data do support this reasoning. Two possible explanations are suggested: (1) the mechanism that generally mediates the refractive state is out of synchrony, which could account for the tendency of amblyopic eyes to show a myopic shift; and (2) the mechanism itself is sound but ocular component growth simply occurs at different rates in the two eyes.

If the second explanation is correct, then it would be anticipated that comparison of the progression rates for the two eyes, during rapid adolescent progression,

Table 10.3. Mean Rates of Refractive Error Progression for Juvenile (6 to 15 years) and Adult (16 to 25 years) Anisometropes*

| | Anisometropia category | | | | | |
| | Maintained anisometropia | | Lost anisometropia | | Developed anisometropia | |
	Myopes	Hyperopes	Myopes	Hyperopes	Myopes	Hyperopes
Juvenile Group						
Smaller change	0.142	0.014	0.128	−0.014†	0.152	0.090
Larger change	0.314	0.018	0.134	0.160	0.230	0.292
Ratio‡	0.452	0.777	0.955	0.088	0.661	0.308
Adult Group						
Smaller change	0.052	0.030	0.066	−0.001†	0.096	0.052
Larger change	0.098	0.022	0.078	0.020	0.156	0.192
Ratio‡	0.531	1.364	0.846	0.050	0.615	0.271

*Mean progression (D/year) is given for both the eye showing the smaller change and the eye showing the larger change.
†Minus sign indicates a hyperopic shift in refractive error.
‡Ratio of progression for eye having the smaller change to progression for eye having the larger change.

Table 10.4. Prevalence of Anisometropia and Amblyopia in Various Conditions

Investigator(s)	Condition	Condition and prevalence	Prevalence	No. subjects
Merriam (1980)	Blepharoptosis	Anisometropia	12%	65
Pratt et al. (1984)	Marcus Gunn syndrome	Anisometropia	25%	71
Tredici and von Noorden (1985)	Duane's syndrome (congenital)	Anisometropia	17%	70
O'Malley and Urist (1982)	Duane's syndrome	Anisometropia	16%	97
Isenberg (1977)	Duane's syndrome	Anisometropic amblyopia	67%	101
Morin and Bryars (1980)	Congenital glaucoma	Anisometropic amblyopia	12%	51

should correlate with those accompanying residual progression in adulthood. The mean rates of refractive changes and the associated interocular ratio (progression for the eye with the smaller rate of change as compared to that of the eye with the greater rate of change) are presented in Table 10.3. When assessed in the manner shown in this table, the comparative refractive progression rates correlate highly (r = 0.856, $P < .025$), suggesting that anisometropia develops as a consequence of an asymmetry in the ocular growth rates.

To put the discussion into perspective, it is necessary to consider the refractive changes in terms of component growth. For example, if we assume that the progression in anisomyopia is due entirely to an increase in axial length, it follows that a progression of 0.25 D per year is the equivalent of an axial length increase of 0.083 mm per year, or a percentage change of 0.35% per year. This is calculated on the basis of an initial axial length of 24 mm (Borish 1970, 63), with 0.25 D of myopia represented by .083 mm of axial elongation. If the companion eye was advancing at half this rate, as the mean rate implies (Table 10.3), the asymmetry in growth rate would be only 0.175% per year.

The analogy with axial length is appropriate because anisometropia and its progression are unique for another reason: Sorsby et al. (1967) have shown that axial length makes a significant contribution in most cases of anisometropia of 2.00 D or more; although in isometropia, axial length does not become a significant factor until the error exceeds 4.00 D of myopia or 6.00 D of hyperopia. Reanalysis of the Sorsby et al. (1967) data provides a correlation of 0.94 ($P < .001$) between the calculated axial length and the vertical meridian anisometropia for sixty-seven anisometropes ranging from 2.00 to 15.4 D of interocular difference, with a median value of 3.50 D. When van der Torren's results (1985) (Table 10.1) are reanalyzed, the ultrasound axial length differences correlate well with the anisometropia (r = 0.71, $P < .025$) for the nine subjects with refractive differences ranging from 6.00 to 11.5 D. The regression equation ($Y = 0.34X - 0.09$) suggests that 1 mm of axial elongation is associated with 3.00 D of anisomyopia.

Anisometropia greater than 2.00 D would appear to present a bilateral asymmetry beyond the range expected in the normal human, but not manifesting the characteristics of hemihypertrophy. Mascie-Taylor (1981) reports from a sample of 146 individuals that the mean left foot length was greater than mean right foot length by a mere 0.3%. The mean foot length standard deviation was 0.56%. This highlights the accuracy of normal bilateral skeletal growth. In comparison, anthropomorphic measurements by Silver et al. (1953) from children of about 6 years of age with the syndrome of congenital hemihypertrophy revealed asymmetries of about 9.5%. Hemihypertrophy tends to be unilaterally disclosed, which does not appear to be the case in anisometropic growth patterns. Overall foot measurements of 23 anisometropes show large but nondirectional asymmetries ranging from 1 to 15 mm (mean 5.7 mm). Martinez (1977) found that anisometropes tend to have asymmetric monocular nasopupillary distances, although they are not consistently lateralized relative to the degree of ametropia. He also reported a greater frequency of facial asymmetry in anisometropia, particularly in cases of anisomyopia.

REFRACTIVE CHANGES IN
AMBLYOPIC EYES

The changes in refraction of amblyopic eyes are not well understood. Friedman et al. (1985) showed a statistically significant relationship between amblyopic and nonamblyopic eyes of nonstrabismic patients treated with spectacles before age 3 years and reassessed at age 7 years. The nonamblyopic eyes showed a statistically significant higher frequency of myopic shift (seventeen of twenty-one patients) than did the amblyopic eyes (six of sixteen patients). A similar result was obtained by Lepard (1975) for fifty-five strabismic amblyopes between the mean ages of 4 and 14 years.

In view of the small number of anisometropic amblyopes in the present study, nothing definitive can be stated; however, the trends are certainly interesting. Amblyopes in the group that developed anisometropia showed the greater myopic shift in the dominant (nonamblyopic) eye in all eleven subjects. The situation for the other two groups was quite different. Five of the seven amblyopes who lost their anisometropia had their greatest myopic shift in the amblyopic and more hyperopic eye, which accounted for their isometropization. Subjects who retained their anisometropia either showed the greater myopic shift in their amblyopic eye for the anisomyopes or showed relatively symmetrical changes in the case of the anisohyperopes. From the limited data, it would be speculative to imply that the amblyopia was involved in the observed trends.

DEPRIVATION-INDUCED
ANISOMYOPIA

A reasonable body of evidence indicates that anisomyopia or isomyopia may be induced in young humans due to visual or image deprivation. An increased incidence of myopia in eyes with ptosis was recorded by O'Leary and Millodot (1979) and by Till (1983). This finding is consistent with reports of anisometropia associated with a number of conditions, which are listed in Table 10.4. Collectively, these reports show that the effects of deprivation during infancy would appear to predispose the eye to the development of myopia. This finding is counter to the results mentioned where the influence of amblyopia (a consequence of early deprivation) tends to reduce the myopic changes in the affected eye during the adolescent growth phase.

■

CLINICAL MANAGEMENT: SPECTACLES OR CONTACT LENSES?

On the basis of Knapp's law we may conclude that in anisometropia due to a difference in the axial lengths of the two eyes, less aniseikonia will be induced when spectacle lenses, rather than contact lenses, are worn. However, several reports have demonstrated a *higher* degree of aniseikonia when axial anisometropia is corrected with spectacles rather than with contact lenses. Rabin et al. (1983) and Bradley et al. (1983) review this work (Figure 10.7) and demonstrate significant residual aniseikonia when differing levels of anisometropia were corrected with spectacle lenses of identical form and positioned at the same vertex distance. Their explanation for this deviation from Knapp's law was that the myopic anisometrope has *optical magnification* (due to an elongated eye), and this is accompanied by *neural minification* (due to reduction in the number of photoreceptors per unit area, associated with retinal stretching). Furthermore, retinal stretching around the fovea may increase by a greater proportion than the axial length of the eye. Rabin et al. (1981) illustrated this with fundus photographs for two 7 D ani-

Figure 10.7. Graph demonstrating the significant residual aniseikonia that is present when differing levels of anisometropia were corrected with spectacle lenses of identical form. The regression line represents the data of Rabin et al. (1983), whereas the circles and triangles indicate the data of other researchers. The open triangles represent cases for which the spectacle lenses were fitted at a distance closer than the anterior focal plane. (From Rabin et al. 1983.)

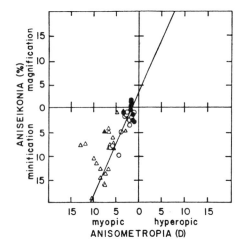

somyopes whose aniseikonia differed by a factor of two. As anticipated, the subject with the greater aniseikonia also had significantly more stretching, which would account for the overall minification.

Because the degree of anisometropia correlates well with both the interocular difference in axial length and the resultant aniseikonia, it should be possible to determine if the combined effects of retinal stretch and relative spectacle magnification can account for the experimental results. The effect of retinal stretch is to deform the shape of the vitreous chamber of the eye and to reduce the density of the retinal elements per unit area.

Kronfeld (1969) describes the vitreous chamber as approximating a hemisphere having a vertical diameter of 23 mm. Since the scleral coat is approximately 0.5 mm thick at the equator, the radius of the retina is about 11 mm. If it is assumed that the globe elongates and deforms into an ellipsoid configuration as a result of the progression of myopia, this will permit the calculation of the relative change in the density of the retinal elements.

If density of the retinal elements is stated as the number of retinal elements per unit of surface area,

$$D = \text{Density for a hemispheric retina} = \frac{N}{2\pi b^2}$$

$$D' = \text{Density for a semi-ellipsoid retina} = \frac{N}{2\pi b^2(a/b)}$$

$$= \frac{N}{2\pi(ab)}$$

where a is the axial length of the posterior segment, measured from the equator, and $2b$ is the vertical diameter of the retina.

If it is assumed that 0.33 mm change in axial length results in 1.00 D of anisometropia, then

$$a = b + 0.33 = 11.33.$$

Hence, the change in relative density per diopter of myopia is equivalent to

$$\frac{D'}{D} = \frac{\dfrac{N}{2\pi(ab)}}{\dfrac{N}{2\pi b^2}} = \frac{b}{a} = \frac{11.00}{11.33} = 0.9709.$$

This implies that if there is uniform retinal stretch, it is accompanied by neural magnification of -2.91% for each diopter of axial myopia. If the stretching should be nonuniform, there would be variations from this predicted value. Stretching confined to the equator would produce less minification, whereas the formation of a posterior staphyloma would result in more stretching.

Optical magnification of the retinal image is introduced when axial myopia is corrected with spectacles or contact lenses. Bennett (1974) provides a simple formula for calculating the relative spectacle magnification accompanying the correction of axial ametropia:

$$RSM = \frac{1}{1 + pF},$$

where F is the power of the correcting lens, and
p is the distance of the lens from the anterior focal point of the eye.

If we assume that p is equal to zero for a spectacle lens and 16 mm for a contact lens, and that F is equal to -1.00 D, the magnification accompanying optical correction with a spectacle lens and a contact lens would be

$$\text{Spectacle Lens } RSM_{SL} = 1.00, \text{ and}$$

$$\text{Contact Lens } RSM_{CL} = \frac{1}{1 - 0.016}$$

$$= 1.0163.$$

The method of correction influences the retinal image size, such that a contact lens produces a magnification of $+1.63\%$ for each diopter of myopia while a spectacle lens would not significantly alter the image size. The latter result is described by Knapp's law.

The overall magnification, which determines the resultant aniseikonia, can be calculated by combining the influence of optical magnification and neural magnification.

$$M_{SL} = 1.00 \ (0.9709) = 0.9709 = -2.91\%/D$$

$$M_{CL} = 1.0163 \ (0.9709) = 0.9869 = -1.33\%/D.$$

These estimates can be compared to the experimental results of Bradley et al. (1983), Rabin et al. (1983), and van der Torren (1985). Rabin et al. (1981) determined that -2.2 to -2.4% residual aniseikonia accompanied the correction of anisometropia with spectacles. When contact lenses were used, van der Torren (1985) found a value of $-0.65\%/D$. These experimental values can be compared in relative terms with the theoretical estimates.

$$\text{Experimental results: } \frac{M_{CL} \text{ (van der Torren 1985)}}{M_{SL} \text{ (Rabin et al. 1983)}} = \frac{0.9935}{0.9770} = 1.0169.$$

$$\text{Theoretical results: } \frac{M_{CL}}{M_{SL}} = \frac{0.9867}{0.9709} = 1.0163.$$

When compared in this manner, there is very close agreement, with the overestimation implying that retinal stretching is nonuniform. This infers that more stretching occurs at the equator, which could be expected because the sclera is much thinner there than at the posterior pole (Kronfeld 1969). In addition, the relative agreement between experimental and theoretical values shows that there is, on average, no significant refractive (as compared to axial) contribution in the development of anisomyopia.

Van Alphen (1986) has demonstrated that not only the retina but also the choroid tends to stretch nonlinearly, with the greatest stretch in the equatorial region. It is unlikely that the stretching in anisomyopia is due to a difference in the steady-state intraocular pressure between the two eyes. Bonomi (1982) found no difference in the intraocular pressure between the two eyes of 137 myopic anisometropes. The myopic eye (or the eye with the greater myopia) showed a lower scleral rigidity and a higher outflow facility, but no difference in intraocular pressure.

From a clinical standpoint these results are very important. They illustrate gross stretching of the retina, approximately 12% more stretching in the eye with the greater ametropia, for a 5.00 D anisomyope. This elongation of the globe does not appear to be accompanied by retinal growth or a compensation for the reduction in receptor density. The major role played by this stretching in determining the final degree of aniseikonia suggests a serious challenge to the conventional wisdom of managing anisometropia, for these results illustrate that aniseikonia is minimized if the patient is corrected using contact lenses rather than spectacles as is generally recommended. This opinion is supported by Winn et al. (1986).

NEURAL COMPENSATION

Fortunately, there are indications that the visual system is able to achieve significant neural compensation for the anomalies introduced by anisomyopia and anisometropic amblyopia. Mamedov (1977) identified binocular instability in virtually all cases of anisometropia beyond 2.00 D. Below this level, instability was related to the degree of anisometropia.

Goodwin and Romano (1985) demonstrated that monocular blur degrades stereoacuity in normals more severely than binocular blur. However, three of five anisometropic amblyopes performed better than would be expected on the basis of the acuity of their amblyopic eye.

Oculomotor adaptation accompanies the differential prism associated with an anisometropic spectacle prescription. Several researchers (Allen 1974, Henson and Dharamshi 1982) have demonstrated that it is the rate of change of prismatic effect with eye position and not the amount of the prismatic effect, which is important when adapting to an anisometropic prescription. Henson and Dharamshi (1982) induced artificial anisometropia of 1.5, 3.0, and 4.5 D with a contact lens/spectacle combination. The subjects initially exhibited a phoria whose amount depended on eye position. After 2½ hours of binocular experience this incomitant phoria had largely disappeared for the two lower levels of anisometropia. There was a very low degree of adaptation to the induced imbalance of 4.5 D. Substantial neural compensation is suggested to occur above threshold for the anisometropic amblyope in the upper contrast range. Hess and Bradley (1980) show that the amblyope's performance in this range exceeds that obtained from simply blurring the image.

These results explain how some people with high degrees of anisometropia are able to manifest such remarkably good binocular vision with better than average stereoacuity and tolerate significant increases in their anisometropia. The gradual progression and occasional regression of anisometropia also explain why many researchers failed to find a significant correlation between the degree of anisometropia and the degree of binocularity or amblyopia.

——■————————————————————————————

SUMMARY

Anisomyopia is seldom outgrown and tends to increase into adulthood at approximately 0.05 D of difference per year. Using 2.00 D difference in the spherical equivalent refraction of the two eyes as a criterion for anisometropia, the relative prevalence of anisomyopia increases with age from about 20% of anisometropes at age 10 years or below to 75% at age 30 (see Figure 10.3). Progression rates, in both eyes, for adult anisomyopes exceed the 0.05 D per year reported by Goss et al. (1985) for adult isomyopes older than 18 years.

It is proposed that the development and advancement of anisomyopia could be explained by a small difference in intraocular growth/stretch rates. This is supported by a significant correlation of interocular progression rates between adolescent and adult phases of development. In addition, the residual aniseikonia accompanying optical correction of anisometropia can be accounted for by this stretch-deformation model. No doubt, many of the individual differences and resulting confusion in explaining anisomyopia depend on age of onset. For example, instances of late-onset (post-adolescence) anisomyopia would manifest few, if any, of the skeletal asymmetries that have been reported (Martinez 1977), whereas their alterations in axial length (Sorsby et al. 1962, van der Torren 1985) would be primarily a consequence of stretch rather than growth.

The advancement of anisometropia with age explains the clinical enigma associated with the patient who has an excellent quality of binocular vision in the presence of high anisometropia. These patients epitomize the amazing adaptability of the visual system's sensorimotor functions, as well as providing an insight into the retinal stretch that accompanies high myopia. However, despite this ability to adapt to the imposed influences of aniseikonia and differential prism, the conventional philosophy of recommending spectacles in anisometropia must be reviewed, for it appears that most anisometropes manifest less aniseikonia if their axial ametropia is corrected with contact lenses.

REFERENCES

Allen DC. Vertical prism adaptation in anisometropes. Am J Optom Physiol Opt 1974; 51:252.

Bennett AG. Optics of Contact Lenses, 4th ed. London: Association of Dispensing Opticians, 1974;57.

Blum H, Bettman J, Peters HB. Vision Screening for Elementary Schools: The Orinda Study. Berkeley: University of California Press, 1959.

Bonomi L, Mecca E, Massa F. Intraocular pressure in myopic anisometropia. Int Ophthalmol 1982;5:145–148.

Borish IM. Clinical Refraction, 3rd ed. Chicago: Professional Press, 1970;9, 63, 258.

Bradley A, Rabin J, Freeman RD. Nonoptical determinants of aniseikonia. Invest Ophthalmol Vis Sci 1983;24:507–512.

Charman WN. The accommodative resting point and refractive error. Ophthalmic Optn 1982;22:469–473.

Curtin BJ. The Myopias: Basic Science and Clinical Management. Philadelphia: Harper and Row, 1985.

Dobson V, Fulton AB, Manning K, et al. Cycloplegic refractions of premature infants. Am J Ophthalmol 1981;91:490–495.

de Vries J. Anisometropia in children: analysis of a hospital population. Br J Ophthalmol 1985;69:504–507.

Ebenholtz SM. Accommodative hysteresis: a precursor for induced myopia? Invest Ophthalmol Vis Sci 1983;24:513–515.

Fiorentini A, Maffei L, Pirchio M, Spinelli D. An electrophysiological correlate of perceptual suppression in anisometropia. Vis Res 1978;18:1617–1621.

Fledelius HC. Prevalence of astigmatism and anisometropia in adult Danes. With reference to presbyope's possible use of super market standard glasses. Acta Ophthalmol 1984;62:391–400.

Flom MC, Bedell HE. Identifying amblyopia using associated conditions, acuity, and nonacuity features. Am J Optom Physiol Opt 1985;62:153–160.

Friedman Z, Neumann E, Abel-Peleg B. Outcome of treatment of marked ametropia without strabismus following screening and diagnosis before the age of three. J Pediatr Ophthalmol Strabismus 1985;22:54–57.

Fulton AB, Dobson V, Salem D, et al. Cycloplegic refractions in infants and young children. Am J Ophthalmol 1980;90:239–247.

Fulton AB, Manning K, Salem D, et al. Cycloplegic refractions of premature infants. Am J Ophthalmol 1981;91:490–495.

Giles GH. The distribution of visual defects. Br J Physiol Opt 1950;7:179–208.

Goss DA, Winkler RL. Progression of myopia in youth: age of cessation. Am J Optom Physiol Opt 1983;60:651–658.

Goss DA, Erickson P, Cox VD. Prevalence and pattern of adult myopia progression in a general optometric practice population. Am J Optom Physiol Opt 1985;62:470–477.

Goodwin RT, Romano PE. Stereoacuity degradation by experimental and real monocular and binocular amblyopia. Invest Ophthalmol Vis Sci 1985;26:917–923.

Harwerth RS, Smith III EL. Binocular summation in man and monkey. Am J Optom Physiol Opt 1985;62:439–446.

Hendrickson P, Rosenblum W. Accommodation demand and deprivation in kitten ocular development. Invest Ophthalmol Vis Sci 1985;26:343–349.

Henson D, Dharamshi BG. Oculomotor adaptation to induced heterophoria and anisometropia. Invest Ophthalmol Vis Sci 1982;22:234–240.

Hess RF, Bradley A. Contrast perception above threshold is only minimally impaired in human amblyopia. Nature 1980;287:463–464.

Hirsch MJ. Visual anomalies among children of grammar school age. J Am Optom Assoc 1952;23:663–671.

Hirsch MJ. Anisometropia: a preliminary report of the Ojai longitudinal study. Am J Optom Arch Am Acad Optom 1967;44:581–585.

Ingram RM. Refraction of one year old children after atropine cycloplegia. Br J Ophthalmol 1979;63:343–347.

Ingram RM, Walker C. Refraction as a means of predicting squint or amblyopia in preschool siblings of children known to have these defects. Br J Ophthalmol 1979;63:238–242.

Ingram RM, Barr A. Changes in refraction between ages 1 and 3½ years. Br J Ophthalmol 1979;63:339–342.

Isenberg S, Urist MJ. Clinical observations in 101 consecutive patients with Duane's retraction syndrome. Am J Ophthalmol 1977;84:419–425.

Jampolsky A, Flom BC, Weymouth FW, Moses LE. Unequal corrected visual acuity as related to anisometropia. Arch Ophthalmol 1955;54:893–905.

Kehoe JC. Frequency of vertical anisometropia. Am J Optom Arch Am Acad Optom 1942; 19:1.

Kirkham TH. Anisometropia and amblyopia in Duane's syndrome. Am J Ophthalmol 1970; 69:774–777.

Kronfeld PC. The gross anatomy and embryology of the eye. In: Davson H, ed. The Eye, vol. 1. London: Academic Press, 1969;5–7.

Laatikainen L, Erkkila H. Refractive errors and ocular findings in school children. Acta Ophthalmol 1980;58:129–135.

Lebensohn JE. The management of anisometropia. Ear Nose Throat J 1957;36:4.

Lepard CW. Comparative changes in the error of refraction between fixing and amblyopic eyes during growth and development. Am J Ophthalmol 1975;80:485–490.

Mamedov MD. Binocular vision in uncorrected myopic anisometropia. Oftalmol Zh 1977; 32:285–289.

Martinez JB. The naso-pupillary distance in anisometropia. Arch Soc esp Oftal 1977; 37:923–934.

Mascie-Taylor CGN, MacLarnon AM, Lanigan PM, McManus IC. Foot-length asymmetry, sex and handedness. Science 1981;212:1416–1417.

Mayer DL, Fulton AB, Hansen RM. Preferential looking acuity obtained with a staircase procedure in pediatric patients. Invest Ophthalmol Vis Sci 1982;23:538–543.

Merriam WM, Forest DE, Helveston EM. Congenital blepharoptosis, anisometropia and amblyopia. Am J Ophthalmol 1980;89:401–407.

Morin JD, Bryars JH. Causes of loss of vision in congenital glaucoma. Arch Ophthalmol 1980;98:1575–1576.

O'Leary DJ, Millodot M. Eyelid closure causes myopia in humans. Experientia 1979; 35:1478.

O'Malley ER, Helveston EM, Ellis FD. Duane's retraction syndrome. J Pediatr Ophthalmol Strabismus 1982;19:161–165.

Ong, J, Burley WS. Effect of induced anisometropia on depth perception. Am J Optom Physiol Opt 1972;49:333–335.

Persson HE, Wanger P. Pattern-reversal electroretinograms in squint amblyopia, artificial anisometropia and simulated eccentric fixation. Acta Ophthalmol 1982;60:123–132.

Phillips CI. Strabismus, anisometropia and amblyopia. Br J Ophthalmol 1959;43:449.

Pratt SG, Beyer CK, Johnson CC. The Marcus Gunn phenomenon. A review of 71 cases. Ophthalmology 1984;91:27–30.

Rabin J, van Sluyters RC, Malach R. Emmetropisation: a vision-dependent phenomenon. Invest Ophthalmol Vis Sci 1981;20:561–564.

Rabin J, Bradley A, Freeman RD. On the relation between aniseikonia and axial anisometropia. Am J Optom Physiol Opt 1983;60:553–558.

Rosner J. Pediatric Optometry. Boston: Butterworth, 1982;344.

Sanfilippo S, Muchnick RS, Schlossman A. Preliminary observations on high anisometropia. Am Orthoptic J 1978;28:127–129.

Schapero M. Amblyopia. Philadelphia: Chilton Books, 1971.

Seniakina AS. Characteristics of refractogenesis and the development of acquired anisometropia. Oftalmol Zh 1979;34:7–11.

Silver HK, Kiyasu W, George J, Deamer WC. Syndrome of congenital hemihypertrophy, shortness of stature, and elevated urinary gonadotropias. Pediatrics 1953;12:368–376.

Simons K. Effects on stereopsis of monocular versus binocular degradation of image contrast. Invest Ophthalmol Vis Sci 1984;25:987–989.

Sorsby A, Leary GA, Richards MJ. The optical components in anisometropia. Vis Res 1962; 2:43–51.

Sorsby A. Modern Ophthalmology, vol. 3, Topical Aspects. London: Butterworths, 1972; 346–349.

Tanlamai T, Goss DA. Prevalence of monocular amblyopia among anisometropia. Am J Optom Physiol Opt 1979;56:704–715.

Till P. Anisometropia in congenital unilateral ptosis — a survey. Br Orthop J 1983;40:63–65.

Tredici TD, von Noorden GK. Are anisometropia and amblyopia common in Duane's syndrome? J Pediatr Ophthalmol Strabismus 1985;22:23–25.

van Alphen GWHM. Choroidal stress and emmetropization. Vis Res 1986;27:723–738.

van der Torren K. Treatment of amblyopia in strongly anisometropic eyes. Doc Opthalmol 1985;59:99–104.

von Noorden GK. Burian-von Noorden's binocular vision and ocular motility. St. Louis: CV Mosby, 1985.

Winn B, Ackerley RG, Brown CA, et al. The superiority of contact lens in the correction of all anisometropia. Trans Br Cont Lens Assc Annu Clin Conf 1986;95–100.

Zonis S, Miller B. Refraction in the Israeli newborn. J Pediatr Ophthalmol Strabismus 1974;2:77.

___11___

Optical Components Contributing to Refractive Anomalies

Paul Erickson

□

The human eye is an enclosed two-lens optical system that focuses light on its posterior inside surface (the retina). The eyeball is filled with an aqueous fluid whose optical density is slightly greater than that of water. At the eye's anterior surface is the cornea, a thin powerfully converging lens. Within the eye are an approximately circular aperture stop of variable diameter (the pupil) and a converging lens with variable power (the crystalline lens).

The unaccommodated eye tends to exhibit positive spherical aberration. As the eye accommodates by increasing the refracting power of the crystalline lens, spherical aberration shifts to become less positive or even negative. The magnitude of this aberration varies significantly among human eyes (Koomen et al. 1949, Ivanoff 1956). Other high-order monochromatic aberrations of the eye can be demonstrated (Howland and Howland 1976), although these off-axis effects are of little consequence in considering the refractive error of the eye. The eye also produces approximately 2 D of chromatic aberration across the visible spectrum (Wald and Griffin 1947).

In the unaccommodated emmetropic eye, parallel wavefronts of light incident on the cornea along the visual axis are brought into focus in the plane of the foveal retinal receptors. In myopia, parallel wavefronts are brought into focus anterior to the retina, and these wavefronts are again diverging at the retinal plane. Conversely, in hyperopia, parallel wavefronts are still converging at the plane of the retina. The astigmatic eye causes light to converge to two separate foci, either of which may be anterior or posterior to the retina. Thus the presence of astigmatism complicates the characterization of both the magnitude and the type of refractive error.

The refractive error is defined with the eye having its minimum possible refracting power; this is the case when the crystalline lens has assumed a configuration in which it makes minimal possible contribution to the refracting power of the eye.

Limiting consideration to paraxial optics eliminates concern over off-axis aberrations. The effects of spherical aberration can be controlled by the size of the pupil. For high spatial frequency targets, the subjective refraction is relatively insensitive to pupil diameters above 4 mm. However, for large diameters, the optimum refraction for high and low spatial frequencies can differ by 0.5 D (Green and Campbell 1965, Charman et al. 1978). For pupil diameters less than 3 mm, the increased depth of focus (Campbell 1957) diminishes the reliability of the subjective refraction.

A substantial variation in refractive error measurement will result as the spectral composition of the target is varied across the visible spectrum (Wald and Griffin 1947). In white light, for the purpose of refraction, the eye is assumed to respond as if the source were composed of energy at approximately 555 nm, the region of maximum sensitivity for photopic adaptation (Wald 1945). Under these conditions, Bedford and Wyszecki (1957) found that chromatic aberration is negligible for pupil diameters of 5 mm or less. If the eye is dark adapted, maximum sensitivity shifts to approximately 505 nm (Wald 1945). This can effect an apparent shift toward myopia of 0.25 D to 0.5 D.

O'Leary and Millodot (1978) demonstrated that the retinoscopic reflex has a specular and a diffuse component. The specular reflection occurs at the vitreous/retina surface (anterior to the receptors) and produces an objective measurement of refractive error that is approximately 0.4 D less myopic than the subjective refractive error. The diffuse reflection is produced in the vicinity of the pigment epithelium (posterior to the receptors). Thus it results in an objective refractive error very slightly more myopic than the subjective refraction. Through the first three decades, the specular portion predominates. As the eye ages, the diffuse reflection gains prominence, causing the discrepancy between objective and subjective measures of refractive error to diminish by approximately 0.1 D per decade (Millodot and O'Leary 1978).

The conditions under which the refractive error is defined are summarized in Table 11.1 in their approximate order of importance. The pupil size selected pro-

Table 11.1.   Conditions for Defining Refractive Error

Factor	Required condition
Eye	
Accommodation	Zero
Adaptation*	Photopic
Pupil diameter	3 to 4 mm
Target	
Spectral composition	White or 555 nm
Spatial composition*	30 cpd or greater

*Not required for objective measurement.
cpd = cycles per degree

vides insurance against contamination of measurements by aberrations without creating an excessive depth of focus. Note that although cycloplegia insures against accommodative artifacts, the accompanying pupillary mydriasis increases the risk of artifacts due to geometric aberrations.

THE COMPONENTS OF OCULAR REFRACTION

The components of refraction are those individual features of the eye whose collective optical properties alter the vergence of light to produce the refractive error. To understand the contributions of these elements, it is helpful to consider the eye as a system of coaxial spherical refracting surfaces (Duke-Elder and Abrams 1970). Each surface forms an interface between transparent media of different refractive index. By knowing the relative indices of refraction, the radii of curvature at these surfaces, and their position relative to the retina, the refractive error of the eye can be calculated.

Unfortunately, these values are not all as easily obtained as the refraction itself. An understanding of the methods and problems associated with measuring the components is essential in the interpretation of component data and their contributions to refractive errors.

□ Index of Refraction

It is generally assumed that physiologic variation of refractive indices for the transparent media of the eye is negligible. The validity of this assumption depends chiefly on intraspecies variation of the composition and concentration of substances dissolved in the ocular fluids and the proportional water content of the cornea and crystalline lens. The refractive index of the crystalline lens is heterogeneous, varying monotonically from its surface to its center. It is most optically dense in its center (the nucleus) and the least dense at its surface.

Whereas the refractive index of a homogeneous section of a transparent substance can be measured quite easily in vitro, no method is available to directly assess this property for the optical media of the living eye. Index values can be determined indirectly by calculation if measurements for all other component variables are known.

Fatt and Harris (1973) derived a relationship whereby a change in corneal thickness due to a change in its hydration could be used to calculate its refractive index. This function has value in assessing refractive changes due to edema.

Because of its optical complexity, characterization of the refractive index of the crystalline lens has been difficult, even in the laboratory. Early methods (Nakao et al. 1968, Philipson 1969) involved freezing and sectioning lens specimens. Campbell (1984) developed a nondestructive method for determining the refractive index distribution of the lens. Angular deviations of a laser beam were measured as they passed through successive transverse layers of the extracted whole lens. These data were then integrated to provide a continuous distribution for the indices of the lens. Variation in index for the surface layers of the specimens was less than 2%. Because the distribution of lens protein concentration appears to be closely related to refractive index distribution (Philipson 1969), refractive index distributions of the lens within a species should be similar to the same extent that protein concentrations are similar.

Nevertheless, the refractive indices of the optical media of the living eye remain essentially inaccessible to investigation. Their effects on the development of refractive error, although presumably minor, have not been documented.

☐ Radius of Curvature

An optically smooth surface produces specular reflection. This in turn results in images whose position and size can be used to calculate the radius of curvature of the surface. For optically transparent substances, the amount of light reflected is a function of the illumination and obliquity of the incident light and the refractive index differential at the surface. The reflected image at the cornea/air surface is easily discernible. Images reflected by the remaining surfaces are substantially dimmer and difficult to measure along the visual axis.

The curvature of the anterior corneal surface is usually measured with a keratometer. The other surface curvatures are usually determined from photographs of the reflected images. The underlying assumptions are that each surface is spherical or toroidal over the area measured, that the surfaces are coaxial to the visual axis, and that values for refractive indices used in the calculations are correct. The validity of these assumptions has been questioned (Ludlam and Wittenberg 1966, Ludlam 1967). Because the weaker reflected images cannot be viewed without oblique projection of the target, an unknown and potentially significant error in measurement can be expected due to oblique astigmatism at the measured and interposing surfaces. Ludlam (1967) suggested that errors up to 3.00 D could result from this factor.

Flaws in analytic methodology can also result in incorrect values for curvature measurements. Most biometric studies of the components of refraction have failed to analyze data by meridian (Ludlam and Wittenberg 1966), thus masking the effects of astigmatism and component toricity on refractive error. In addition, most of the curvature values reported in these studies were not independent measurements (Ludlam et al. 1965). Thus, errors in one measurement were propagated to subsequent measurements and calculations.

It has also been suggested that component curvature information could be derived from Scheimpflug photography or ultrasonic B-scan of the eye. Surface contours thereby obtained could be fit by circular templates (Hockwin et al. 1983) or mathematical curve-fitting routines (Fonda et al. 1982, Richards et al. 1988). Their results may be too coarse for refractive component analysis.

Brungardt (1975) noted that the *effective* curvature of the anterior corneal surface could be determined by refracting the eye with and without a rigid contact lens of known curvature and power in place. Unfortunately, this parsimonious technique is not readily applied to other refracting surfaces in the eye.

□ Axial Position

Several methods have been used successfully to determine axial positions of the components of refraction. Total axial length can be determined by taking advantage of the retinal phosphene to x-rays in the dark-adapted eye (Rushton 1938). This technique locates the position of the receptors themselves and requires no assumptions about the optical or sonic density of the ocular tissues. Reliability is not high, however, with the standard error expected to be 0.2 mm (Ludlam 1967).

Optical methods, such as optical pachometry, ophthalmophakometry, and Scheimpflug photography, make use of the diffuse reflection of light by cross sections of the cornea and crystalline lens. Standard principles of geometric optics and trigonometry are used to calculate surface positions from biomicroscopic images. These methods can locate the positions of the major refracting surfaces, but not that of the retina. The concerns noted previously for these techniques with regard to curvature apply here as well. Measurements are quite reliable, with an expected standard error of about 0.02 mm (Hockwin et al. 1983). Accuracy can be further enhanced by digitizing techniques (Richards et al. 1988).

A-scan ultrasonography has gained widespread clinical use in predicting appropriate intraocular lens power after cataract extraction. Reflections from the major ocular component surfaces, including the retina, can be generated with a 20 MHz transducer. The variable measured is time between reflections. Distance traversed is the product of time and acoustic velocity for the tissue traversed. Standard distance errors near 0.02 mm can be expected (Coleman 1979). Even greater reliability was reported for corneal thickness measurements (Ling et al. 1986).

In spite of this reliability, intraocular lens powers based on ultrasonic measurements of axial length have resulted in significant ametropias (greater than 2.00 D) in 10% of recipient eyes (Hoffer 1981a). These deviations from predictions have been attributed to erroneously short axial length measurements caused by corneal applanation (Oguchi et al. 1974, Hoffer 1981b) and unpredictable acoustic velocities in cataractous lenticular tissue (Coleman et al. 1977, Lindstrom et al. 1979). This uncertainty associated with acoustic velocity variance among individuals is analogous to that postulated for refractive index. Clearly, more information is needed on the distribution of acoustic velocities for the tissues of the eye. Nevertheless, ultrasonography is the most versatile and reliable method currently available for obtaining axial position data. In addition, these measurements are independent of those for other refractive parameters.

☐ Component Alignment

Wavefronts obliquely striking a spherical refracting surface will be brought to an astigmatic focus. Since the angles of incidence in both the tangential and sagittal planes are greater than when incidence is perpendicular, the effect is additional refracting power in all meridians. In the eye, this effect is present *paraxially* when a refracting surface is decentered with respect to the visual axis or is tilted from perpendicular to the axis. These special cases of oblique astigmatism are directly related by

$$d = r \sin \alpha \tag{1}$$

where r is the radius of curvature of the refracting surface, d is the lateral decentration of the visual axis from the optical axis of the surface, and α is the angle of tilt of the surface about its intersection with the visual axis.

This relationship can be verified by inspection of Figure 11.1. For large amounts of misalignment, this relationship breaks down, because the refracting surfaces of

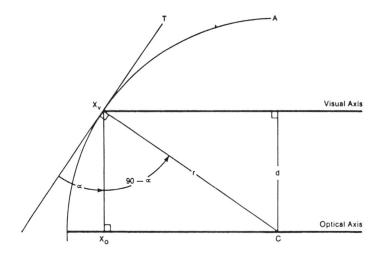

Figure 11.1. The relationship between oblique astigmatism due to lens tilt and that due to lateral decentration. Arc A is a spherical refracting surface of radius r whose center of curvature is at c. Line T is tangent to A at X_v, its intersection with the visual axis. Thus, A is tilted with respect to the visual axis by angle α. An arbitrary optical axis is selected parallel to the visual axis and displaced laterally by distance d. From triangle X_vX_oC, it can be seen that $\cos (90 - \alpha) = d/r$. Thus, $d = r \sin \alpha$.

the eye are aspheric, flattening in the periphery. Although this effect has long been identified as a source of refractive astigmatism in the crystalline lens (Tscherning 1890) and the cornea (Gullstrand 1966), it is not generally recognized that it also contributes to a more myopic refractive error.

ANALYSIS OF REFRACTIVE ERROR BY VARYING COMPONENTS

□ Previous Model Eyes

Previously proposed model eyes have varied greatly in complexity. Listing's reduced eye (Helmholtz 1924) was one of the least complicated, having only three component parameters; Lotmar's model eye (1971) sought to account for the aberrations of the eye; the large aperture model eye developed by Pomerantzeff et al. (1971) included sixteen parameters for the crystalline lens alone; and other models (Erickson 1978, Blaker 1980) incorporated features designed to analyze the component changes occurring during accommodation.

The most widely accepted model — the standard on which most subsequent model eyes have been based — is Gullstrand's "exact" schematic eye (1924). Values for the optical components of this eye are shown in Table 11.2. For this eye, Gullstrand specified both the radii and axial positions of the various refracting surfaces including front and back corneal surfaces and the surfaces of the lens cortex and nucleus, in addition to specifying indices of refraction for the cornea, aqueous, lens cortex and nucleus, and vitreous. Gullstrand also described a "simplified" schematic eye in which the cornea was defined as a single surface having a radius of curvature of 7.8 mm, and a single refractive index of 1.413 was used for the crystalline lens.

Whereas in a theoretical analysis the modeller can study the effects of the variation of any component, biometric data do not permit such an analysis. When dealing with actual eyes, the indices of refraction are not measured, and neither the cornea-aqueous surface nor the internal crystalline lens surfaces are generally evaluated. To account for these "missing values," several strategies may be used: Refractive indices are replaced by constants based on previously published information, functions can be derived that define the missing data in terms of measurable variables (as in the case of crystalline lens power), and the model can be simplified in such a manner that the missing values are not required.

In traditional model eyes, the refractive error and its components are described in terms of the principal points, the nodal points, and the focal points. Once defined, these cardinal points provide an efficient means for quantifying geometric image formation by the eye's optical system: Focal lengths and refracting power

Table 11.2.   Gullstrand's Schematic Eye

Indices of refraction		
Cornea	1.376	
Aqueous	1.336	
Lens Cortex	1.386	
Lens Nucleus	1.406	
Vitreous	1.336	

| Surface | Refractive surfaces | |
	Radius of Curvature (mm)	Axial Position (mm)
Air/cornea	7.7	0
Cornea/aqueous	6.8	0.5
Aqueous/lens cortex	10.0	3.6
Lens cortex/nucleus (ant.)	7.911	4.146
Lens nucleus/cortex (post.)	5.76	6.565
Lens cortex/vitreous	6.0	7.2
Retina	—	24.0

After Gullstrand A. Appendices to part I. In: Southall JPC, ed. Helmholtz's treatise on physiological optics, vol. 1. New York: Optical Society of America, 1924;261–282.

are defined relative to the calculated principal planes. Unfortunately, these traditional models are of limited use when dealing with ametropia: The positions of the principal planes vary from one eye to another and are not clinically determinable; refractive error is specified in reference to the spectacle plane or the corneal plane, neither of which can be directly derived from principal plane values; and the principal planes have different axial locations for the two principal meridians of an astigmatic eye.

COMPONENT ANALYSIS BASED ON CLINICAL MEASURES: A NEW APPROACH

The model proposed here has two important properties: (1) Axial positions are considered in terms of the actual optical surfaces rather than in terms of the car-

Table 11.3.   Basic Equations for Model Eye

Symbols	Subscripts
n = refractive index	o = air
r = radius of curvature	c = cornea
P = surface refractive power	l = crystalline lens
V = vergence exiting refracting surface	a = aqueous
t = intersurface distance (thickness, depth)	v = vitreous

Surface power equations	Reduced vergence equations
$P_{lv} = (n_l - n_v)/r_{lv}$	$V_{lv} = P_{lv} - n_v/t_v$
$P_{la} = (n_l - n_a)/r_{la}$	$V_{la} = P_{la} + n_l/(n_l/V_{lv} - t_l)$
$P_{ca} = (n_a - n_c)/r_{ac}$	$V_{ca} = P_{ca} + n_a/(n_a/V_{la} - t_a)$
$P_{co} = (n_c - 1)/r_{co}$	$V_{co} = P_{co} + n_c/(n_c/V_{ca} - t_c)$

After Erickson P. Mathematical model for predicting dioptric effects of optical parameter changes in the eye. Am J Optom Physiol Opt 1977;54:226–33.

dinal points of the system; and (2) light is considered to emanate from the retina, passing backward through the eye.

The desired properties can be achieved by a simple paraxial wavefront tracing model (Erickson 1977). The retinal fovea is treated as the real object to be imaged by the paraxial optics of the eye. The vergence of the emerging wavefronts at the anterior corneal surface is equivalent to the refractive state of the eye. The position at which these wavefronts come to focus in image space is equivalent to the far point of the eye. All refractive values are thus defined at, or referred to, a single invariant and clinically identifiable landmark; the paraxial apex of the cornea. Mathematically, this is accomplished by systematically calculating the reduced vergence of wavefronts emanating from the retinal object through to each optical surface in the model. The stepwise equations for these calculations are given in Table 11.3. The sign convention used requires that all values for radius, axial distance (thickness, depth), and refractive index be positive. The crystalline lens model shown in Table 11.3 is for a single index structure. The number of refracting surfaces in the model can be increased or decreased by adding or deleting a reduced vergence and a surface power equation for each surface added or deleted.

The quantity V_{co} is the refractive state of the eye. The quantity $-V_{co}$ is referred to as the refractive error. This value is measured clinically in the refraction. For refractive errors greater than 4 D, adjustments to the spectacle plane refractions are required when referring them to the corneal apex. This is accomplished by the formula

$$F_c = \frac{F_s}{1 - dF_s} \qquad (2)$$

where F_s is the spectacle plane refraction, d is the vertex distance, and F_c is the corneal apical plane refraction equivalent to $-V_{co}$.

To incorporate astigmatic surfaces, the wavefront trace is done in specific meridians. In those special cases where only one surface is astigmatic or where all astigmatic surfaces have common principal meridians, the trace is completed for the principal meridians. The two values for V_{co} thereby obtained can be converted directly to a standard form for expressing astigmatic refractive errors.

In the general case, the principal meridians of the various astigmatic refracting surfaces may all be different. Keating and Carroll (1976) showed that arbitrary meridians of the astigmatic eye can be treated as having a "refractive error" whose value is determined by the equation

$$P_\theta = P_s + P_c \sin^2 (\alpha - \theta) \qquad (3)$$

where P_s is the spherical refractive error (or surface power), P_c is the cylinder, α is the cylinder axis, and θ is any arbitrary meridian.

Brubaker et al. (1969) showed that knowledge of this value in any three meridians is theoretically sufficient to calculate the astigmatic refractive error of the eye in standard form. Improved analyses of this technique were subsequently made by Long (1974) and Worthey (1977).

The preceding equation can also be applied to individual astigmatic surfaces. By calculating meridional surface power for each of at least three selected meridians for each refracting surface in the eye, then tracing wavefronts separately along those meridians, a meridional refraction for the eye can be calculated. This technique is explained elsewhere in more detail along with a computing algorithm for performing the tedious calculations (Erickson 1981). Each meridional trace provides a value for refractive error referred to the corneal apex. The results are equally valid for astigmatism due to surface toricity or to component misalignment.

To incorporate misalignment of spherical surfaces into the model, separate calculations for the sagittal and tangential meridians must be made (Morgan 1978). The sagittal image vergence, V_s', is determined by

$$V_s' = K + V_s \qquad (4)$$

where V_s is the object vergence obliquely striking the sagittal meridian of the refracting surface, and

$$K = \frac{n' \cos\alpha' - n \cos\alpha}{r}. \tag{5}$$

where n is the refractive index of object space, r is the surface radius of curvature, and α is the angle of incidence of the chief ray. In the case of a tilted surface, α is the angle of tilt, n' is the refractive index of image space, and α' is the angle of refraction of the chief ray where

$$n \sin\alpha = n' \sin\alpha'. \tag{6}$$

The tangential image vergence, V_t', is found by

$$V_t' = \frac{K + V_t \cos^2\alpha}{\cos^2\alpha'} \tag{7}$$

where V_t is the tangential object vergence. Where required, vergence values for other meridians can be calculated using the same series of equations (Erickson 1981).

□ Effects of Component Variation

The model described in Table 11.3 was used to study the effects of variation in component values on refractive error. Specific component parameters were varied from the baseline values listed in Table 11.2. Resultant refractive errors were computed for the model eye. All results are reported as changes in refractive error compared to the slightly hyperopic baseline refraction. Negative changes indicate increased myopia. Positive changes indicate increased hyperopia.

□ Refractive Index

The effects of small (0.1%) and large (1%) changes in the refractive indices of the model are shown in Table 11.4. For example, the small increase in corneal index was from the 1.376 baseline to 1.377. The large increase was to 1.390.

This analysis suggests that refractive error is somewhat insensitive to variation in the refractive indices of the cornea and lens cortex. It is quite sensitive to variation in the lens nucleus and vitreous, however, which could confound analysis of the refractive components. The extent of this problem is unknown because information on the physiologic variability of these parameters is not available.

The effects of refractive index change on the refracting power of a thin optical element are relatively independent of the indices of adjacent media (Erickson

Table 11.4. Effects of Refractive Index Change on Refractive Error*

Medium	Percent change			
	−1.0	−0.1	+0.1	+1.0
Cornea	−0.18	−0.02	+0.02	+0.17
Aqueous	+0.81	+0.08	−0.08	−0.82
Anterior lens cortex	−0.24	−0.02	+0.02	+0.23
Lens nucleus	+2.74	+0.28	−0.28	−2.81
Posterior lens cortex	−0.20	−0.02	+0.02	+0.19
Vitreous	−1.72	−0.17	+0.17	+1.67

*In diopters.

1977). Thus, elements such as the cornea and lens cortex, whose physical forms in air are diverging lenses, show increased minus power in air and less plus in situ as their refractive indices increase. In the eye, this results in reduced refracting power.

□ Axial Positions of Refracting Surfaces

The effects on refractive error of small (0.1 mm) changes in axial position of the refracting surfaces of the eye are shown in Table 11.5. They demonstrate the importance of precisely defining component changes when assessing their effects on refraction. It is not uncommon, for example, to see decreases in anterior chamber depth stated to result in decreased hyperopia or increased myopia (e.g., Grosvenor 1987). This assumption is probably attributable to a potentially misleading consideration of the equivalent power of the eye. If the eye is considered a two-lens system, its equivalent power is determined by

$$F_e = F_c + F_1 - t\,F_c F_1 \tag{8}$$

where F_c and F_l are equivalent powers of the cornea and crystalline lens, respectively, and t is the separation between the equivalent lenses.

Because F_c and F_l are both positive, F_e decreases as t increases. Since t is analogous to anterior chamber depth, this analysis suggests that increasing it will increase hyperopia or decrease myopia.

As seen in Table 11.5, the concept of increasing anterior chamber depth is ambiguous as it pertains to refractive error. For a given axial length, moving the lens away from the cornea, thereby increasing anterior chamber depth, results in less

Table 11.5. Effects of Axial Position Change on Refractive Error

Variable increased by 0.1 mm	Method of increase	Accompanying increase in axial length (mm)	Change in refractive error (D)
Anterior chamber depth	Change in cornea position	0.1	−0.14
	Change in lens position	0	+0.13
Vitreous chamber depth	Change in retina position	0.1	−0.28
	Change in lens position	0	−0.13
Crystalline lens thickness	Into anterior chamber	0	−0.04
	Into vitreous chamber	0	+0.09
	No change in chamber depth	0.1	−0.18
Cornea thickness	Into anterior chamber	0	−0.03
	Anterior surface displacement	0.1	−0.17

myopia. If chamber depth increases by growth of the cornea away from the lens, myopia increases. Both changes result in the same equivalent power for the eye.

The same considerations are required when evaluating refractive effects of cornea and lens thickness changes. Anteriorward corneal thickening causes significant increases in myopia. Posteriorward thickening has a negligible effect on refractive error. In the crystalline lens, anteriorward thickening increases myopia, whereas posteriorward thickening decreases myopia. These changes can be qualitatively viewed as simple effectivity changes. If increased lens thickness is associated with greater axial length, as it might be in comparing two eyes, thickness is directly related to myopia.

Changes in vitreous chamber depth can be seen to be highly effective in modifying refractive error. Note that under all of these conditions, equivalent power calculations for the individual elements will give ambiguous information with regard to refractive error.

It should also be emphasized that although all surface position changes that result in increased axial length will be accompanied by increased myopia, the magnitude of the effect depends highly on the component involved. This suggests that undifferentiated axial length values are unjustifiably imprecise gauges of refractive error mechanisms. By emphasizing surface position as a component attribute, the ambiguities described here can be avoided.

□ Component Misalignment

The effects of component misalignment are illustrated in Figure 11.2. The meridian of greatest increase in myopia — that forming the tangential focus — is perpendicular to the meridian about which the refracting surface is tilted or coinci-

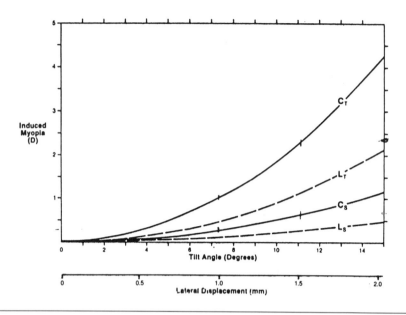

Figure 11.2. Myopia due to oblique astigmatism induced by tilting of the crystalline lens (*L*) and tilting or displacement of the cornea (*C*). The tangential refractive error is denoted by the subscript *T*, sagittal refractive error by the subscript *S*. The scale for displacement applies only to the cornea.

dent to the meridian along which it is displaced. The meridian of least increase in myopia, that forming the sagittal focus, is perpendicular to the tangential meridian.

In terms of refractive error in minus cylinder form, the induced sagittal error is equivalent to the sphere. The cylinder is equal to the difference between sagittal and tangential errors. The minus cylinder axis is in the sagittal meridian. For example, if the cornea is displaced 1 mm nasally, the induced myopia is -0.25 D -0.75 D $\times$ 90 degrees. If the crystalline lens is tipped forward 11 degrees, the induced myopia is -0.25 D -0.87 D $\times$ 180 degrees.

☐ Astigmatism

Because no one value describes the refractive error of the astigmatic eye, the analysis of its components is generally either complicated or compromised. The analysis may be reduced to a single variable for refractive error by averaging the refractive errors of the principal meridians (the spherical equivalent) or by restricting consideration to a particular principal meridian. Alternately, astigmatic eyes might be eliminated entirely from the analysis. The latter two approaches are most likely to bias component and refractive error distributions and their interpretation. The use of spherical equivalents has obvious advantages when the principal meridians of astigmatic surfaces are not orthogonal.

When refractive error changes embody mechanisms that are manifested meridionally, however, a meridional analysis of data is essential.

—— ■ ————————————————————————————————————

COMPONENT CHANGES IN MYOPIA PROGRESSION

Juvenile myopic progression has generally stabilized by age 16, although there is considerable variation in the pattern and rate (Goss and Winkler 1983). In Table 11.6, some reported component changes during juvenile development have been linearized to show the hypothetical effects on the development of myopia.

This example illustrates how an eye might become *more* myopic during development. The absolute magnitude of myopia is also a function of initial component values that could predispose a more myopic refractive error (Leary 1981, Erickson 1984) as shown in Figures 11.3 and 11.4. If the axial positions of the refracting surfaces are held constant, steeper curvatures and surface misalignment will always be associated with greater myopia. If surface curvatures are held constant, axial positions farther from the retina will always be associated with greater myopia.

Table 11.6. Hypothetical Component Changes in Myopic Progression

Component	Approximate annual change	Effect on refractive error (annual)
Corneal power	−0.02 D*	+0.02 D
Anterior chamber depth	−0.01 mm†	−0.01 D
Crystalline lens power	−0.18 D*	+0.14 D
Vitreous chamber depth	+0.15 mm*	−0.42 D
Net effect		−0.27 D

Values derived from:
*Sorsby A et al. Refraction and its components during growth of the eye from the age of three. Medical Research Council Special Report No. 301. London: H.M. Stationary Office, 1961.
†Fontana ST, Brubaker RF. Volume and depth of the anterior chamber in the normal aging human eye. Arch Ophthalmol 1980;98:1803–1808.

Higher amounts of myopia are usually associated with larger increases in vitreous chamber depth (Sorsby et al. 1961). For every 1 mm increase in chamber depth, myopia increases by 2.00 to 3.00 D (Figure 11.3). This relation is not linear. As vitreous chamber depth continues to increase, the rate of myopic increase diminishes. This nonlinearity can be demonstrated by comparing the chamber depth and refractive status scales on Figure 11.4.

Meridional changes in refractive error must involve mechanisms other than the axial length components. Such changes can usually be attributed to changes in corneal toricity (Goss and Erickson 1987), but could also be caused by realignment of the eye's refractive components, changes in the toricity of the crystalline lens, or the onset of inhomogeneities in refractive index of the ocular media. The closer to the retina that these changes occur, the less effect they have on the refractive error. For example, a 1.00 D change in the cylindrical power of the crystalline lens results in an astigmatic refractive error change of approximately 0.75 D

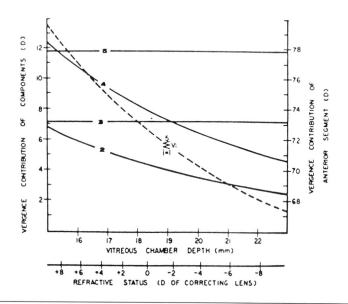

Figure 11.3. Vergence contributions in diopters (left scale) of the components of the anterior segment as a function of vitreous chamber depth. Components are identified as follows: 1 = corneal power, 2 = anterior chamber vergence change, 3 = anterior lens surface power, 4 = lens thickness vergence change, 5 = posterior lens surface power. The right scale applies to the combined vergence contribution of the anterior segment (dotted line). (Reprinted by permission of the publisher from Erickson P. Complete ocular component analysis by vergence contribution. Am J Optom Physiol Opt 1984;61:469–472. © The Am Acad of Optom 1984.)

Figure 11.4.
Contributions of the components as a percentage of the total contribution of the anterior segment. Component numbers are as in Figure 11.3. (Reprinted by permission of the publisher from Erickson P. Complete ocular component analysis by vergence contribution. Am J Optom Physiol Opt 1984;61:469–472. © The Am Acad of Optom 1984.)

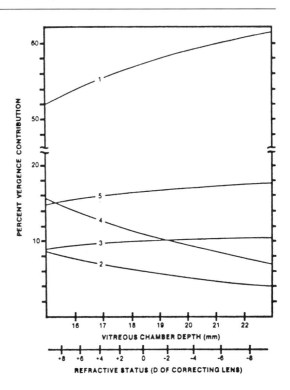

(Erickson 1978). A 1.00 D change in corneal toricity, on the other hand, is manifested as a 1.00 D change in astigmatism. This effectivity applies to spherical curvature changes as well.

CONCLUSION

Evaluation of the refractive components requires a mathematical model and system of analysis that preserves the optical characteristics of the components as they actually function in contributing to the refractive error of the eye. The model described in this chapter meets those requirements. It avoids weaknesses of other models that incorporate cardinal point calculations and a mixed metric of linear and reciprocal variables. The results presented emphasize the need for precisely defining the components and the changes they exhibit in the development of refractive errors.

■

REFERENCES

Bedford RE, Wyszecki G. Axial chromatic aberration of the human eye. J Opt Soc Am 1957;47:564–565.

Blaker JW. Toward an adaptive model of the human eye. J Opt Soc Am 1980;70:220–223.

Brubaker RF, Reineke RD, Copeland JC. Meridional refractometry. I. Derivation of equations. Arch Ophthalmol 1969;81:849–852.

Brungardt TF. K readings versus valid corneal curvature values. J Am Optom Assoc 1975; 46:230–233.

Campbell FW. The depth of field of the human eye. Optica Acta 1957;4:157–164.

Campbell MCW. Measurement of refractive index in an intact crystalline lens. Vis Res 1984;24:409–415.

Charman WN, Jennings JAM, Whitefoot H. The refraction of the eye in relation to spherical aberration and pupil size. Br J Physiol Opt 1978;32:78–93.

Coleman DJ. Ultrasonic measurement of eye dimensions. In: Dallow RL, ed. Ophthalmic Ultrasonography: Comparative Techniques. Boston: Little, Brown, 1979.

Coleman DJ, Lizzi FL, Jack RL. Ultrasonography of the Eye and Orbit. Philadelphia: Lea & Febiger, 1977.

Duke-Elder S, Abrams D. Ophthalmic optics and refraction. In: Duke-Elder S, ed. System of Ophthalmology. St. Louis: CV Mosby, 1970;V:96.

Erickson P. Mathematical model for predicting dioptric effects of optical parameter changes in the eye. Am J Optom Physiol Opt 1977;54:226–233.

Erickson P. Crystalline lens position and accommodative efficiency. Am J Optom Physiol Opt 1978;55:571–575.

Erickson P. An algorithm for computing astigmatic refractive errors from ocular parameters. Am J Optom Physiol Opt 1981;58:155–158.

Erickson P. Complete ocular component analysis by vergence contribution. Am J Optom Physiol Opt 1984;61:469–472.

Fatt I, Harris MG. Refractive index of the cornea as a function of its thickness. Am J Optom Arch Am Acad Optom 1973;60:383–386.

Fonda S, Salvadori B, Vecchi D. Analytic reconstruction of the human cornea by means of a slit lamp and digital picture processing. In: von Bally G, Greguss P, eds. Optics in Biomedical Sciences. New York:Springer-Verlag, 1982;221–224.

Fontana ST, Brubaker RF. Volume and depth of the anterior chamber in the normal aging human eye. Arch Ophthalmol 1980;98:1803–1808.

Goss DA, Erickson P. Meridional corneal components of myopia progression in young adults and children. Am J Optom Physiol Opt 1987;64:475–481.

Goss DA, Winkler RL. Progression of myopia in youth: age of cessation. Am J Optom Physiol Opt 1983;60:651–658.

Green DG, Campbell FW. Effect of focus on the visual response to a sinusoidally modulated spatial stimulus. J Opt Soc Am 1965;55:1154–1157.

Grosvenor T. Reduction in axial length with age: an emmetropizing mechanism for the adult eye? Am J Optom Physiol Opt 1987;64:657–663.

Gullstrand A. Appendices to part I. In: Southall JPC, ed. Helmholtz's Treatise on Physiological Optics, vol. I. New York: Optical Society of America, 1924;261–482.

Gullstrand A. Photographic-ophthalmometric and clinical investigations of corneal refraction. Ludlam WM trans. Am J Optom Arch Am Acad Optom 1966;43:143–197.

Helmholtz H von. The dioptrics of the eye. In: Southall JPC, ed. Helmholtz's Treatise on Physiological Optics, vol. I. New York: Optical Society of America, 1924;57–260.

Hockwin O, Weigelin E, Laser H, Dragomirescu V. Biometry of the anterior eye segment by Scheimpflug photography. Ophthalmic Res 1983;15:102–108.

Hoffer KJ. Accuracy of ultrasound intraocular lens calculation. Arch Ophthalmol 1981a; 99:1819–1823.

Hoffer KJ. Intraocular lens calculation: the problem of the short eye. Ophthalmic Surg 1981b;12:269–272.

Howland B, Howland HC. Subjective measurement of high-order aberrations of the eye. Science 1976;193:580–582.

Ivanoff A. About the spherical aberration of the eye. J Opt Soc Am 1956;46:901–903.

Keating MP, Carroll JP. Blurred imagery and the cylinder sine-squared law. Am J Optom Physiol Opt 1976;53:63–69.

Koomen M, Tousey R, Scolnik R. The spherical aberration of the eye. J Opt Soc Am 1949; 39:370–376.

Leary GA. Ocular component analysis by vergence contribution to the back vertex power of the anterior segment. Am J Optom Physiol Opt 1981;58:899–909.

Lindstrom RL, Lindstrom CW, Harris WS. Accuracy of lens implant power determination using A-scan. Contact Intraocular Len Med J 1979;5:61–66.

Ling T, Ho A, Holden BA. Method of evaluating ultrasonic pachometers. Am J Optom Physiol Opt 1986;63:462–466.

Long WF. A mathematical analysis of multimeridional refractometry. Am J Optom Physiol Opt 1974;51:260–263.

Lotmar W. Theoretical eye model with aspherics. J Opt Soc Am 1971;61:1522–1529.

Ludlam WM. Human experimentation and research on refractive state — an evaluation of in vivo ocular component metrology. In: Hirsch MJ, ed. Synopsis of the Refractive State of the Eye. A Symposium. Minneapolis: Burgess Publishing Co., 1967;13–25.

Ludlam WM, Wittenberg S. Measurements of the ocular dioptric elements utilizing photographic methods. Pt II. Cornea — theoretical considerations. Am J Optom Arch Am Acad Optom 1966;43:249–267.

Ludlam WM, Wittenberg S, Rosenthal J. Measurements of the ocular dioptric elements utilizing photographic methods. Pt I. Errors analysis of Sorsby's photographic ophthalmophakometry. Am J Optom Arch Am Acad Optom 1965;42:394–416.

Millodot M, O'Leary D. The discrepancy between retinoscopic and subjective measurements: effect of age. Am J Optom Physiol Opt 1978;55:309–316.

Morgan MW. The Optics of Ophthalmic Lenses. Chicago: Professional Press, 1978.

Nakao S, Fujimoto S, Nagata R, Iwata K. Model of refractive-index distribution in the rabbit crystalline lens. J Opt Soc Am 1968;58:1125–1130.

Oguchi Y, van Balen ATM. Ultrasonic study of the refraction of patients with pseudophakos. Ultrasound Med Biol 1974;1:267–273.

O'Leary D, Millodot M. The discrepancy between retinoscopic and subjective refraction: effect of light polarization. Am J Optom Physiol Opt 1978;55:553–556.

Philipson B. Distribution of protein within the normal rat lens. Invest Ophthalmol Vis Sci 1969;8:258–270.

Pomerantzeff O, Fish H, Govignon J, Schepens CL. Wide angle optical model of the human eye. Ann Ophthalmol 1971;3:815–819.

Richards DW, Russell SR, Anderson DR. A method for improved biometry of the anterior chamber with a Scheimpflug technique. Invest Ophthalmol Vis Sci 1988;29:1826–1835.

Rushton RH. The clinical measurement of the axial length of the living eye. Trans Ophthalmol Soc UK 1938;58:136–142.

Sorsby A, Benjamin B, Sheridan M, Stone J, Leary GA. Refraction and its components during growth of the eye from the age of three. Medical Research Council Special Report No. 301. London: H.M. Stationary Office, 1961.

Tscherning M. Étude sur la position du cristallin de l'oeil humain. In: Javal E, ed. Memoires d'Ophthalmometrie. Paris: Masson Publishers, 1890.

Wald G. Human vision and the spectrum. Science 1945;101:653–658.

Wald G, Griffin DR. The change in refractive power of the human eye in dim and bright light. J Opt Soc Am 1947;37:321–336.

Worthey JA. Simplified analysis of meridional refraction data. Am J Optom Physiol Opt 1977;54:771–775.

__12_____

Optical Adaptations of the Vertebrate Eye

Jacob G. Sivak

☐

The vertebrate eye is a sophisticated optical instrument that appeared after millennia of evolutionary development. Its optical components (cornea, lens, and humors) transmit and focus light energy on a photosensitive transducing element, the retina. The last two decades have witnessed an asymptotic increase in the number of studies addressing various aspects of visual science, and considerable progress in understanding the molecular and neural events associated with photochemistry and neural processing has taken place. However, much less attention has been paid to the eye's optical performance, especially to questions relating optical adaptations to evolutionary development. At the same time, there has been a marked increase in interest in experimentally produced refractive error, especially myopia.

Theories concerning a possible relationship between environmental factors such as nearwork (reading and writing) and the development of myopia are not new, dating back at least to Donders (1864). The nearwork hypothesis has been the most prominent and controversial approach of the past century. Numerous studies carried out by a variety of workers, using either human epidemiologic data or experimental methods involving nonhuman primates, have attempted to relate myopia to prolonged attention to the near visual field (see Baldwin 1981, Goss and Criswell 1981, and Criswell and Goss 1983 for comprehensive reviews).

The more recent experimental work dealing with myopia can be characterized as involving (1) more direct manipulation of the visual environment, including study of such factors as form vision deprivation (for example, Wiesel and Raviola 1977, 1979), increased body temperature (Maurice and Mushin 1966, Lauber et al. 1980) and increased intraocular pressure (Maurice and Mushin 1966, Lauber et al. 1961); (2) more attention to the immediate postnatal period of ocular development; and (3) a broader range of vertebrates, including birds (e.g., Bercovitz et

The author's research reported in this review was supported by the Natural Sciences and Engineering Research Council of Canada.

al. 1972, Wallman et al. 1978, Yinon et al. 1980, Hodos and Kuenzel 1984) and a wide variety of nonprimate mammals (Tokoro 1970, Rose et al. 1974, Sherman et al. 1977). This diversity of approach and developmental interest makes it important to appreciate the normal refractive diversity of the vertebrate eye. The discussion that follows reviews the effects of two prime environmental factors, terrestrial vs aquatic life and nocturnal vs diurnal vision, on visual optics. In addition, because of interest in the possible role of accommodation in the development of myopia (for example, Young 1963, Greene 1980), a brief review of current views on vertebrate accommodative mechanisms will be included.

VISUAL OPTICS IN WATER AND AIR

The cornea is a relatively thin, avascular, transparent structure consisting of two curved and fairly parallel surfaces. Its refractive function depends on the existence of media of unequal refractive index in front and in back — a condition met when the eye is in air but not when it is in water (Figure 12.1). Clearly, the aquatic

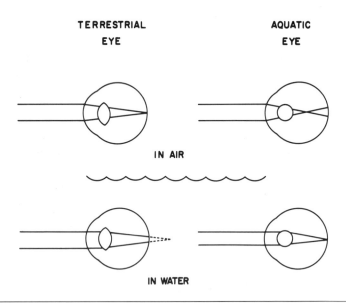

Figure 12.1. Schematic representation of the optical effect of air on an aquatic eye and the effect of water on an aerial eye. (Reproduced with permission from Sivak 1988.)

habitat of ancestral vertebrates limited the original function of the cornea to that of a transparent window.

Present day aquatic species, be they fishes or aquatic mammals (sirenians, cetaceans) possess a spherical or nearly spherical crystalline lens of high refractive index (an equivalent index of 1.65 is commonly quoted for fish; Walls 1942, Kreuzer and Sivak 1984). Underwater the lens is the only refractive structure of the eye. The typical aquatic cornea has a relatively flat shape, presumably an adaptation related to the need for streamlining body shape in a dense medium such as water (Jamieson 1971). The variety of accommodative mechanisms described or suggested for aquatic vertebrates always involve lens movement (Beer 1894, Franz 1934, Walls 1942, Sivak 1980).

When the cornea is exposed to air, as in the case of vertebrate evolution to a terrestrial life-style, it often becomes the dominant refractive element, simply due to the substantial refractive index difference between air and the aqueous humor of the eye. In addition, the radius of curvature of the terrestrial cornea is relatively short, often shorter than that of the globe as a whole, as in humans. This factor may be related to the need for a significant arched configuration to maintain a smooth refractive surface in air. Whatever the reason, it adds to the refractive importance of this structure.

The crystalline lens, on the other hand, is in an optically more difficult position. That the lens is a cellular ectodermal structure located within the eye and that new growth takes place around the equator throughout life mean that older tissue is compressed toward the center rather than being disposed of. These factors have enormous consequences in terms of physical changes associated with presbyopia and cataract. It is appropriate to note that the lens, which never stops developing, is one of the first structures of the body to show significant loss of function with age. An additional and related point is that the lens must have an elevated refractive index in order to function as a refractive element within the fluid-filled eye, presumably by maintaining one of the highest protein concentrations of any bodily tissue (Spector 1982).

The spherical shape and even higher refractive index of the fish lens is indicative of an impressive biologic and optical achievement. The equatorial location of new lens growth, as well as the fact that lens cells must taper anteriorly and posteriorly in order to articulate with the tips of adjacent cells, makes it reasonable to expect the lens to assume a more elliptical shape as it grows (Figure 12.2). Indeed, this is the common developmental description of the human lens (Scammon and Hesdorffer 1937, Duke-Elder 1958, Tripathi and Tripathi 1983), and no other explanation for lens shape is given. How the fish lens maintains the spherical shape of the embryonic nucleus is a mystery.

There are numerous examples in the comparative literature indicating that lens shape is in fact determined by the overall refractive needs of the species. Perhaps the most obvious example is the change in shape of the amphibian lens during metamorphosis (Figure 12.3) from aquatic larvae to terrestrial forms (Sivak and Warburg 1980, 1983, Sivak et al. 1985b). These studies examine the rate and

A   B   C

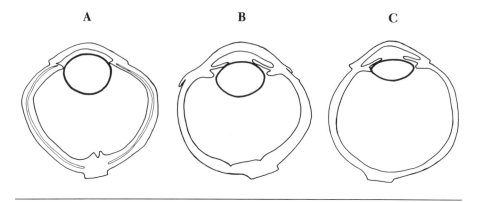

Figure 12.2.   Drawings of the human eye A, at 5 months of embryo development; B, at birth; C, as an adult. (Reproduced with permission from Sivak and Dovrat 1984.)

extent of ocular metamorphic change in five species with widely varying life histories. Ocular effects and, in particular, lens shape changes were found from measurements of gross anatomy at various metamorphic stages using a freeze-sectioning technique. In addition, refractive states were measured retinoscopically in air and water.

The results (Sivak and Warburg 1980, 1983; Sivak et al. 1985b) show that the larval eye is aquatic in form in all species. The lens is spherical or nearly so in shape, and it is in close proximity to the relatively flat cornea (Figure 11.3). There is no obvious optical difference between larval amphibian eyes and those of a typical fish. However, the adults of the same species show widely varying metamorphic change, both in rate and extent of change. For example, the lens of the toad *Pelobates syriacus* is flattened (equatorial diameter 21% greater than axial), and the eye is subject to a long (20-week) metamorphic period. By comparison, the lens of the bullfrog (*Rana catesbeiana*) is less flattened in the adult (12.5%), but the change takes place over a short 24-hour period just before the animal moves on to land. A similar rapid change is found in *Salamandra salamandra*. In *Notophthalmis viridescens*, a urodele that undergoes a second metamorphosis back to water after a land period, the lens changes shape twice (spherical – flattened – spherical). Finally, in the clawed frog (*Xenopus laevis*), which remains aquatic as an adult, the lens maintains its spherical shape.

As already noted, the mechanism of lens shape variation is not known. It may be due entirely to new lens growth, as brought about by a temporary increase in the rate of equitorial cell mitosis, or it may be the result of a change in volume and configuration of existing cells. The fact that the adult lens of certain species is not larger than that of the larval form supports the latter explanation or possibly a combination of both.

This discussion has emphasized metamorphic lens change because the change from spherical to nonspherical shape is very obvious. However, such changes are

Figure 12.3. Frozen sections of the eyes and head of a larval (top) and adult (bottom) amphibian (*Salamandra salamandra*). Note change in shape of lens. (Reproduced with permission from Sivak and Warburg 1980.)

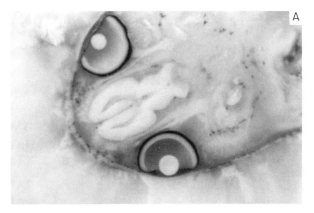

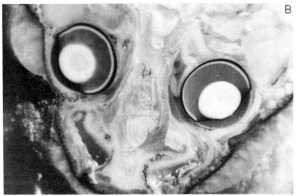

accompanied by change in corneal curvature, anterior chamber depth, and lens-to-retina distance. In other words, the entire refractive plan of the eye is altered. What triggers these changes? What molecular growth factors are responsible, and how are messages related to growth disseminated to the various ocular tissues involved? How are changes to the various optical parameters of the eye integrated?

NOCTURNAL VS DIURNAL VISION

The foregoing description draws attention to two refractive considerations. First, the principal optical problem faced by the vertebrate eye during its evolution was the change from life in water to life in air. Second, the refractive components of the eye are adjusted to suit the refractive needs of the animal in question. This approach assumes a uniform interest in having a sharply focused image fall on the retinas of the eyes of all vertebrates. The duplex nature of the human eye offers a clue to the contrary, for the refractive performances of nocturnal visual systems may differ extensively from those of diurnal ones. Whereas acute resolution ability is of prime importance in the latter, sensitivity to low light levels is the primary concern of the former. It may not be a serious overgeneralization to state that adaptations that enhance visual acuity, be they optical or neural, reduce sensitivity and vice versa (Franz 1934, Walls 1942). The rat eye, for example, may be characterized as having a large, almost spherical, lens with a relatively small vitreal chamber (Powers and Green 1978, Gur and Sivak 1979). Corneal radius of curvature is relatively large, and the corneal arch occupies close to 50% of the circumference of the whole eye (Figure 12.4). These adaptations are believed to enhance the light-gathering ability of the eye (Walls 1942). However, the optical performance of the eye and lens is poor when measured by such parameters as spherical aberration or ganglion cell response to retinal defocus (Powers and Green 1978, Campbell and Hughes 1981, Sivak et al. 1983). Postnatal measurements indicate that the lens at birth is similar to that of diurnal species in terms of shape and control of spherical aberration. However, it rapidly assumes the characteristics of the adult after birth (Sivak and Dovrat 1984). At birth, for example, the difference between axial and equatorial lens diameters is about equal to that of a newborn human. However, the rat lens becomes much more spherical after birth, and, as in adults, the lens occupies most of the intraocular space by 16 days. Furthermore, the lens of the newborn rat is relatively free of the large negative spherical aberration found in adult lenses. Large amounts of negative spherical aberration appear 5 days after birth.

It is pertinent to note that Walls (1942) referred to an indifference to optical quality in an effort to explain the hyperopia reportedly noted in measurements of refractive state of small-eyed mammals. It is also useful to point out that the mammals, as a vertebrate class, first developed during the Triassic period, the golden age of the dinosaurs. The earliest mammals are believed to have been nocturnal secretory species, a trait still characteristic of the group today (Romer 1970). With a few exceptions, such as the ground squirrels, truly diurnal forms did not appear until the evolution of the higher primates. Mammalian nocturnality is characterized visually by the predominance of all rod or nearly all rod retinas, poor resolution ability, poor image-forming ability, the common existence of a tapetum, and the absence or near absence of an effective accommodative mechanism. Refractive comparisons between the human eye and common laboratory species, such as rats, cats, and rabbits, must take this factor into account. Thus, two studies dealing with the optical performance of the small eye of the ground squirrel show little or no evidence of the hyperopia normally associated with other small-eyed mammals (Gur and Sivak 1979, McCourt and Jacobs 1984). In both studies, refractive measures, as well as the electrophysiologic response of retinal ganglion cells to grating targets, indicate near emmetropia. Refractive state may not only be related to eye size per se, but also to whether the animal is nocturnal or diurnal (Glickstein and

Figure 12.4. Frozen section of the eye of a nocturnal mammal (rat — top) and a diurnal mammal (ground squirrel — bottom). Note relative difference in size, shape, and location of lens. (From Gur and Sivak 1979. © The Am Acad of Optom 1979. Reprinted by permission.)

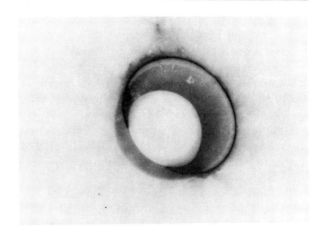

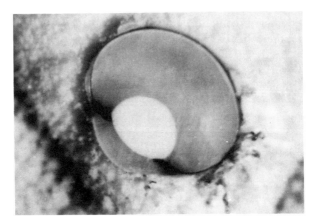

Millodot 1970). Although not as obvious as the mammal example, all vertebrate classes show this dichotomous relationship.

ACCOMMODATION

Accommodation has been referred to in two contexts: First, aquatic vertebrates accommodate by means of lens movement. Second, accommodation is an ocular feature that is associated with diurnal vision. In fact, ocular accommodation is a prominent example of convergent evolution.

The wide variety of accommodative adaptations may be summarized from past and recent surveys as follows (Walls 1942, Duke-Elder 1958, Sivak 1980): The teleosts, or modern bony fishes, which form the majority of aquatic vertebrate species, accommodate by moving the rigid spherical lens toward the retina by means of an autonomically innervated ectodermal muscle. The size and direction of movement can be related to diet and feeding behavior (Tamura 1957, Sivak 1973). Nocturnal species, such as bullheads, show little or no accommodative response.

Additional mechanisms proposed for lens movement in lampreys (Franz 1932), sharks (Franz 1931) and dolphins (Herman et al. 1975) remain speculative and unconfirmed. Similarly, the question of amphibian accommodation is a matter of uncertainty.

The peak of accommodative development among species with aerial vision appears in reptiles (lizards) and birds. In brief, the force of contraction of a large striated ciliary muscle is transmitted directly to the lens by means of a series of morphologic adaptations, including an annular lens pad, which increases lens equatorial diameter; large ciliary body folds; and an obvious corneoscleral indentation or sulcus, which is maintained by a ring of scleral ossicles (Figure 12.5).

An exaggerated form of accommodation takes place in certain diving birds as a means of compensating for the refractive neutralization of the cornea when the eye enters water (Levy and Sivak 1980, Sivak et al. 1985a). In these instances, the effect of ciliary muscle contraction is augmented by contraction of the iris sphincter, a massive striate muscle in diving species. The result is the formation of an anterior lenticonus of very short radius of curvature (Figure 12.5). Certain authors have implicated both the cornea and the lens in avian accommodation (for exam-

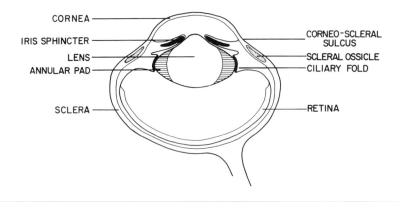

Figure 12.5. Drawing of avian intraocular morphology and lens shape with accommodation in certain aquatic species. (Reproduced with permission from Sivak 1988.)

ple, Gundlach et al. 1945). However, recent work with pigeons (Levy 1979) and chickens (Sivak et al. 1985a) does not support the view that the cornea participates in accommodation. Further, new data suggest that avian accommodation decreases with age (Sivak et al. 1986). Presumably this is due to the same cause as human presbyopia, that is, age-related change in mechanical properties of the crystalline lens (Weale 1962).

The nocturnal preferences of ancestral and most living mammals have already been noted. The diminished importance of acute resolution ability is reflected in the appearance of a less effective accommodative mechanism. The principal difference is that the ciliary body and the lens are not in direct contact with each other. The effect of ciliary muscle contraction is transmitted indirectly to the lens via the suspensory ligaments by a process still not completely understood. It is interesting to note that vestigial remnants of the scleral ossicles are found in the eyes of monotremes, the most primitive group of living mammals (Walls 1942).

Current understanding of human accommodation is based on the writing of Helmholtz (1855), Fincham (1937), Weale (1962), and Fisher (1969, 1971). Briefly, the effect of ciliary muscle contraction is to relax the tension exerted by the suspensory ligaments on the lens. The ensuing change in lens shape, involving mainly its anterior surface, depends on the elastic properties of the acellular lens capsule and the lens itself. More recently, Rafferty and Scholz (1985) have described a network of actin filaments in the apical area of lens epithelial cells. It is suggested that the epithelial cells of the lens may be contractile.

Walls' emphasis on the evolutionary relation between mammalian and reptilian accommodation is supported by the results of studies dealing with the anatomy and physiology of the ciliary muscle. An electron microscopic examination of the human ciliary muscle (Ishikawa 1962) reveals many striate muscle characteristics. These include an organized relationship between myofilaments and the presence of numerous motor nerve endings and cell organelles (mitochondria, endoplasmic reticulum). According to Ripps et al. (1962), the functional organization of the ciliary muscle of the cat is of the type associated with striate muscle. The muscle is organized in discrete motor units rather than as a syncytium. Interruption of a proportion of ciliary nerves results in an equal proportion of loss of accommodation. Westheimer and Blair (1973) show that the motor pathway to the ciliary muscle (monkey) is not interrupted by a synapse in the ciliary ganglion (Figure 12.6). Thus, messages from the central nervous system travel directly to the muscle in the manner characteristic of somatomotor organization. Although this last conclusion is still being disputed (Ruskell and Griffiths 1979), there is no question that the neuromuscular organization of the accommodative apparatus of higher mammals is somewhat between conventional smooth and striate descriptions.

Although it is commonly assumed that the human accommodative mechanism is representative of all mammals (for example, Tansley 1965), the comparative literature in this area is sparse and contradictory. Substantial amounts of accommodation (10.00 D or more) are typically found only in humans or other primates. In the rodents, as exemplified by the rat, a ciliary muscle is absent or underde-

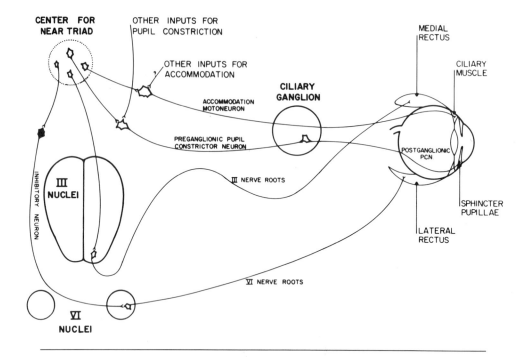

Figure 12.6. Motor pathways subserving accommodation, pupil constriction, and convergence. (Reproduced with permission from Westheimer and Blair 1973.)

veloped and accommodation is not considered to exist (Lashley 1932, Hughes 1977). Nor has an accommodative response been confirmed in the rabbit (Meyer et al. 1972). Accommodation appears to be absent in hoofed mammals (Walls 1942, Duke-Elder 1958), although a well-developed ciliary muscle has been noted to exist (Woolf 1956) and small variations in refractive state (about 1.00 D) noted over time (Sivak and Allen 1975).

The cat has received considerable attention because of its popularity as an experimental animal. However, the results of several studies are variable and indicate accommodative ranges from 2.00 D (Hess and Heine 1898, Ripps et al. 1962) to 15.00 D (Hartridge and Yamada 1922, Lovasik 1979). A growing body of evidence indicates that the accommodative ability of the cat involves lens movement rather than change in shape (Vakkur and Bishop 1963, Lovasik 1979), and this view is supported by Fisher (1971) who notes that measurements of cat (and rabbit) lens polar elasticity preclude the possibility of shape change. This point warrants intensive investigation, for confirmation of an accommodative change in lens position will indicate a greater diversity of adaptive visual development than previously considered.

Accommodative data for other nonprimates include ranges such as 3.00 D for a large-eyed bat, the flying fox (Murphy et al. 1983), and 2.00 D for ground squirrels (Gur and Sivak 1979). The latter is a very diurnal animal and some accommodation is to be expected. Data on the Indian mongoose, another diurnal species, shows up to 12.00 D of accommodation (Nellis et al. 1989).

Otters are believed to be capable of the large amounts of accommodation needed to counteract the neutralization of the cornea in water, presumably using the iris and ciliary body, as described previously for certain aquatic birds (Walls 1942). Such a mechanism would be a major departure from the typical mammal eye. Behavioral measures with otters show that visual acuity in air and water are equal (Schusterman and Barret 1973). Anatomical and optical data also indicate that otters are capable of extraordinary amounts of accommodation (Ballard et al. 1989). This review of vertebrate accommodation emphasizes the diversity of mechanisms and the danger of generalizing from one species to another, even those within a single class.

■

SUMMARY AND CONCLUSIONS

The effects of two prime environmental factors, terrestrial vs aquatic life and nocturnal vs diurnal vision, on the refractive make-up of the vertebrate eye have been described. Whereas the cornea is normally the main refractive structure of the terrestrial eye it is of little or no refractive importance when the eye is in water. As a result, the terrestrial eye differs morphologically and physiologically from its aquatic precursor. For example, the latter has a spherical lens of high refractive index, whereas the lens of a terrestrial eye is elliptical in shape and softer in consistency.

Good resolving power is important to diurnal vision, but sensitivity to low light levels is the primary concern in nocturnal conditions. Adaptations that enhance visual acuity, be they optical or neural, reduce sensitivity and vice versa. The rat eye for example, may be characterized as having poor resolving power, a large, nearly spherical, lens with substantial amounts of spherical aberration, a cornea with relatively large radius of curvature, and the virtual absence of an accommodative mechanism.

Vertebrate accommodative mechanisms differ widely, in terms of both mechanism and efficiency. Lens motion, as exemplified by the accommodative response of teleost fishes, is the mechanism common to aquatic species, and a change in lens shape describes the usual terrestrial mode of accommodation. Accommodation in terrestrial species usually involves the contraction of a mesodermal ciliary muscle. However, the effect of the ciliary muscle may be direct or indirect, depending on whether the ciliary body and lens are in contact.

The extensive optical diversity of the vertebrate eye described in the preceding sections is a fine example of evolutionary adaptation to differing needs. Put simply, each species has an eye that is of maximum advantage to its own survival. The principal reason for reviewing this diversity is to emphasize the difficulty that can arise from anthropocentric generalizations based on human perceptions of the nature of refractive anomalies. After all, experimental myopia research is generated by human interest in what is perceived as a human malfunction, namely myopia. It is tempting to suggest, in the comparative context, that myopia may be a desirable condition in certain cases.

Myopia may be defined as an ocular refractive condition in which a point in space between optical infinity and the eye in question is in conjugate focus with the retina. In fact, myopia was considered a standard refractive condition in fish by Beer (1894) and Walls (1942) to explain the accommodative mechanism of this group. Because the direction of accommodative lens movement is toward the retina and because the distance light travels in water is restricted, it seemed reasonable to expect myopia in the unaccommodated state and a refractive shift toward emmetropia with accommodation. More recent studies show that accommodative lens motion and refraction in fish are quite variable in terms of visual direction and, therefore, a single characteristic refractive description is not possible (Sivak 1980). Nevertheless, the refractive direction of accommodative change is opposite to that of the human eye, and the existence of alternative evolutionary approaches should be considered.

Some of the questions that those interested in myopia should examine have already been mentioned in the context of optical adaptations during normal ocular development. For example, how is lens size and shape controlled, and what molecular or subcellular mechanism is used to bring about such changes? Similar questions can be considered in terms of corneal growth and development.

How messages about the need for refractive change are delivered and interpreted is the overriding question. Is retinal defocus, as in the case of a formerly aquatic amphibian that has metamorphosed and has become exposed to air, the stimulus for such change; or do alterations in the optical structure of the eye anticipate behavioral ones? If the retina is the source of information about optical performance, what are the afferent and efferent paths of this mechanism? Why does a poorly focused image stimulate ocular growth and produce myopia (Hodos and Kuenzel 1984)?

Accommodation may play a key role as the source of information about optical performance, at least in those species within which accommodation is appreciable in size. Accommodation and myopia have been considered in terms of mechanical stress on the lens and globe (Greene 1980). However, a study by Harkness (1977) demonstrates that the state of accommodation is used as a distance cue in chameleons, a species with a well-developed striate ciliary muscle. Accommodation may also signal a lack of sufficient ocular refractive power with resulting change in rate of growth of the lens and globe. An excessive or aberrant amount of accommodation could in turn result in excessive ocular growth (Wallman et al. 1981).

This review has emphasized the diverse optics found among vertebrates and the need to understand this diversity when comparing experimental results from one species to another. This does not rule out the possibility that the same underlying molecular events that lead to myopia are fundamental to all species.

REFERENCES

Baldwin WR. A review of statistical studies of relations between myopia and ethnic behavioral and physiological characteristics. Am J Optom Physiol Opt 1981;58:516–527.

Ballard KA, Sivak JG, Howland HC. Intraocular muscles of the Canadian river otter and Canadian beaver and their optical function. Can J Zool 1989;67:469–474.

Beer T. Die Accommodation des Fischanges. Pfluegers Arch 1894;58:523–650.

Bercovitz AB, Harrison PC, Leary GA. Light induced alterations in growth pattern of the avian eye. Vis Res 1972;12:1253–1259.

Campbell MCW, Hughes A. An analytic gradient index schematic lens and eye for the rat predicts aberrations for finite pupils. Vis Res 1981;21:1129–1148.

Criswell MH, Goss DA. Myopia development in nonhuman primates — a literature review. Am J Optom Physiol Optics 1983;60:250–268.

Donders FC. On the Anomalies of Accommodation and Refraction of the Eye. London: New Sydenham Society, 1864.

Duke-Elder S. System of Ophthalmology, vol. I. The Eye in Evolution. London: Henry Kimpton, 1958.

Fincham EF. The Mechanism of Accommodation. Br J Ophthalmol (Suppl 8) 1937;1–40.

Fisher RF. The significance of the shape of the lens and capsular energy changes in accommodation. J Physiol 1969;201:21–47.

Fisher RF. The elastic components of the human lens. J Physiol 1971;212:147–180.

Franz V. Die Akkommodation des Selachieranges und seine Abblendrungsapparate, nebst Befunden an der Ritina. Zool Jarb Abt Allegm Zool Physiol Tiere 1931;49:323–462.

Franz V. Auge und Akkommodation von Petromyzon (Lampreta) fluviatilis. L Zool Jahrb Abt Allegm Zool Physiol Tiere 1932;52:118–178.

Franz V. Vergleichende Anatomie des Wirbeltierauges. In: Bolk L, Goppert E, Kallius E, Lubosch W, eds. Handbuch der vergleichende Anatomie der Wilbeltiere, vol. 2, Part III. Berlin: Urban Schwartzenberg, 1934;989–1292.

Glickstein M, Millodot M. Retinoscopy and eye size. Science 1970;168:605–606.

Goss DA, Criswell MH. Myopia development in experimental animals — a literature review. Am J Optom Physiol Opt 1981;58:859–869.

Green PR. Mechanical considerations in myopia. Relative effects of accommodation, convergence, intraocular pressure and the extraocular muscles. Am J Optom Physiol Opt 1980;58:528–535.

Gundlach RH, Chard RD, Skahen JR. The mechanism of accommodation in pigeons. J Comp Physiol Psychol 1945;38:27–42.

Gur M, Sivak JG. Refractive state of the eye of a small diurnal mammal: the ground squirrel. Am J Optom Physiol Opt 1979;56:689–695.

Harkness L. Chameleons use accommodation cues to judge distance. Nature 1977; 267:346–349.

Hartridge H, Yamada K. Accommodation and other optical properties of the eye of the cat. Br J Ophthalmol 1922;6:481–492.

Helmholtz H. Uber die Akkommodation des Auges. Albrecht v. Graefes Arch Ophthalmol 1855;1:1–14.

Herman LM, Peacock MF, Yunker MP, Madsen CJ. Bottlenosed dolphin: double slit pupil yields equivalent aerial and underwater diurnal acuity. Science 1975;189:650–652.

Hess C, Heine L. Arbeiten aus dem gebiete der accommodations lahre. Arch Ophthalmol 1898;46:243–276.

Hodos W, Kuenzel WJ. Retinal-image degredation produces ocular enlargement in chicks. Invest Ophthalmol Vis Sci 1984;25:652–659.

Hughes A. The topography of vision in mammals of contrasting lifestyle: comparative optics and retinal organization. In: Crescitelli F, ed. Handbook of Sensory Physiology, vol. VII/5 The Visual System in Vertebrates. Berlin: Springer Verlag, 1977;613–756.

Ishikawa T. Fine structure of the human ciliary muscle. Invest Ophthalmol Vis Sci 1962; 1:587–608.

Jamieson GS. The functional significance of corneal distortion in marine mammals. Can J Zool 1971;49:421–423.

Kreuzer RO, Sivak JG. Spherical aberration of the fish lens: interspecies variation and age. J Comp Physiol 1984;154:415–422.

Lashley KS. The mechanism of vision. V. The structure and image-forming power of the rat's eye. J Comp Physiol Psychol 1932;13:173–200.

Lauber JK, Schutze JV, McGinnis J. Effects of exposure to continuous light on the eye of the growing chick. Proc Soc Exp Biol Med 1961;106:871–872.

Levy B. A study of the accommodative mechanisms in four avian species. Master's Thesis, University of Waterloo, Waterloo, Ontario, Canada, 1979.

Levy B, Sivak JG. Mechanisms of accommodation in the bird eye. J Comp Physiol 1980; 137:267–272.

Lovasik J. Neural control of mechanisms of ocular accommodation in cat. Ph.D. dissertation, University of Waterloo, Waterloo, Ontario, Canada, 1979.

Maurice DM, Mushin AS. Production of myopia in rabbits by raised body temperature and increased IOP. Lancet 1966;2:1160–1162.

McCourt ME, Jacobs GH. Refractive state, depth of focus and accommodation of the eye of the California ground squirrel. (*Spermophilus beecheyi*). Vis Res 1984;24:1161–1266.

Meyer DL, Meyer-Haame S, Schaeffer KP. Electrophysiological investigation of refractive state and accommodation in the rabbit's eye. Pflugers Arch 1972;332:80–86.

Murphy CJ, Howland HC, Kwiecinski GG, et al. Visual accommodation in the flying fox (*Pteropus giganteus*). 1983;23:617–620.

Nellis DW, Sivak JG, McFarland WN, Howland HC. Characteristics of the eye of the Indian mongoose (*Herpestes auropunctatus*). Can J Zool 1989;67:2814–2820.

Powers MK, Green DG. Single retinal ganglion cell responses in the dark-reared rat: grating acuity, contrast sensitivity and defocusing. Vis Res 1978;18:1533–1539.

Rafferty NS, Scholz DL. Identification of actin filaments in the polygonal arrays in intact rabbit lens epithelial cells. Invest Ophthalmol Vis Sci (Suppl) 1985;26:162.

Ripps H, Siegel IM, Getz WB. Functional organization of ciliary muscle in the cat. Am J Physiol 1962;203:851–859.

Romer AS. The Vertebrate Body. Philadelphia: WB Saunders, 1970.

Rose L, Yinon U, Belkin M. Myopia induced in cats deprived of distance vision during development. Vis Res 1974;14:1029–1032.

Ruskell GL, Griffiths T. Peripheral nerve pathway to the ciliary muscle. Exp Eye Res 1979; 28:277–284.

Scammon RE, Hesdorffer MB. Growth in mass and volume of the human lens in post-natal life. Arch Ophthalmol 1937;17:104–112.

Schusterman RJ, Barret B. Amphibious nature of visual acuity in the Asian "clawless" otter. Nature 1973;244:518–519.

Sherman SM, Norton TT, Casagrande VA. Myopia in the lidsutured tree shrew (*Tupaia glis*). Brain Res 1977;114:154–157.

Sivak JG. Interrelation of feeding behavior and accommodative lens movements in some species of North American freshwater fishes. J Fish Res Bd Can 1973;13:1141–1146.

Sivak JG. Accommodation in vertebrates: a contemporary survey. In: Zadunaisky JA, Davson H, eds. Current Topics in Eye Research, vol. 3. New York: Academic Press, 1980; 281–330.

Sivak JG. Optics and diversity of eyes in vertebrates. In: Atema J, Fay RR, Popper AN, eds. Sensory Biology of Aquatic Animals. New York: Springer Verlag, 1988.

Sivak JG, Allen DB. An evaluation of the "ramp" retina of the horse eye. Vis Res 1975; 15:1353–1356.

Sivak JG, Dovrat A. 1984. Early postnatal development of the rat lens. Exp Biol 1984; 43:57–65.

Sivak JG, Warburg M. Optical metamorphosis of the eye of *Salamandra salamandra*. Can J Zool 1980;58:2059–2064.

Sivak JG, Warburg M. Changes in optical properties of the eye during metamorphosis of an anuran, *Pelobates syriacus*. J Comp Physiol 1983;159:329–332.

Sivak JG, Gur M, Dovrat A. Spherical aberration of the lens of the ground squirrel. (*Spermophilis tridecemlineatus*). Ophthalmol Physiol Opt 1983;3:261–265.

Sivak JG, Hildebrand T, Lebert C. Magnitude and rate of accommodation in diving and non-diving birds. Vis Res 1985a;25:925–933.

Sivak JG, Levy B, Weber AP, Glover RF. Environmental influence on shape of the crystalline lens: the amphibian example. Exp Biol 1985b;44:29–40.

Sivak JG, Hildebrand TE, Lebert CG, et al. Ocular accommodation in chickens: corneal vs. lenticular accommodation and effect of age. Vis Res 1986;26:1865–1872.

Spector A. Aging of the lens and cataract formation. In: Sekuler R, Kline D, Dismukes K, eds. Aging and Human Visual Function. New York: Alan R Liss, 1982;27–43.

Tamura T. A study of visual perception in fish especially on resolving power and accommodation. Bull Jpn Soc Scient Fish 1957;22:536–557.

Tansley K. Vision in Vertebrates. London: Chapman and Hall, 1965.

Tokoro T. Experimental myopia in rabbits. Invest Ophthalmol Vis Sci 1970;9:926–934.

Tripathi RC, Tripathi BJ. Lens morphology, aging and cataract. Gerontology 1983;38: 258–270.

Vakkur GJ, Bishop PO. The schematic eye of the cat. Vis Res 1963;3:357–381.

Wallman J, Turkel J, Trachtman J. Extreme myopia produced by modest change in early visual experience. Science 1978;201:1249–1251.

Wallman J, Rosenthal D, Adams JJ, et al. Role of accommodation and developmental aspects of experimental myopia in chicks. In: Fledelius HD, Alsbirk, Goldschmidt E, eds. Doc Ophthalmol Proc Series 28. The Hague: W. Junk, 1981;197–206.

Walls GL. The Vertebrate Eye and its Adaptive Radiation. Bloomfield Hills, Mich: Cranbrook Institute of Science, 1942.

Weale RA. Presbyopia. Br J Ophthalmol 1962;46:660–668.

Westheimer G, Blair SM. The parasympathetic pathways to internal eye muscles. Invest Ophthalmol Vis Sci 1973;12:193–197.

Wiesel TN, Raviola E. Myopia and eye enlargement after neonatal lid fusion in monkeys. Nature 1977;266:66–68.

Wiesel TN, Raviola E. Increase in axial length of the macaque monkey eye after corneal opacification. Invest Ophthalmol Vis Sci 1979;18:1232–1236.

Woolf D. A comparative cytological study of the ciliary muscle. Anat Rec 1956;124:145–163.

Yinon U, Rose L, Shapiro A. Myopia in the eye of developing chicks following monocular and binocular lid closure. Vis Res 1980;20:137–141.

Young FA. The effect of restricted visual space on the refractive error of the young monkey eye. Invest Ophthalmol Vis Sci 1963;2:571–577.

__13

Normal and Induced Myopia in Birds: Models for Human Vision

William Hodos, A.L. Holden,
F.W. Fitzke, B.P. Hayes,
and J.C. Low

☐

There has been considerable interest in animal studies of myopic growth. Yinon (1984) has summarized the literature on avian models. In the newly hatched chick, myopia can be produced rapidly as a consequence of lid suture or after wearing simple visual occluders. Study of the avian eye has several advantages: Vision in birds is a subject of wide neurobiologic interest; birds are highly visual animals, making use of acute spatial vision (in the control of flight and in feeding) and are thus likely to be well suited to cast light on the notion that retinal image quality can regulate eye growth. Further, experiments on normal and experimentally modified eye growth can be carried out over a short time period in numbers sufficient to test a variety of mechanistic hypotheses of neurobiologic and ophthalmic relevance. Our studies of the pigeon (*Columba livia*) and the chick (*Gallus domesticus*) are presented in more detail elsewhere (Fitzke et al. 1985a, 1985b; Hodos et al. 1985; Hayes et al. 1986).

LOWER-FIELD MYOPIA IN THE PIGEON

In human vision, fine details of the visual world are gained only at the fovea. In a panoramic visual system, such as that of the pigeon's, detailed vision is provided

We are grateful for financial support from The Moorfields Eye Hospital, The National Eye Institute (United States), The Royal Society, and The Smith, Kline and French Foundation; for technical assistance from F.H. Sheen, P. West, and D. Goulding; and for the statistical advice of P.K. Clark.

over a wide expanse of visual space. Cell densities remain high over considerable areas of the retina (Pumphrey 1961, Hayes 1982), and there is relatively little decline in acuity passing from the laterally directed optical axis to the frontal periphery (Ulrich 1982). It is interesting to compare the organization of a panoramic and a foveocentric eye. When the pigeon is walking or feeding, it has to view the nearby ground and food, while at the same time remaining visually alert to distant predators and alarm signals.

We report electrophysiological evidence for a regional refractive adaptation in the visual field of the pigeon. Below the horizon, the photoreceptors are near conjugate with the ground. At and above the horizon, the eye is near emmetropic. Nearby and distant objects (on the ground and above the horizon) are seen simultaneously in focus.

The literature contains persistent suggestions of sectorial variations in the refractive state of the pigeon's eye (Catania 1964, Millodot and Blough 1971, Nye 1973, Erichsen 1979), with the frontal visual field specialized for near vision (myopic) and the lateral visual field specialized for distance vision (emmetropic). Only the study of Erichsen (1979) has measured refractive state across wide angles in the visual field with retinoscopy. However, off-axis retinoscopy is an extremely difficult technique. Further, the hypermetropic artifact of retinoscopy (Glickstein and Millodot 1970) varies with eccentricity and precludes absolute measurements of refractive state.

We used an alternative technique to refract the eye, which is objective, can provide absolute readings, and refracts the photoreceptor plane. We have recently developed a Maxwellian-view optometer, using Scheiner's principle (Westheimer 1966, Emsley 1952), where defocus of a grating stimulus is accompanied by lateral image shift. Figure 13.1 shows schematically the optical design of the optometer. The light sources are two light-emitting diodes, S1 and S2, which are driven in counterphase. L1 is a collimating lens, and L2 is the final Maxwellian-view lens. A grating stimulus is carried in the field stop FS and can be moved axially by a micrometer. S1 and S2 are imaged in the pupil plane of the eye (PP). The grating is imaged on the retina. When the grating is at the first principal focus of L2, it is conjugate with the photoreceptors if the eye is emmetropic. If the eye is myopic, the grating becomes conjugate with the photoreceptors at a position closer to the final lens, and this distance from the first principal focus is proportional to refractive error. When the grating is out of focus at the photoreceptors, alternation between the sources S1 and S2 results in image shift on the retina. We detect the response to image shift as a small, focal, electroretinogram (ERG), after averaging. When the grating is conjugate with the photoreceptors, the ERG is minimal, ideally dropping to the level of residual noise. Typically, residual noise is 0.28 μV, SD 0.13 μV. As defocus is introduced, the averaged responses rise on each side of this minimum. A refractive run is carried out by averaging the ERG with a range of optometer settings. The profile is fitted with a V-shaped function to determine the minimum point, which corresponds to the refractive state, as illustrated in Figure 13.2. Repeating such runs provides a measure of the accuracy of the refraction: Three to six repetitions can result in standard errors of the mean

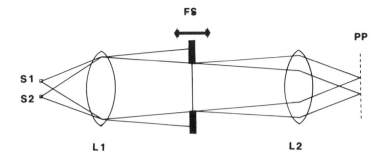

Figure 13.1. Optical design of the maxwellian-view optometer. S1 and S2 are the light sources, two light emitting diodes, driven by counterphase square-waves, and equated in luminance. L1 is a collimating lens. L2 is the final Maxwellian-view lens. A grating stimulus is carried in the field stop FS and can be moved axially by a micrometer. The grating subtends 27 degrees of visual angle. The sources are imaged in the pupil-plane (PP), and the grating is imaged on the retina.

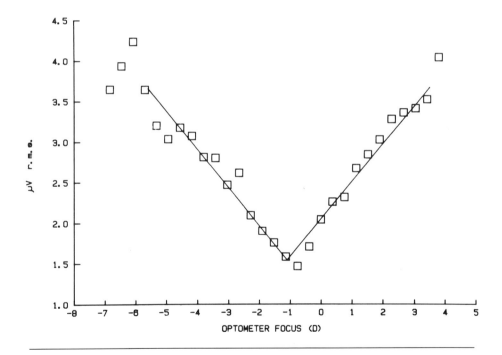

Figure 13.2. Refractive profile of the pattern-shift electroretinogram. The root mean square RMS response amplitude is plotted as a function of optometer focus. The stimulus was a bar grating of spatial frequency 1.47 cycles/degree, subtending 27 degrees of visual angle in maxwellian view. The V-shaped function, whose reflection point gives the refractive state of the retinal photoreceptors, is fitted by computer.

of 0.2 to 0.4 D. In all experiments the beak tip was positioned 35 degrees below
the pupil center, as this head orientation is used in walking and in flight (Hodos
et al. 1984).

The mean refractive state in the lateral field, on the horizon (azimuth 90 degrees), was +0.013 D, SD 0.97, n = 76. This is not significantly different from
emmetropia when Student's *t*-test is applied. All refractive runs taken along the
horizon were also essentially emmetropic. Vertical cuts through the visual field
were made at azimuths 35, 65, and 90 degrees to sample the visual field symmet-
rically in front of and behind the optical axis. The results in each azimuth were
markedly similar and are combined in Figure 13.3. Above the horizon, all refractions are within 2.00 D of emmetropia, and are well fitted by a straight line of
zero slope. Thus, the upper visual field is emmetropic. Below the horizon, however, is a marked deviation from an "all-emmetropic" eye. Refractive states move
to more myopic values at lower elevations.

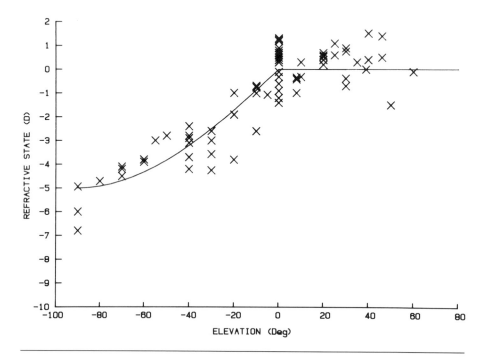

Figure 13.3. Refractive state (D) as a function of elevation in the visual field
of the pigeon. The continuous line from elevation − 90 degrees to elevation
0 degrees (from the ground vertically below the eye to the horizon) is the best-
fitting sine function, and corresponds to an eye where the pupil-center is 20
cm above the ground. The photoreceptors in the upper retina are conjugate
with the ground plane.

Why should this be so? The effect is not due to astigmatism, which we have measured in control experiments, nor can it be due to any aberration of the eye symmetric about the optical axis. We tested the idea that the eye is adapted to be focused on the ground when the bird is walking. This would require lower field myopia to follow a sine curve, with maximal myopia at an elevation of −90 degrees, moving to emmetropia at the horizon. Such a curve is shown in Figure 13.3 as the continuous line. Sine curves were fitted to the data by computer, minimizing the mean squared error for successive values of a parameter H, which was the eye-to-ground distance. The best-fitting value of H was 20 cm. The eye-to-ground distance in ten pigeons, was 18.6 cm, SD 1.93 cm. Although the bird can adopt a range of raised or crouched postures, the agreement of eye-to-ground distance appears reasonable, and suggests that the photoreceptors in the upper retina are conjugate with the ground, for the frontal, axial, and lateral visual field.

Our findings show that there is a regional variation in refractive state in the pigeon eye, with a graded myopia in the lower visual field, and an emmetropic horizon and upper visual field. We find that the eye is emmetropic in frontal vision at and above the horizon (that is, 35 degrees above the eye-beak axis). Because the pigeon flies and walks with its beak held 35 degrees down (Hodos et al. 1984), forward vision is subserved by an emmetropic sector of the visual field. In frontal vision the eye must be emmetropic in the upper part of its binocular field (Martin and Young 1983, Martinoya et al. 1981), and myopic in the lower part. Figure 13.4 shows diagrammatically how this lower field myopia brings the ground con-

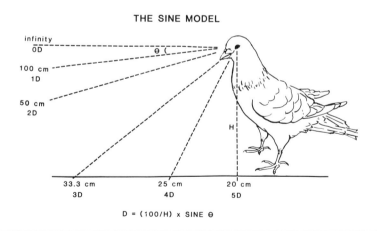

THE SINE MODEL

$$D = (100/H) \times SINE\ \theta$$

Figure 13.4. Diagram shows how lower-field myopia brings the entire ground-plane conjugate to the photoreceptors of the upper retina, when the pigeon is walking on the ground. A pigeon with eye-ground distance of 20 cm would need graded myopia following a sine-curve to attain 5 D of myopia at 90 degrees below the horizon.

jugate to the photoreceptors in the upper retina, when the bird is walking on the ground.

We do not know whether lower-field myopia is unique to the eyes of granivorous birds. We suspect that it may be present in terrestrial animals, which preserve optical quality and retinal grain in peripheral vision. We speculate that a comparable organization may exist in animals specialized for frontal vision, such as the cat or the burrowing owl. In these animals, the vertical horopter is at or close to ground level (Cooper and Pettigrew 1979), and the use of precise binocular machinery might be enhanced if the photoreceptors of the upper retina were near conjugate to the ground plane.

Many fascinating problems remain in the study of lower-field myopia in the pigeon, including a morphologic and optical study of its basis. Is it the result of a well-controlled gene plan, or is it locally regulated or fine-tuned during development by visual feedback? Does a comparable situation exist in the chick, which carries out foraging from its earliest post-hatching days, over a period in time when eye-ground height varies from a few centimeters to the adult state?

EXPERIMENTAL MYOPIA IN THE CHICK

We have applied the technique of objective electroretinographic refraction to the study of experimental myopia in the chick. Recent interest in this myopia model has been stimulated by the important observations of Wallman et al. (1978). Our intention was to follow-up the finding that the application of simple devices to the eye of the young chick can produce an increase in eye size (Hodos and Kuenzel 1984). We wished to establish whether these large eyes were indeed myopic, using a technique free from the small-eye artifact of retinoscopy, and to provide a morphologic description of eye dimensions in normal and myopic eyes of sufficient precision for a ray-tracing analysis. We hoped that the morphology of the anterior segment, including the outflow apparatus and the accommodatory system, might supply clues as to the cause of overgrowth. Our program of experiments is not complete, but the results of refractive studies and of eye morphology are summarized below.

Three devices — domes, arches, and rings — were applied to 3-day-old chicks. The domes degraded the image over the entire visual field of one eye. The arches degraded only the lateral visual field, leaving unobstructed vision in the frontal and posterior visual field. The rings did not occlude the visual field at all, but served as a control for possible mechanical impediments to growth of the other devices. Untreated chicks served as a fourth, control group.

We used devices as an alternative to lid suture because they allow several further experimental designs to be carried out. The devices can carry ophthalmic lenses and can be constructed so as to occlude only part of the visual field. It would be worthwhile to establish whether the sign or the magnitude of refractive error control the extent of induced myopia and to know whether partial occlusion of the visual field (as with the arch device) results in myopia in only part of the eyeball.

Chicks were refracted in the lateral visual field at ages of 3 to 7 weeks; if they had worn devices, they were refracted after the device was removed. Statistical analysis of the refractive states of the four groups was carried out by one-way analysis of variance, followed by Dunnett's test for comparing experimental group means to the mean of a control group. The results are summarized in Table 13.1, where n equals the number of refractions in each group.

The mean refractive states of normal and ring eyes did not differ significantly from each other, nor from emmetropia. Thus, the application of the ring device produced no discernible effect on refractive state. The means of the arch and dome groups, however, differed significantly from each other, from emmetropia, and from the mean of the normal eyes ($P = < 0.005$). The dome device, in particular, produced a large shift to myopic refraction.

Morphologic measurements were made from macrophotographs of the intact and hemisected eyes fixed as for electron microscopy. Effects of the devices on eye dimensions were analyzed from the mean differences between the treated (left) and untreated control (right) eyes, by analysis of variance. The rings did not affect eye growth. The arch significantly increased the dorsoventral equatorial diameter of the eye. This effect suggests that myopia may be restricted to the sector of the retina undergoing visual deprivation: The view of the anterior and posterior retina was left unobstructed by the arch device.

The dome device had the most dramatic effects on eye morphology and resulted in increases in both axial and equatorial dimensions. Dome eyes had a bulging cornea, increased anterior chamber depth, a more open angle, and a greater corneal diameter than control eyes. Axial length of the posterior segment was also increased. Figure 13.5 illustrates the morphology of a normal and a dome eye.

We have modeled an average dome eye with ray tracing. The main structural change is a 13% increase in the length of the posterior segment, which in itself

Table 13.1.   Refraction States of the Three Experimental Groups and Untreated, Normal Chicks

	Normals	Rings	Arches	Domes
Mean refraction	−0.20 D	−0.19 D	−4.11 D	−14.88 D
SD	1.3 D	0.88 D	3.0 D	8.03 D
n	45	32	33	30

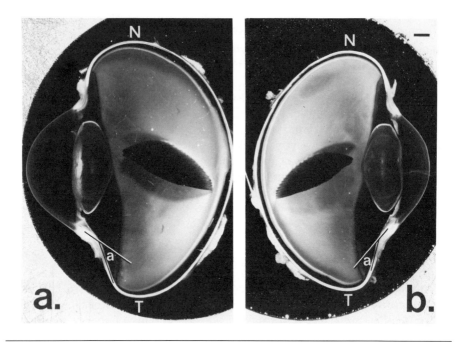

Figure 13.5. The ventral halves of (a) dome-treated, (b) control eyes from a chick treated with the dome device for 30 days, age 36 days. The axial length of the left eye is 2 mm greater than that of the right eye. The dome-treated eye shows bulging of the anterior segment, and the drainage angle is more open than the control. Ossicle angle (a) is increased by 14 degrees in the left eye. The posterior segment is more rounded in the left eye and the lens-to-photoreceptor distance is increased by 0.8 mm (13%). Swelling of the choroid can be seen in the dome eye. N, nasal; T, temporal (Scale line, 1 mm; × 6).

introduces 18.00 D of myopia. This effect is counteracted by the increase in anterior chamber depth, which reduces the net myopia to about − 15 D. We have noted no change in lenticular dimensions, nor in the accommodation apparatus.

In addition to the dimensional changes noted, several features were observed, particularly in dome eyes, which suggested that inflammatory responses may have occurred. There was an increased thickness of the choroid and a cloudiness of the anterior vitreous, which extended from the ciliary body to the base of the pecten. These inflammatory reactions and the swollen appearance of the circumorbital skin suggested that elevated temperature might play a role in the development of this form of experimental myopia. The role of temperature in the development of myopia in children was of interest to Hirsch (1957). Elevated ocular temperatures during periods of eye growth could encourage scleral growth, which could result in an elongated globe and a myopic refractive error.

To determine whether elevated eye temperatures occur during the development of experimental myopia, chicks were reared with domes, rings, or as untreated controls (Hodos et al. 1987). At the end of the rearing period, they were anesthetized, and a thermoprobe (a thermocouple in a 29-gauge needle) was inserted into the eye along the optic axis. Temperature readings were made at 1 mm intervals to a depth of 12 mm. Temperature readings of the circumorbital skin and the air inside the dome showed that the temperature of the circumorbital skin was nearly 1°C warmer than the comparable contralateral tissue. The air temperature inside the dome, close to the cornea, was nearly 4°C warmer than the air at the control cornea. The internal temperatures of the dome eyes were elevated from 2.8 to 5.2°C at the cornea, and 0.7 to 2.0°C at the axial sclera. Smaller elevations were found in the ring eyes. Two dome chicks that had lost their devices 24 to 48 hours before temperature measurement had thermal gradients nearly identical to those from untreated control eyes. The results suggest that the domes contribute to the development of this type of experimental myopia by trapping heat radiated from the eye. We have observed further that when chicks are raised in the dark with domes, arches, crescents, or rings, only the dome chicks develop an enlargement of the globe, which is equivalent to about one third of the enlargement of light-reared chicks (Hodos et al., unpublished data).

Our experiments on the chick show that we have a convenient and reproducible model for producing large myopic shifts in a period shorter than 2 months. We are currently measuring intraocular pressure in normal and experimentally myopic chick eyes, for it is clearly important to test how intraocular pressure is involved in the eye enlargement. The morphologic changes we observe in dome eyes are unilateral, and do not resemble the flattening of the cornea and reduction in anterior chamber depth found in avian glaucoma produced by rearing in continuous illumination. However, because clinical observations in humans suggest some intersection of myopic and glaucomatous changes, it is reasonable to expect some analogous overlap in the chick, and dome-produced myopia provides an ideal model to test this theory rigorously.

Our results with the arch device are compatible with myopia being restricted to the visually deprived sectors of the retina. Others have pursued this idea (Gottleib et al. 1987), showing that wearing a device such as a partial dome, with a removed sector giving clear vision to one part of the retina, gives an increased lens-retina distance only in the deprived portion of the retina. This experimental myopia persists after optic nerve section (Troilo et al. 1987). Thus, the effect may be local and need involve no visual feedback from brain to eye (via accommodation or via the efferent system). A simple explanation could be that retinal cells sensitive to image quality can produce trophic substances that modify scleral growth or relaxation. If the effect, which is under investigation in a number of laboratories, is chiefly exerted on relaxation of the sclera, then there may be fascinating analogies between experimental myopia in birds and myopia in humans, both in its low-grade and pathologic forms.

---■---

SUMMARY

We have used a newly developed electroretinographic optometer, which determines the refractive state at the plane of the photoreceptors, to refract normal pigeon eyes, as well as the eyes of normal chicks and chicks rendered myopic by wearing circumorbital devices.

Our results with normal pigeon eyes show that although the eye of this species is emmetropic for stimuli on the horizon or in the upper visual field, it becomes progressively myopic for stimuli below the horizon. This myopia varies quantitatively with retinal location, showing that the photoreceptors in the upper retina are conjugate to the ground plane. This natural lower-field myopia has adaptive value for a granivorous, ground-feeding animal.

Electroretinographic refraction of the eyes of chicks rendered myopic by wearing arch and dome circumorbital devices revealed the development of moderate and extreme amounts of myopia during the first few weeks of life. Histologic examination of normal and myopic eyes showed that the myopia resulted from posterior segment elongation.

---■---

REFERENCES

Catania AC. On the visual acuity of the pigeon. J Exp Anal Behav 1964;7:361–366.

Cooper ML, Pettigrew JD. A neurophysiological determination of the vertical horopter in the cat and owl. J Comp Neurol 1979;184:1–26.

Emsley HH. Visual Optics, vol. 1. London: Hatton Press, 1952.

Erichsen JT. How birds look at objects. D.Phil. Thesis, Oxford University, 1979.

Fitzke FW, Hayes BP, Hodos W, Holden AL. Electrophysiological optometry using Scheiner's principle in the pigeon eye. J Physiol 1985a;369:17–31.

Fitzke FW, Hayes BP, Hodos W, et al. Refractive sectors in the visual field of the pigeon eye. J Physiol 1985b;369:33–44.

Glickstein M, Millodot M. Retinoscopy and eye size. Science 1970;168:605–606.

Gottlieb MD, Fugate-Wentzek LA, Wallman J. Different visual deprivations produce different ametropias and different eye shapes. Invest Ophthalmol Vis Sci 1987;28:1225–1235.

Hayes BP. The structural organisation of the pigeon retina. Prog Ret Res 1982;1:197–226.

Hayes BP, Fitzke FW, Hodos W, Holden AL. A morphological analysis of experimental myopia in young chickens. Invest Ophthalmol Vis Sci 1986;27:981–991.

Hirsch M. The relationship between measles and myopia. Am J Optom Arch Am Acad Optom 1957;34:289.

Hodos W, Erichsen JT, Bessette BB, Phillips SJ. Head orientation in pigeons: postural, locomotor and visual determinants. Neurosci Abstr 1984;10:397.

Hodos W, Kuenzel WJ. Retinal image degradation produces ocular enlargement in chicks. Invest Ophthalmol Vis Sci 1984;25:652–659.

Hodos W, Fitzke FW, Hayes BP, Holden AL. Experimental myopia in chicks: ocular refraction by electroretinography. Invest Ophthalmol Vis Sci 1985;26:1423–1430.

Hodos W, Revzin AM, Kuenzel WJ. Thermal gradients in the chick eye: a contributing factor in experimental myopia. Invest Ophthalmol Vis Sci 1987;28:1859–1866.

Hodos W, Kuenzel WJ, Bessette BB. Ocular enlargement in dark reared chicks with image degrading optical devices. Unpublished data.

Martin GR, Young SR. The retinal binocular field of the pigeon (*Columba livia*; English Racing Homer). Vis Res 1983;23:911–915.

Martinoya G, Rey J, Bloch S. Limits of the pigeon's binocular field and direction for best binocular viewing. Vis Res 1981;21:1197–1200.

Millodot M, Blough P. The refractive state of the pigeon eye. Vis Res 1971;11:1019–1022.

Nye PW. On the functional differences between frontal and lateral visual fields of the pigeon. Vis Res 1973;13:559–574.

Pumphrey RJ. Sensory organs: vision. In: Marshall AJ, ed. Biology and Comparative Physiology of Birds. New York: Academic Press, 1961.

Troilo D, Gottleib MD, Wallman J. Eye growth is controlled both by the retina and the brain. Invest Ophthalmol Vis Sci (ARVO Suppl) 1987;28:263.

Ulrich DJ, Blough PM, Blough DS. The pigeon's distant visual acuity as a function of viewing angle. Vis Res 1982;22:429–431.

Wallman J, Turkel J, Trachtman J. Extreme myopia produced by modest change in early visual experience. Science 1978;201:1249–1251.

Westheimer G. The maxwellian view. Vis Res 1966;6:669–682.

Yinon U. Myopia induction in animals following alteration of the visual input during development: a review. Curr Eye Res 1984;3:677–690.

14

Experimentally Induced Refractive Anomalies in Mammals

Earl L. Smith III

□

In a wide variety of animal species, abnormal visual experience during early development interferes with the normally coordinated growth of ocular components and produces anomalous refractive states (Goss and Criswell 1981, Criswell and Goss 1983, Yinon 1984). Research is currently directed toward identifying the environmental factors that influence the emmetropization process and the mechanisms by which these factors affect the eye's refractive status. This chapter will examine the consequences of one type of abnormal visual experience — form deprivation — on the eye's refractive status, and explore how this abnormal visual experience adds to our understanding of ocular development.

From a clinical point of view, this research is particularly exciting because with the knowledge derived from these investigations, it may be possible to manipulate environmental factors to minimize or eliminate refractive errors in humans. Certainly it should be possible to modify visual environments or management procedures that would otherwise promote the development of anomalous refractive states.

Investigations involving three of the most frequently studied mammalian species — the monkey, the cat, and the tree shrew — are considered in this chapter. As experimental subjects, there are limitations and advantages to each of these species. In many instances, the macaque monkey is studied because the visual systems of humans and monkeys are quantitatively and qualitatively similar (Boothe et al. 1985, Harwerth and Smith 1985). Therefore, data obtained from monkeys can be extrapolated to the human population with a high degree of confidence. The tree shrew is a valuable subject because it is a prototypic primate that matures in a comparably short time and develops large refractive errors in response to anomalous visual experience (Sherman et al. 1977, Marsh and Norton 1983). Although its visual system is somewhat different from that of primates (Rodieck 1979), the cat is a desirable subject in refractive error studies because of the wealth of anatomic and physiologic knowledge that is available for the feline's visual system.

FORM DEPRIVATION

Pattern or form deprivation is a term that refers to a type of anomalous visual experience that is characterized by an absence of patterned visual stimulation of the retina. The most common experimental manipulation employed to produce form deprivation involves surgically suturing the eyelids together. Eyelid closure severely degrades the spatial characteristics of the retinal image and reduces retinal illumination in a wavelength-dependent manner (Crawford and Marc 1976, Loop and Sherman 1977). It has been demonstrated that lid suture performed early in the life of an experimental animal is one of the most effective means of disrupting the emmetropization process; however, there is substantial intersubject and interspecies variability in the resulting refractive errors.

□ Induced Myopia in Monkeys

Figures 14.1 and 14.2 illustrate the mean interocular refractive-error differences and axial-length ratios, respectively, for monocularly deprived monkeys from five different investigations. Assuming that the subjects were not anisometropic before lid suture, the mean data demonstrate, as first reported by Wiesel and Raviola (1977), that lid suture in the immature monkey results in a relative axial myopia. In twenty-nine of the thirty-three cases presented in the investigations considered in Figures 14.1 and 14.2, monocular lid suture caused the deprived eye to assume

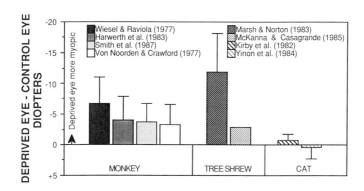

Figure 14.1. Mean interocular refractive error differences obtained in different laboratories for monocularly lid-sutured monkeys, tree shrews, and cats. The error bars indicate one standard deviation.

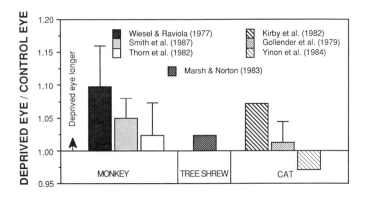

Figure 14.2.   Mean interocular axial length ratios obtained in different laboratories for monocularly lid-sutured monkeys, tree shrews, and cats. The error bars indicate one standard deviation.

a longer axial length or to become more myopic and less hyperopic than the non-deprived control eye (Wiesel and Raviola 1977, von Noorden and Crawford 1978, Thorn et al. 1982, Harwerth et al. 1983, Smith et al. 1987a).

The refractive-error alterations produced by form deprivation in the developing monkey are axial in nature (Figure 14.2). The abnormal axial elongation can be attributed primarily to a selective increase in the depth of the vitreous chamber (Wiesel and Raviola 1977, Thorn et al. 1982). In most cases, the magnitude of relative myopia correlates well with the axial length alterations (Smith et al. 1987b). There is no evidence that lid closure causes any systematic alterations in corneal curvature, anterior chamber depth, or lens thickness in the developing monkey (Raviola and Wiesel 1985).

As the error bars in Figures 14.1 and 14.2 denote, a substantial amount of inter-subject variability in the magnitude of refractive error alterations is produced by form deprivation. Based on interocular comparisons in monocularly deprived monkeys, the range of refractive-error alterations associated with lid suture is approximately 17.00 D, extending from 3.25 D of hyperopia to 13.50 D of myopia. Much of the intersubject variability can be attributed to differences in age of onset and the duration of deprivation (Raviola and Wiesel 1985, Greene and Guyton 1986, Smith et al. 1987a, 1987b).

The influence of the period of deprivation on the magnitude of the induced refractive error is illustrated in Figure 14.3, where the age at onset and the duration of deprivation are indicated for a selected subset of individual monocularly deprived monkeys. In general, the earlier the deprivation was initiated and the longer it was maintained, the higher the degree of relative myopia produced in the deprived eye. Regression analyses indicated that both the age at onset and the duration of deprivation have a significant impact on the magnitude of the relative myopia and that the combination of these two variables can account for as

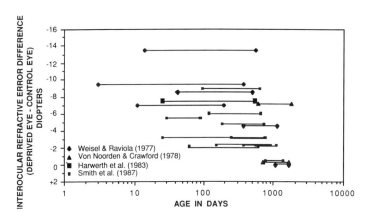

Figure 14.3. The period of monocular deprivation (age of onset and duration of treatment) plotted as a function of the magnitude of the relative myopia for individual monocularly lid-sutured monkeys. Only monkeys deprived for a minimum of 2 months and that developed a relative myopia were included.

much as 30% of the variance in monkeys that develop a relative myopia in their deprived eyes (Smith et al. 1987a, 1987b).

A general property of visual system development is that there are restricted critical or sensitive periods in early life during which adverse environmental factors can disrupt the normal developmental process (Mitchell and Timney 1985, Harwerth et al. 1986). The data in Figure 14.3 illustrate that there is a critical period within which there is a decreasing susceptibility of refractive mechanisms to the influence of form deprivation. During early development, form deprivation causes the monkey's eye to become relatively myopic; however, equivalent periods of form deprivation fail to alter the refractive status of adult monkeys (Wiesel and Raviola 1977, von Noorden and Crawford 1978). The critical period for the effects of form deprivation appear to begin very early in life, essentially at birth, and to be largely complete by about 2 to 3 years of age (Greene and Guyton 1986, Smith et al. 1987b). The end of the critical period coincides approximately with the completion of the rapid growth phase in axial length (Kiely et al. 1986). However, Young (1961) has reported that small refractive errors (<1.00 D) can be produced by altered visual environments in 4- to 6-year-old monkeys. Normal axial growth in the monkey is not complete until about 5 years of age (Kiely et al. 1986).

The duration of deprivation influences the magnitude of the induced myopia because the anomalous axial growth produced by lid suture ceases and the formerly deprived eye assumes a normal growth rate when form deprivation is discontinued (Raviola and Wiesel 1985). At any given age, some minimum period of deprivation is likely required to alter significantly the eye's refractive status. It is important to note, however, that, at an early age, this minimum period can be quite short. Relatively brief periods of lid suture (for example, 1 to 2 weeks) before about 1 month of age can produce a substantial myopic refractive error (for example, 4.00 to 5.00 D; von Noorden and Crawford 1978, Smith et al. 1987a).

In contrast to the relative myopia observed in the great majority of form-deprived monkeys, a small proportion of the total number of monkeys that were lid sutured early in life (four of fifty monocularly lid-sutured monkeys reported in the literature) developed a relative axial hyperopia in their deprived eyes (Thorn et al. 1982, Harwerth et al. 1983, Smith et al. 1987a). It is not known why these exceptions fail to develop an axial myopia; their early visual history was not obviously different from that of the majority of monkeys that became myopic as a result of form deprivation. Nevertheless, these exceptions suggest that factors other than form deprivation are important in the development of lid-suture myopia. It is possible that these exceptions occur because of unidentified, individual differences between monkeys or because of unrecognized procedural differences between subjects studied within the same laboratory.

☐ Induced Myopia in Tree Shrews

The tree shrew is a promising animal model for the development of anomalous refractive errors. Neonatal lid suture in the tree shrew reliably produces refractive errors that have many similarities with refractive anomalies in more advanced primates. Moreover, the relative time course of ocular and refractive development in the tree shrew is similar to that of macaque monkeys; however, ocular growth occurs approximately four times faster in the tree shrew (McBrien and Norton 1987, Kiely et al. 1986).

Several laboratories have reported that, without exception, long-term neonatal lid suture in the tree shrew produces a relative myopia in the deprived eye (Sherman et al. 1977, Marsh and Norton 1983, McBrien and Norton 1987). If the lid suture is initiated just before natural eye opening (about 20 to 21 days of age), a relative myopia can first be detected after about 30 days of deprivation. Thereafter, the magnitude of relative myopia increases with age until the subjects are between 3- to 4-months-old, the age at which normal eye growth is typically complete. When neonatal lid suture is maintained throughout ocular development, the deprived eye usually develops a relative myopia of about 10.00 D, but, as observed in monkeys and humans, there is a substantial degree of intersubject variability in the magnitude of the induced refractive error (see Figure 14.1) (McBrien and Norton 1987).

Lid-suture myopia in the tree shrew is predominantly axial in nature (Figure 14.2) and is due primarily to an elongation of the vitreous chamber (Marsh and Norton 1983). The absolute axial length increase is comparatively small (about 0.2 to 0.5 mm for long-term, neonatal lid suture), but in relative terms the axial changes in tree shrew are equivalent to those in the monkey (3 to 5%; Sherman et al. 1977, Marsh and Norton 1983).

□ Induced Refractive Errors in Cats

Most, though not all, studies have found that prolonged lid suture disrupts the normal emmetropization process in developing kittens. In comparison to the refractive abnormalities observed in primates, the magnitudes of the deprivation-induced refractive errors in kittens are small, and there are marked interlaboratory inconsistencies in the type of refractive errors exhibited by lid-sutured kittens (Figure 14.1).

The most consistent myopic-like changes were observed by Kirby et al. (1982). They found that all kittens (n = 20) that were monocularly lid-sutured between 13 and 80 days of age for periods of 275 to 663 days developed longer axial lengths is their deprived eyes. The interocular axial-length differences varied from 0.9 to 1.9 mm; on average, the deprived eye was 1.37 mm longer than the fellow control eye (about 7%; see Figure 14.2). Only ten of twenty kittens, however, demonstrated a relative myopic refractive error in the deprived eye (from −0.5 to −3.0 D). The magnitudes of the induced abnormalities were not correlated with either the age of onset or the duration of deprivation.

Kirby et al. (1982) also reported that many of the deprived eyes (ten of sixteen kittens) had flatter corneal curvatures than their fellow control eyes. In some cases, the resulting reduction in corneal power compensated for the increase in axial length; in most instances, however, predictions based on changes in axial length and corneal curvature overestimated the relative myopia that was actually manifested in the deprived eye, suggesting that other ocular components helped to minimize the magnitude of the induced refractive errors.

Gollender et al. (1979) reported that monocular lid fusion had a tendency to produce axial elongation in developing kittens, but that some deprived eyes had shorter axial lengths than their fellow control eyes. In seven of their ten monocularly deprived kittens, the deprived eyes had longer axial lengths; interocular differences were observed in both the anterior and vitreous chambers. Of the three deprived kittens that exhibited shorter axial lengths in their deprived eyes, two were subjected to the shortest periods of deprivation (from 11 to 69 days of age; the durations of deprivation for the other kittens ranged between 140 and 858 days). The shorter axial lengths in these kittens were attributed primarily to dramatic reductions in the anterior chamber. It is possible that the duration of deprivation was too short to produce axial elongation in these kittens. The relative rate of development of anomalous refractive errors has not been studied in the cat; but in a systematic study of refractive-error development in tree shrews, McBrien and Norton (1987) discovered that axial elongation, particularly of the vitreous chamber of the deprived eye, did not begin until after 30 days of deprivation. Possibly these two kittens would have developed an axial elongation if the duration of deprivation had been longer. Taken together, the results of Kirby et al. (1982) and Gollender et al. (1979) indicate the kitten responds to form deprivation in manner similar to that of primates; specifically, neonatal lid fusion in the great majority of kittens causes the deprived eye to develop a longer axial length and, in many cases, a myopic refractive error.

■
_____

FACTORS ASSOCIATED WITH
LID-SUTURE MYOPIA

As a rearing procedure for form-depriving developing animals, lid suture offers several advantages. It is a relatively simple surgical procedure, well tolerated by infant subjects. After the lids have been successfully fused, little time or effort is required to monitor the treatment and no adjustments are required as the subject matures. On the other hand, a number of inherent side effects are associated with lid suture. In addition to reducing pattern visual stimulation, lid suture alters the retinal image in a number of other ways. Moreover, fusing the eyelids physically changes the ocular environment in ways that may, by themselves, influence ocular development. All of the factors associated with lid suture must be taken into account before the induced changes in refractive error described earlier can be properly interpreted.

□ Visual vs Mechanical Factors

Lid closure elevates the temperature of ocular tissue (Hodos et al. 1987) and reduces the level of oxygen available at the corneal surface (Efron and Carney 1979). By the nature of the surgical procedure, lid fusion alters lid tension and possibly exerts abnormal mechanical pressure on the globe. It has also been suggested that lid suture, presumably by interfering with the drainage of intraocular fluids, may indirectly elevate intraocular pressure (Raviola and Wiesel 1978). These mechanical and physical factors can modify the eye's refractive status (Robb 1977, Greene and McMahon 1979, Mohan et al. 1977) and must be considered to analyze the role of lid suture in the genesis of experimentally induced refractive errors.

A useful strategy that has been used to evaluate the contribution of mechanical factors involves rearing monocularly lid-sutured animals in total darkness. Dark rearing obviously eliminates visual stimulation of both eyes so that subsequent interocular comparisons provide an opportunity to determine if the nonvisual aspects of lid suture are capable of altering the eye's refractive status. Studies of both monkeys and tree shrews that have been raised in total darkness after monocular lid suture have shown that the refractive errors and axial lengths of the deprived and nondeprived eyes of dark-reared subjects were virtually identical (Figure 14.4). Lid closure, by itself, did not alter the refractive status of primates (Raviola and Wiesel 1978, McKanna et al. 1983). These results demonstrate that the anomalous visual experience associated with lid closure is necessary for the genesis of lid-suture myopia.

The dark-rearing experiments, however, did not rule out the possibility that altered visual experience affects the eye's refractive status only when it occurs in conjunction with the nonvisual effects of lid suture. Wiesel and Raviola (1979)

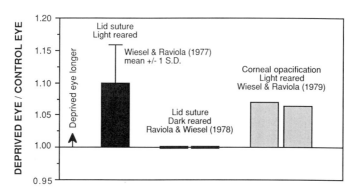

Figure 14.4. Interocular axial length ratios for monocularly form deprived monkeys.

tested this possibility by form depriving young monkeys using a method that avoided many of the potentially confounding, nonvisual factors associated with lid suture. They prevented patterned retinal stimulation to one eye by opacifying the cornea with multiple stromal injections of an inert suspension of latex particles. The latex injections rendered the cornea opaque and reduced light transmission by about 1 log unit, but avoided the mechanical and thermal complications of lid closure. After the opacification procedures, treated eyes assumed a faster growth rate than their fellow control eyes. The resulting axial elongation was restricted to the vitreous chamber and appeared comparable to that produced by lid suture in light-reared monkeys (Figure 14.4). This experiment suggests that axial myopia produced by lid suture is caused, or at least initiated, by abnormal visual experience. Nevertheless, our understanding of experimental ametropias is not sufficient to discard totally the idea that some of the nonvisual factors contribute to the refractive errors produced by lid suture. The corneal curvature changes observed in lid-sutured cats (Kirby et al. 1982) and tree shrews (McBrien and Norton 1987) could possibly be secondary to mechanical factors.

□ Critical Visual Factors

Lid fusion has three major effects on the retinal image: (1) decreased image contrast at all spatial frequencies, particularly high spatial frequencies; (2) reduced retinal illumination; and (3) altered spectral composition of the retinal image (Crawford and Marc 1976, Loop and Sherman 1977). The contribution that the alterations in the spectral characteristics of the retinal image makes to the development of lid-suture myopia has not been examined directly. However, studies of animals reared in total darkness and investigations of animals that had one eye defocused during development provide some insight into the possible consequences that a decrease in retinal illumination and a reduction in image contrast have on the eye's refractive status.

□ Selective Spectral Absorption

Comparisons of the effects of lid suture and corneal opacification in the developing monkey suggest that the specific spectral changes in the retinal image associated with lid suture are not essential for the induction of experimental myopia. Eyelid transmittance decreases as a function of wavelength; as a result, with lid fusion, the retinal image is dominated by relatively long wavelength light. Although the spectral transmittance of corneas opacified by injections of polystyrene latex has not been measured, the resulting reduction in transmission probably does not vary in a wavelength-dependent manner similar to that caused by lid suture. The similarity in the axial elongation observed in lid-sutured monkeys and monkeys with opacified corneas suggest that alterations in the spectral content of the retinal image are not required to trigger the development of lid-suture myopia. However, the ocular consequences of restricting the spectral characteristics of the retinal image to specific wavelengths during development have not been investigated in primates or cats.

□ Reduced Retinal Illumination

In avian species, reduced periods of light exposure (including total dark rearing) have been shown to induce abnormal axial elongation (Osol et al. 1986). Therefore, reduction in retinal illumination should be considered a potential factor in the genesis of the anomalous refractive errors associated with lid suture. As yet, the influence on the eye's refractive status of a reduction in retinal illumination, comparable to that produced by lid fusion, has not been directly evaluated in primates or cats. Observations on the refractive status of dark-reared animals shed some light on the possible consequences of a reduction in retinal illumination.

In cats and monkeys, the consequences of dark rearing appear to be consistent and can be interpreted in a more straightforward manner. Regal et al. (1976) dark-reared 2-week-old monkeys for either 3 (n = 2) or 6 months (n = 1) and found that all of the subjects' eyes exhibited hyperopic refractive errors that ranged from + 4.25 to + 6.00 D. The two monocularly lid-sutured monkeys that Raviola and Wiesel (1978) dark reared starting either at 9 days or 12 weeks of age for periods of 12 and 10 months, respectively, both had hyperopic refractive errors (+ 2.00 D in both eyes). In cats, dark rearing from about 1 to 2 weeks of age for periods ranging from 6 to 11 months leads to hyperopia and relatively shorter axial lengths (n = 19; Yinon et al. 1984). The hyperopia observed in these dark-reared animals suggests that decreased retinal illumination is not likely to precipitate the myopia observed in lid-sutured monkeys and cats.

□ Reduced Image Contrast

Degraded spatial vision associated with reduced image contrast appears, almost by default, to be the most likely aspect of lid closure that triggers the onset of lid-suture myopia. To examine the role that reduced image contrast plays in the genesis of the refractive errors produced by lid suture, several investigators have used lens-rearing procedures to produce optical defocus in developing cats and monkeys. Optical defocus, like lid closure, reduces image contrast in a spatial-frequency-dependent fashion. The greater the degree of optical defocus, the greater the reduction in image contrast and the greater the range of spatial frequencies that are affected. Unlike lid suture, the amount of optical defocus to which an animal is subjected can be controlled in a relatively straightforward manner by adjusting the power of an external ophthalmic lens. Moreover, optical defocus is a potentially valuable rearing strategy because it provides a means for evaluating the effects of degraded form vision without the possible confounding effects of either light deprivation or the potential mechanical and thermal effects of lid closure.

The goal of most lens-rearing strategies has been to create an optical imbalance between the two eyes. Typically high-powered ophthalmic lenses, either spectacle lenses held in goggles or contact lenses, have been secured in front of one eye, with zero-powered lenses in front of the fellow eye. Viewing through the high-powered lenses simulated a large refractive error in the "treated" eye. Kittens, and presumable monkeys, reared with this optically induced anisometropia postured their accommodation for the eye viewing through the zero-powered lens (Eggers and Blakemore 1978) and, thus, the high-powered minus lens before the fellow "treated" eye resulted in a habitually defocused retinal image.

In the first investigation of the effects of optical defocus, Smith et al. (1980) reared kittens with goggles that secured a high-powered minus spectacle lens in front of one eye (-10.0 to -16.0 D) and a zero-powered lens before the fellow eye. The kittens wore the anisometropic goggles for 2 to 3 hours each day beginning at 4 weeks of age for 8 weeks. When the kittens were not wearing the goggles, they were kept in total darkness. At the end of the treatment period, the mean refractive error for the defocused eyes was significantly more myopic (-1.12 D) than that for control eyes ($+1.06$ D). All eight of the lens-reared kittens exhibited a relative myopic refractive error in the defocused eye and, in five of the eight subjects, the defocused eye had a longer axial length than its fellow control eye. The similarity in the refractive errors produced by optical defocus and, in some kittens, by lid closure suggests that retinal image blur is the key factor in the development of lid-suture myopia.

In a subsequent investigation, Nathan et al. (1984) used hard contact lenses ($+6.0$, -3.0 to -16.0 D) to defocus developing kittens from 3 to 8 to 16 weeks of age. Although they failed to observe any systematic alterations in refractive error, axial length measurements indicated that in seven of the eight monocularly treated animals subjected to at least 6.0 D of optical defocus, the defocused eye was longer than the control eye. The interocular axial length differences in four of these seven subjects exceeded the range of differences observed in control kittens. The defocused eye in the remaining kitten was significantly shorter than the control eye. It was concluded that myopia could not be induced reliably in kittens by retinal image degradation.

Procedural differences may have contributed to the apparent inconsistencies between the studies of Smith et al. (1980) and Nathan et al. (1984). The rearing procedures used in the two studies were substantially different. With the goggle-rearing procedures used by Smith et al., the magnitude of the interocular imbalance could be confidently specified; but in addition to blurring one eye, the goggle-rearing procedure restricted the visual fields of both eyes. In comparison, the contact lenses used by Nathan et al. (1984) did not restrict the subjects' field of view, but the effective powers of the lenses depended on the relationship between the corneal curvature and the base curve of the contact lens. The base curves used by Nathan et al. (1984) were flatter than the corneal curvatures reported for normally developing kittens (Thorn et al. 1976, Freeman et al. 1978). The flatter base curves would alter the effective power of their contact lenses and possibly, by exerting mechanical force, alter the shape of their kittens' corneas.

In a recent investigation, Ni and Smith (1989) have taken into account many of the experimental variables that may have led to the conflicting results in previous studies. They used both goggle-held spectacle lenses and extended-wear soft contact lenses to produce varying degrees of optical defocus in one eye of developing kittens ($+10.0$ to -13.0 D). The results of their study indicated that when the degree of defocus was large (≥ 10.0 D), the defocused eyes developed a relative axial myopia. Goggles and contact lenses were equally effective in producing abnormal refractive errors. Small amounts of optical defocus (3.00 to 4.00 D), however, failed to produce consistent changes in either axial length or the kitten's refractive status (Figure 14.5).

Considered together, the results of the investigations of image degradation in kittens demonstrate that a substantial amount of optical defocus is required to disrupt the emmetropization process. It is apparent that the vision-dependent mechanisms that influence the kitten's refractive status can function adequately in the presence of moderate degrees of optical defocus. Because defocus acts as a high spatial frequency filter, it is likely that these mechanisms do not require high spatial frequency information and/or high image contrast to mediate normal ocular development. From retrospective studies of low-vision patients, it has been observed that visual disorders that led to myopia are associated primarily with peripheral retinal impairment (Nathan et al. 1985). If a peripheral retinal mechanism were responsible for the myopic refractive errors found in lid-sutured kittens, it would be expected that a high degree of optical defocus would be required to disrupt the emmetropization process and produce a myopic refractive error (Ikeda and Wright 1972).

The role of retinal image degradation in the development of the myopia observed in lid-sutured monkeys is still in question. As in the cat, both spectacle lens and contact lens regimens have been used to defocus the retinal image in developing monkeys. Crewther et al. (1986, 1988) reared monkeys from ages of 8 to 46 weeks for periods of up to 15 months with soft, continuous-wear contact lenses on one eye (+6, −6, or −9 D). Although all of the animals experienced interruptions in lens wear due either to loss of the lens or because of alterations in corneal integrity, four of the ten monkeys developed significant interocular refractive error differences. However, in contrast to lid-sutured subjects, the lens-reared monkeys developed a relative hyperopia in the treated eye (Figure 14.6). The relative hyperopia was associated with a decrease in the vitreous chamber

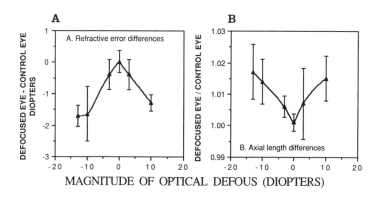

Figure 14.5. Mean (+/− 1 SD) interocular refractive error **(A)** and axial length differences **(B)** for kittens reared with varying degrees of optically induced anisometropia. Both goggle-reared and contact-lens reared animals are included. (From Ni J, Smith EL. Effects of chronic optical defocus on the kitten's refractive status. Vision Res 1989: 29:929–938.)

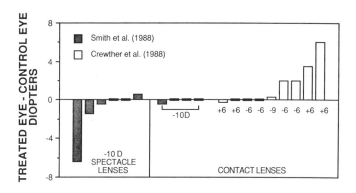

Figure 14.6. Interocular refractive error differences for individual monkeys reared with an optically induced anisometropia.

depth. The age of onset, duration of lens wear, and the power of the contact lens did not appear to influence the incidence or magnitude of the relative hyperopia.

Smith and his colleagues (1985, unpublished data) have used both continuous-wear contact lenses and a helmet-rearing procedure to defocus one eye of infant monkeys. The optical defocus (-9.0 or -10.0 D) was initiated at 30 days of age and continued for periods of 30, 60, or 90 days. There were no substantial interruptions (that is, more than 2 to 3 hours) in the anisometropic rearing procedures for any of the monkeys. Of the six helmet-reared monkeys, two subjects (one treated for 60 days and the other for 90 days) exhibited a significant degree of relative myopia in the defocus eye (Figure 14.6). None of the four monkeys reared with continuous-wear contact lenses demonstrated any significant interocular refractive error differences.

It is interesting that none of the contact-lens reared monkeys in either study became myopic and that some developed a relative hyperopic refractive error in their defocused eyes. Crewther et al. (1988) have suggested that the type of refractive error observed in contact-lens reared monkeys may depend on the age when the defocus is initiated. In this respect, Nathan et al. (1985) have reported that humans who experienced visual impairment that was not congenital but that occurred before 3 years of age tended to become hyperopic. Based on relative rates of ocular development in humans and monkeys (Kiely et al. 1987), the treatment periods used by Crewther and her co-workers corresponded to the age period when humans tend to become hyperopic in response to visual impairment. However, lid suture has been shown to be effective in producing axial myopia during treatment periods that were equivalent to those used by both Smith et al. (unpublished) and Crewther et al. (1988) in their contact-lens rearing procedures (see Figure 14.3).

One of the most likely explanations for the failure to produce a consistent myopia with continuous-wear contact lenses is that the degree of optical defocus was not sufficient to trigger the process responsible for lid-suture myopia. If this speculation is correct, then the mechanisms in the monkey that regulate normal ocular development can function quite adequately with low-contrast and relatively low-spatial frequency information.

SPECULATION ABOUT DIFFERENCES BETWEEN CATS AND PRIMATES

In general, the refractive-error alterations produced by lid closure in cats are smaller in magnitude and more variable in nature than those observed in primates. Differences in ocular anatomy and physiology between cats and primates suggest several possible explanations for the variance observed in experimental refractive errors.

Dark-rearing experiments on monocularly lid-sutured monkeys clearly demonstrate that some degree of abnormal visual stimulation is necessary to trigger the development of abnormal myopic refractive errors (see Figure 14.4). In primates, the eyelids are relatively thin and apparently, under typical housing conditions, transmit a sufficient amount of light to produce myopic alterations; but that may not always be the case in the cat (Yinon 1984). In comparison to primates, cats have thicker and more heavily pigmented eyelids. In addition, the cat's eyelids are covered with fur and their tarsal plates are more substantial than those in the primate. Consequently, the fused eyelids of some cats transmit only a fraction of the incident light (about 0.01% over much of the visible spectrum, Loop and Sherman 1977). It is possible that the density of the eyelids in some cats does not afford adequate visual stimulation to initiate the process that produces myopia in lid-sutured monkeys. If that is the case, it is also reasonable to speculate that intersubject differences between the optical density of eyelids, which can be substantial in cats (Crawford and Marc 1976), may contribute to the intersubject variability observed in some studies of lid-sutured cats (Gollender et al. 1979). Moreover, some of the interlaboratory inconsistencies reported for the effects of lid suture could be due to differences in the lighting levels in animal housing areas.

Differences in the physical characteristics of the eyelids may also be responsible for the differences in the prevalence of corneal curvature changes in monkeys and cats. Whereas, lid closure typically results in a flattening of the cat's cornea (Kirby et al. 1982, Yinon et al. 1984), the monkey's cornea appears to be unaffected (Raviola and Wiesel 1985). The thicker eyelids and the more robust tarsal plates of cats may exert significant mechanical pressure on the developing cornea, resulting in changes in curvature that are not produced by the more flimsy eyelids of monkeys.

Nathan et al. (1984) have hypothesized that differences in the structure of the eye between cat and primate may contribute to the different responses produced by lid suture in these species. In both the monkey and cat, the structural changes associated with abnormal refractive errors produced by lid suture occur primarily in the vitreous chamber; however, the vitreous chamber in the cat occupies a smaller proportion of the axial dimensions of the globe than it does in monkeys or humans (40% vs 65 to 70% of the total axial length; Nathan et al. 1984). In addition, the cat's crystalline lens is larger and occupies some of the equatorial portions of the globe that undergo the greatest changes during the development of lid-suture myopia in primates. It is reasonable to speculate that the relative size of the vitreous chamber and the location of the crystalline lens in the cat may limit, to a greater extent than in primates, the magnitude of the structural changes produced by the mechanisms responsible for lid-suture myopia.

■

MECHANISMS RESPONSIBLE FOR LID-SUTURE MYOPIA

The research described in the preceding sections of this chapter indicates that there is a vision-dependent mechanism(s) that, in response to the altered retinal image associated with lid closure, can modify the eye's refractive status. The mechanisms that mediate the influence of abnormal visual experience on the refractive status of a developing animal are not well understood. Although the neural signals that influence the eye's growth originate in the retina, the site or sites that receive these signals and then, based on the incoming visual information or lack of information, affect the eye's refractive status have not been identified.

Reduction strategies have dominated the investigation of the pathways and mechanisms that are responsible for lid-suture myopia. Typically a pharmacological or surgical manipulation that disrupts a specific neural pathway or some aspect of ocular physiology is paired with lid closure. If the experimental manipulation prevents or interferes with the development of the expected abnormal refractive error, it is assumed that the relevant structure or pathway is involved in mediating the influence of anomalous visual experience on the eye's refractive status. Most of this research has concentrated on structures or mechanisms that have historically been considered to be associated with environmentally mediated visual system alterations.

Anomalous binocular interactions associated with interocular asymmetries in retinal image quality are often responsible for many of the dramatic neuroanatomical alterations produced by abnormal visual experience early in life (Sherman and Spear 1982). Comparisons of the anomalous refractive errors in monocularly and binocularly form-deprived monkeys suggest that the myopia produced by lid suture is not the result of interocular asymmetries in visual stimulation. The magnitude and the nature of the myopic refractive errors produced by bilateral lid closure are equivalent to those observed in monocularly treated monkeys (Wiesel and Raviola 1977, Thorn et al. 1982, Greene and Guyton 1986). In addition, the time course for the development of myopia in binocularly and monocularly deprived monkeys appears to be comparable (Greene and Guyton 1986). These results demonstrate that an interocular imbalance in image quality is not necessary for the development of lid-suture myopia and suggest that the influence of form deprivation is mediated by independent mechanisms for each eye.

Excessive accommodation has frequently been implicated in the genesis of myopic refractive errors. Epidemiologic studies have consistently found associations between myopia and visual demands that require accommodation. For example, professions that require much nearwork tend to be occupied by myopic individuals (Goldschmidt 1968). Moreover, animal studies have demonstrated that subjects raised in restricted "near" visual environments develop myopic refractive errors (Young 1961). Although other interpretations are possible, these types of studies are often interpreted to indicate that excessive accommodation contributes to the development of myopia. A number of hypotheses have been developed to explain how prolonged or excessive accommodation might produce alterations in ocular structures that lead to myopic refractive errors (McBrien and Barnes 1984).

The hypothesis that the myopic refractive errors produced by lid closure can be attributed to excessive accommodation deserves consideration. According to this idea (although it is not typically stated formally), form deprivation leads to excessive or prolonged accommodation. It has been demonstrated that when the eye encounters a structureless visual field, the eye assumes a positive accommodative posture (Leibowitz and Owens 1975). Thus, it is reasonable to speculate that the degraded retinal image associated with lid closure may elicit a similar accommodative response and that lid-sutured eyes may habitually adopt a positive accommodative posture. It is possible that the visual system is constantly adjusting accommodation in an attempt to compensate for the blurred retinal image associated with lid suture. However, since monocular lid closure is very effective in producing a relative myopia in the deprived eye, this hypothesis implies that the two eyes of infant subjects must be capable of adopting different accommodative states; that is, during early development, accommodation is not always yoked and symmetrical in the two eyes. No evidence indicates that infants are capable of differential accommodation. However, if, as some investigators have reasoned, accommodation is involved in regulating the emmetropization process (McKanna and Casagrande 1978a), differential accommodation early in life might be an advantage to a developing infant by providing a means of eliminating small interocular differences in refractive error and ensuring an iosmetropic refractive balance. Presumably as the animal aged, accommodation would become yoked. One manner in which accommodation could regulate the emmetropization process is summarized in the schematic of McKanna and Casagrande's (1981) intersection feedback loop hypothesis shown in Figure 14.7.

The possibility that accommodation plays a role in the development of lid-suture myopia has attracted a substantial amount of attention. The potential contribution of accommodation to lid-suture myopia has typically been assessed by determining whether disruption of normal accommodative function prevents or modifies the expected effects of early form deprivation on the eye's refractive status. The results of several studies using pharmacologic procedures to disrupt accommodation have indicated that in the cat (Hendrickson and Rosenblum 1985), tree shrew (McKanna and Casagrande 1981, 1985), and stump-tailed macaque monkey (*Macaca arctoides*; Raviola and Wiesel 1985) chronic cycloplegia prevents the axial elongation and relative myopia typically produced by degradation of the retinal image. These studies suggest that normal accommodative function is an essential component in the eye's response to form deprivation and support the hypothesis that excessive positive accommodation causes lid-suture myopia.

Related studies have demonstrated that normal accommodative function may also be necessary for the normal emmetropization process. Infant monkeys

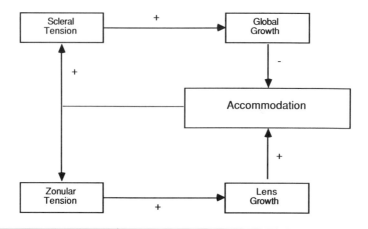

Figure 14.7. Schematic of McKanna and Casagrande's (1981) intersecting feedback loop hypothesis linking ocular growth and accommodation. Positive accommodation, which is driven by visual stimuli, is assumed to promote axial elongation by increasing scleral tension and to retard lens growth by reducing zonular tension. Both the resulting axial elongation and reduction in lens size (presumably increasing lens power) decrease the positive accommodative demand associated with a given visual task. Under ordinary viewing conditions, this system would fine-tune the eye for its visual environment. It is hypothesized that lid-suture myopia occurs because either appropriate visual feedback fails to reduce the amount of positive accommodation or that the degraded retinal image acts as a continuous stimulus for positive accommodation.

(*Macaca nemistrina* and *Macaca arctoides*) that undergo chronic unilateral atropinization, but are otherwise reared normally, and monkeys (*Macaca mulatta*) that are surgically rendered aphakic early in life develop shorter axial lengths and relative hyperopic refractive errors in their treated eyes (Raviola and Wiesel 1985, Kiorpes et al. 1987, Wilson et al. 1987).

Although the results of the preceding studies suggest that the disruption of accommodative function prevents myopia, it must be kept in mind that chronic atropinization, particularly in infants, may have some indirect effect on emmetropization and the development of abnormal refractive errors. It has been reported that chronic atropinization produces alterations in the retinal vasculature of developing kittens (Crewther et al. 1985). Therefore, the effects of alternative procedures for disrupting accommodative function should be evaluated before the contribution of accommodation to lid-suture myopia is firmly established. These experiments are particularly important because pharmacologic stimulation of accommodation with a parasympathomimetic agent during development does not facilitate the development of lid-suture myopia (Raviola and Wiesel 1985).

There are some puzzling contradictions concerning the role of accommodation in lid-suture myopia. These inconsistencies are particularly distressing because they were found in the same laboratory using essentially identical procedures in two very similar species of monkeys. As mentioned earlier, Raviola and Wiesel (1985) have reported that chronic atropinization prevents lid-suture myopia in the *M. arctoides* monkeys. In contrast, chronic atropinization fails to prevent lid-suture myopia in the closely related, Old World monkey, the rhesus monkey (*M. mulatta*). To rule out the possibility that this inconsistency was due to interspecies differences in the efficacy of atropine, accommodative function was disrupted by surgically removing the ciliary ganglion in a monocularly lid-sutured rhesus monkey. Nevertheless, interruption of the parasympathetic innervation to the deprived eye did not prevent the development of a 10.00 D relative myopia. Apparently, accommodation plays a role in lid-suture myopia in *M. arctoides*, but not in *M. mulatta*.

Some evidence suggests that local retinal mechanisms may be involved in the development of abnormal refractive errors in the rhesus monkey. The most compelling argument that lid-suture myopia is mediated by local retinal mechanisms in the rhesus monkey comes from the observation in one animal that intracranial section of the optic chiasm failed to prevent the development of lid-suture myopia (Raviola and Wiesel 1985). It has been speculated that mechanisms and their activity in the retina of the rhesus monkey influences ocular growth directly by releasing regulatory molecules. In line with this idea, Stone et al. (1988) have observed an increase in the immunohistochemical reactivity of form-deprived retinas for vasoactive intestinal polypeptide (VIP). Although the significance of this finding is not known, it was speculated that VIP may play a part in the regulation of ocular growth.

In contrast to its effects in the rhesus monkey, optic nerve section stopped the development of lid-suture myopia in an *M. arctoides* monkey (Raviola and Wiesel 1985). This observation concurs with the hypothesis that the central nervous system, acting through accommodative mechanisms, plays a dominant role in the genesis of refractive errors in the stump-tailed monkeys. It is difficult, however, to imagine that the rhesus and stump-tailed monkeys, two closely related primate species, would exhibit such dramatic differences in the manner in which abnormal visual experience influences ocular development. These apparent differences must be clarified before the results of these experiments can be extrapolated to the human population with any degree of confidence.

CLINICAL RELEVANCE

The clinical relevance of research on refractive errors produced by form deprivation in animals depends on several issues. It is critical that the nature of the experimentally induced refractive error is similar to that which occurs in the human population, and that the factors responsible for the genesis of experimental refractive errors be equally effective in altering the refractive status of humans. In this respect, the myopic refractive errors produced by form deprivation in sub-human mammals, particularly monkeys, exhibit several features that are common to some myopic refractive errors in humans. Lid-suture myopia is associated primarily with an elongation of the vitreous chamber. This abnormal axial growth results in fundus alterations in lid-sutured monkeys (for example, myopic crescents on the temporal aspect of the optic disk) that are characteristic of large myopic errors in humans (Raviola and Wiesel 1985). Moreover, numerous studies of humans suffering from conditions that prevented patterned retinal stimulation at an early age have demonstrated that form deprivation is effective in producing large axial myopias in human infants (Robb 1977, O'Leary and Millodot 1979, Rabin et al. 1981, Hoyt et al. 1981). Even the atypical hyperopic responses to lid suture observed in a relative few infant monkeys have been observed in a small proportion of humans that suffered from early form deprivation (von Noorden and Lewis 1987). Therefore, it appears that the refractive errors produced by form deprivation in experimental animals have a clinical counterpart in the human population.

The extent to which knowledge gained from form-deprived monkeys can be applied to human myopia must be resolved through future research. Human studies have revealed distinguishing features between individuals with myopia clearly suggesting that myopia is not simply a single entity (McBrien and Millodot 1986, 1987). Undoubtedly, multiple factors are involved in the genesis of the spectra of myopias found in the human population. It will be important to determine if the principles discovered in studies of lid-suture myopia will be applicable to human myopia that occurs in the absence of overt form deprivation. It is obvious that alterations in form vision produced by lid suture are drastic. Consequently, one must be cautious in applying knowledge gained from studies of lid suture to human myopia. However, it should also be kept in mind that the drastic visual alterations produced by lid suture have been used successfully to reveal amblyopiogenic mechanisms in form deprivation amblyopia that also appear to be involved in the more common and milder forms of amblyopia. Thus, it is likely that continued study of lid-suture myopia will increase our general understanding of all forms of myopia.

___■___

REFERENCES

Bloom M, Berkley MA. Visual acuity and the near point of accommodation in cats. Vis Res 1977;17:723–730.

Boothe RG, Dobson V, Teller DY. Postnatal development of vision in humans and non-human primates. Annu Rev Neurosci 1985;8:495–545.

Crawford MLJ, Marc RE. Light transmission of cat and monkey eyelids. Vis Res 1976; 16:323–324.

Crewther DP, Crewther SG, Cleland BG. Is the retina sensitive to the effects of prolonged blur? Exp Brain Res 1985;58:427–434.

Crewther SG, Nathan J, Kiely PM, et al. Axial hypermetropia induced in primates. ARVO Abstracts. Invest Ophthalmol Vis Sci 1986;27:202.

Crewther SG, Nathan J, Kiely PM, et al. The effect of defocusing contact lenses on refraction in cynomolgus monkeys. Clin Vis Sci 1988;3:221–228.

Criswell MH, Goss DA. Myopia development in nonhuman primates — a literature review. Am J Optom Physiol Opt 1983;60:250–268.

Efron N, Carney LG. Oxygen levels beneath the closed eyelid. Invest Ophthalmol Vis Sci 1979;18:93–95.

Eggers HM, Blakemore C. Physiological basis of anisometropic amblyopia. Science 1978; 201–203.

Freeman RD, Wong S, Zezula S. Optical development of the kitten cornea. Vis Res 1978; 18:409–414.

Goldschmidt E. On the Etiology of Myopia, an Epidemiological Study. Copenhagen: Munksgaard, 1968.

Gollender M, Thorn F, Erickson P. Development of axial ocular dimensions following eyelid suture in the cat. Vis Res 1979;19:221–223.

Goss DA, Criswell MH. Myopia development in experimental animals — a literature review. Am J Optom Physiol Opt 1981;58:859–869.

Greene PR, Guyton DL. Time course of rhesus lid-suture myopia. Exp Eye Res 1986; 42:529–534.

Greene PR, McMahon TA. Scleral creep vs temperature and pressure in vitro. Exp Eye Res 1979;29:527–537.

Harwerth RS, Smith EL III, Boltz RL, et al. Behavioral studies on the effect of abnormal early visual experience in monkeys: spatial modulation sensitivity. Vis Res 1983; 23:1501–1510.

Harwerth RS, Smith EL III, Duncan GC, et al. Multiple sensitive periods in the development of the primate visual system. Science 1986;232:235–238.

Harwerth RS, Smith EL III. Rhesus monkey as a model for normal vision of humans. Am J Optom Physiol Opt 1985;62:633–641.

Hendrickson P, Rosenblum W. Accommodation demand and deprivation in kitten ocular development. Invest Ophthalmol Vis Sci 1985;26:343–349.

Hodos W, Revzin AM, Kuenzel W. Thermal gradients in the chick eye: a contributing factor in experimental myopia. Invest Ophthalmol Vis Sci 1987;28:1859–1866.

Hoyt CS, Stone RD, Fromer C, Billson FA. Monocular axial myopia associated with neonatal eyelid closure in human infants. Am J Ophthalmol 1981;91:197–200.

Ikeda H, Wright MJ. Differential effects of refractive errors and receptive field organization of central and peripheral ganglion cells. Vis Res 1972;12:1465–1476.

Kiely PM, Crewther SG, Nathan J, et al. A comparison of ocular development of the cynomolgus monkey and man. Clin Vis Sci 1987;1:269–280.

Kiorpes L, Boothe RG, Hendrickson AE, Movshon JA, Eggers HM Gizzi M. Effects of early unilateral blur on the macaque's visual system. I. Behavioral observations. J Neurosci 1987;7:1318–1326.

Kirby AW, Weiss H. Elongation of kitten and monkey eyes following neonatal lid suture. ARVO Abstracts. Invest Ophthalmol Vis Sci 1979;18(suppl):158.

Kirby AW, Sutton L, Weiss H. Elongation of cat eyes following neonatal lid suture. Invest Ophthalmol Vis Sci 1982;22:274–277.

Leibowitz HW, Owens DA. Night myopia and the intermediate dark focus of accommodation. J Opt Soc Am 1975;65:1121–1128.

Loop MS, Sherman S. Visual discrimination during eyelid closure in the cat. Brain Res 1977;128:329–339.

Marsh WL, Norton TT. Measures of refractive state, ocular length and corneal curve in experimentally myopic tree shrews. ARVO Abstracts. Invest Ophthalmol Vis Sci 1983; 24:226.

McBrien NA, Barnes DA. A review and evaluation of theories of refractive error development. Ophthalmol Physiol Opt 1984;2:201–213.

McBrien NA, Millodot M. Amplitude of accommodation and refractive error. Invest Ophthalmol Vis Sci 1986;27:1187–1190.

McBrien NA, Millodot M. The relationship between tonic accommodation and refractive error. Invest Ophthalmol Vis Sci 1987;28:997–1004.

McBrien NA, Norton TT. The development of ocular growth and refractive state in normal and monocularly deprived tree shrew (*Tupaia belangeri*). Soc Neurosci Abstr 1987; 13:1535.

McKanna JA, Casagrande VA. Reduced lens development in lid-suture myopia. Exp Eye Res 1978a;26:715–723.

McKanna JA, Casagrande VA. Zonular dysplasia in lid-suture myopia. In: Yamaji R, ed. The Second International Conference on Myopia, Proceedings. Tokyo: Kannehara Shuppan, Ltd, 1987b;21–26.

McKanna JA, Casagrande VA. Atropine affects lid-suture myopia development: experimental studies of chronic atropinization in tree shrews. Doc Ophthalmol 1981;28:187–192.

McKanna JA, Casagrande VA. Chronic cycloplegia prevents lid-suture myopia in tree shrews. ARVO Abstracts. Invest Ophthalmol Vis Sci 1985;26:331.

McKanna JA, Casagrande VA, Norton TT, Marsh W. Dark-reared tree shrews do not develop lid-suture myopia. ARVO Abstracts. Invest Ophthalmol Vis Sci 1983;24:226.

Mitchell DE, Timney B. Postnatal development of function in the mammalian visual system. In: Brookhart JM, Mountcastle VB, eds. Handbook of Physiology. Am Physiological Soc, Bethesda, 1985;12:507–555.

Mohan M, Rao VA, Dada VK. Experimental myopia in the rabbit. Exp Eye Res 1977; 25:33–38.

Nathan J, Crewther SG, Crewther DP, Kiely PM. Effects of retinal image degradation on ocular growth in cats. Invest Ophthalmol Vis Sci 1984;25:1300–1306.

Nathan J, Kiely PM, Crewther SG, Crewther DP. Disease-associated visual image degradation and spherical refractive errors in children. Am J Optom Physiol Opt 1985;62: 680–688.

Ni J, Smith EL III. Effects of optical defocus on the kitten's refractive status. Vision Res 1989;29:929–938.

O'Leary DJ, Millodot M. Eyelid closure causes myopia in humans. Experientia 1979; 35:1478–1479.

Osol G, Schwartz B, Foss DC. The effects of photoperiod and lid suture on eye growth in chickens. Invest Ophthalmol Vis Sci 1986;27:255–260.

Rabin J, Van Sluyters RC, Malach R. Emmetropization: a vision-dependent phenomenon. Invest Ophthalmol Vis Sci 1981;20:561–564.

Raviola E, Wiesel TN. Effect of dark-rearing on experimental myopia in monkeys. Invest Ophthalmol Vis Sci 1978;17:485–488.

Raviola E, Wiesel TN. An animal model of myopia. N Engl J Med 1985;312:1609–1615.

Regal DM, Boothe R, Teller DY, Sackett GP. Visual acuity and visual responsiveness in dark-reared monkeys. (*Macaca nemestrina*). Vis Res 1976;16:523–530.

Robb RM. Refractive errors associated with hemangiomas of the eyelids and orbit in infancy. Am J Ophthalmol 1977;83:52–58.

Rodieck RW. Visual pathways. Annu Rev Neurosci 1979;2:193–225.

Sherman SM, Norton TT, Casagrande VA. Myopia in the lid-sutured tree shrew (*Tupaia glis*). Brain Res 1977;124:154–157.

Sherman SM, Spear PD. Organization of visual pathways in normal and visually deprived cats. Physiol Rev 1982;62:738–855.

Smith EL III, Harwerth RS. Behavioral measurements of accommodative amplitude in rhesus monkeys. Vis Res 1984;24:1821–1827.

Smith EL III, Harwerth RS, Crawford MLJ, von Noorden GK. Observation on the effects of form deprivation on the refractive status of the monkey. Invest Ophthalmol Vis Sci 1987;28:1236–1245.

Smith EL III, Harwerth RS, Crawford MLJ, von Noorden GK. The influence of the period of deprivation on experimental refractive errors. In: Lennerstrand G, von Noorden GK, eds. Strabismus and Amblyopia — Experimental Basis for Advances in Clinical Management. Houndsmills, England: Macmillan Press, 1988.

Smith EL III, Maguire GW, Watson JT. Axial lengths and refractive errors in kittens reared with an optically induced anisometropia. Invest Ophthalmol Vis Sci 1980;19:1250–1255.

Sommers D, Kaiser-Kupfer MI, Kupfer C. Increased axial length of the eye following neonatal lid suture as measured by A-scan ultrasonography. ARVO Abstracts. Invest Ophthalmol Vis Sci 1978;17(Suppl):295.

Stone RA, Laties AM, Raviola E, Wiesel TN. Increase in retinal vasoactive intestinal polypeptide after eyelid fusion in primates. Proc Natl Acad Sci USA 1988;85:257–260.

Thorn F, Gollender M, Erickson P. The development of the kitten's visual optics. Vis Res 1976;16:1145–1149.

Thorn F, Doty RW, Gramiak R. Effect of eyelid suture on development of ocular dimensions in macaques. Curr Eye Res 1982;1:727–733.

von Noorden GK, Crawford MLJ. Lid closure and refractive error in macaque monkeys. Nature 1978;272:53–54.

von Noorden GK, Lewis RA. Ocular axial length in unilateral congenital cataracts and blepharoptosis. Invest Ophthalmol Vis Sci 1987;28:750–752.

Wiesel TN, Raviola E. Myopia and eye enlargement after neonatal lid fusion in monkeys. Nature 1977;266:66–68.

Wiesel TN, Raviola E. Increase in axial length of the macaque monkey eye after corneal opacification. Invest Ophthalmol Vis Sci 1979;18:1232–1236.

Wilson JR, Fernandes A, Chandler CV, Tigges M, Boothe RG, Gammon JA. Abnormal development of the axial length of aphakic monkey eyes. Invest Ophthalmol Vis Sci 1987; 28:2096–2099.

Wilson JR, Sherman SM. Differential effects of early monocular deprivation on binocular and monocular segments of cat striate cortex. J Neurophysiol 1977;40:891–903.

Yinon U. Myopia induction in animals following alteration of the visual input during development: a review. Curr Eye Res 1984;3:677–690.

Yinon U, Koslowe EC, Rassin MI. The optical effects of eyelid closure on the eyes of kittens reared in light and dark. Curr Eye Res 1984;3:431–439.

Young FA. The effect of restricted visual space on the primate eye. Am J Ophthalmol 1961; 52:799–806.

___15_____

Retinal Factors in Myopia and Emmetropization: Clues from Research on Chicks

Josh Wallman

☐

In humans, the length of the eye is highly correlated with the refractive state over a wide range of refractive errors (Van Alphen 1961), suggesting that failures of ocular growth regulation during development may underlie most refractive errors. Conversely, the generally successful regulation of eye growth may be responsible for the much higher frequency of refractive states near emmetropia in adults than in neonates, who are generally hyperopic. How might this growth regulation be achieved? One can imagine the eye growing in three ways.

1. The growth of each of the components of the eye could be regulated autonomously. This option does not seem to be the case in humans, as shown by the facts that the axial length and corneal curvature are correlated and that refractive error is much more highly correlated with axial length than with corneal curvature.

2. The growth of the vitreous chamber and cornea could involve some interaction, mediated either by a humoral agent secreted by one affecting the other or by mechanical stresses. Such interactions could account for the correlated growth observed and for approximate emmetropization, but seem unlikely to be precise enough to assure emmetropia unless the eye somehow "knew" the lens equations so that a given degree of corneal curvature and anterior chamber depth would elicit the appropriate amount of increase in vitreous length.

3. Finally, visual feedback could guide the growth of the eye so that emmetropia is reached and maintained. One can envision two types of visual feedback. In the simpler of the two, the eye grows in length more rapidly than the cornea

I am grateful to F.A. Miles, M.D. Gottlieb, D.L. Nickla, and C. Harris for careful reading of this chapter. The data shown in Figure 15.2 are from the undergraduate thesis of Jeffrey Winseman. Supported by NIH Research Grant EYO2727.

decreases in curvature, thereby reducing the hyperopia. When the eye became emmetropic, the increased sharpness of the retinal image, which might be detected by the increased activity of retinal neurons sensitive to fine details in the visual world or by a general increase in the level of neural activity at any level in the visual system, would cause the eye to stop elongating. The more complicated type of feedback control would be one in which the eye responded to a signal proportional not only to the magnitude of ametropia, but also to its direction, i.e., whether the eye was hyperopic or myopic. A signal proportional to the difference between the axial length of the eye and the focal length of its optics (the "signed" refractive error), rather than one based on sharpness of the retinal image, would be sufficient. An example of such an error signal would be the average level of accommodation. Because hyperopic eyes have greater average levels of accommodation than myopic eyes, if axial elongation depended on the level of accommodation, hyperopic eyes would elongate more rapidly than would myopic eyes, thereby reducing either ametropia. Although accommodation is used in this example, any error signal having different values in myopic and hyperopic eyes would suffice.

This chapter first describes studies of chick eyes visually deprived by a variety of manipulations. These studies argue that the elongation of the eye can be controlled by the retina. Next, it presents other studies demonstrating that the eye can sense its refractive error and direct its growth toward emmetropia.

STUDIES ON EXPERIMENTAL MYOPIA

□ Effects of Visual Form Deprivation

Evidence in favor of a visual feedback hypothesis comes from observations in several species that visual form deprivation causes ocular elongation and myopia. The literature in this area has been reviewed by Smith in Chapter 14.

In chicks, these effects are particularly large, rapid, and consistent (Wallman et al. 1978, Yinon et al. 1983, Hodos and Kuenzel 1984, Hayes et al. 1986, Lauber and Oishi 1987, Wallman and Adams 1987, Picket-Seltner et al. 1988). (In our laboratory six days of form deprivation produces 18 D of myopia and a 16% increase in vitreous chamber length.) In most of the animal studies, an increase in the variability of refractions is as prominent a finding as the general shift toward myopia, suggesting a failure of regulation of eye growth, rather than simply an increased rate of elongation.

It appears clear that the change in ocular growth is a consequence of the form deprivation, rather than mechanical or thermal disturbances to the eyes. In chicks, covering the eyes with translucent occluders that do not touch the cornea results in ocular elongation, as does closing the lids (Wallman et al. 1978, Hodos and Kuenzel 1984). In addition, in chicks raised in darkness, there is no significant difference between occluded and nonoccluded eyes (Gottlieb et al. 1987).

Raising animals in the dark is a potentially important manipulation as it offers a means of distinguishing between complete deprivation of light and form vision alone. Several papers suggested that darkness "protects" mammals against lid-suture myopia or that it induces hyperopia (Regal et al. 1976; Yinon and Koslowe 1984, 1986; Raviola and Wiesel 1978).

In chicks, darkness causes both increased elongation of the vitreous chamber and corneal flattening (increased radius of curvature), each with different time scales: At first the effect of the elongation of the vitreous chamber dominates, making the eye slightly myopic. Then by four weeks, the corneal flattening dominates, leading to a substantial hyperopia (Gottlieb et al. 1987, Troilo 1989). This temporal difference between the two processes means that there is a point (after two weeks of dark-rearing) at which the eyes are emmetropic, and the effect of darkness could thus be interpreted as having protected the eye from the deprivation myopia. This finding argues for caution in making such assertions in other species without having data at several time points.

Because diffuse light is more effective than darkness in producing eye enlargement, more specific visual deprivations may reveal what aspect of vision is involved in the control of eye growth. In chicks, several manipulations of the visual environment, other than deprivation, have been shown to yield eye enlargements. Chicks raised in dim light, either white (Chiu et al. 1975) or confined to narrow spectral regions (Bercovitz et al. 1972), show eye enlargement, although it has not been shown that specific classes of photoreceptors were stimulated by these illuminants. Chicks raised in bright light for 23 or 24 hr/day also show eye enlargement, which is associated with very shallow anterior chambers and flat corneas (Oishi et al. 1987). The fact that both continuous light and continuous darkness cause these effects suggests that circadian rhythms may have been disrupted and this disruption influenced eye growth.

□ Local Control of Eye Growth in Chicks

Myopia has generally been viewed as a "global" phenomenon in that one would expect that, if the subjective clinical refraction of a patient were myopic (meaning that the fovea is myopic), the rest of the retina would be myopic as well. Furthermore, until recently, one would have been inclined to suspect that if visual experience affects the refractive status of the eye, this effect must be mediated by the brain. Recent work brings both of these assumptions into question. In humans, the pattern of refractions at different angles to the visual axis varies among individuals (Ferree et al. 1932), with characteristic patterns for myopes, emmetropes, and hyperopes (Millodot 1981), implying differences in the shape of the back of the eye.

Furthermore, if we cover one eye of a young chick with a white translucent plastic dome that has an opening so that approximately half the retina has an unrestricted field of view while the other half can only look into the white occluder, the deprived part of the eye becomes enlarged and myopic, while the seeing part is normal (Wallman et al. 1987). The clearest depiction of the differences in the shape of the eyes is obtained by aligning tracings of the eyes (seen from above) and averaging them (Figure 15.1A). To permit quantitative comparisons, we measured the "radius" of the eye from the approximate center of the pupil (close to the second principal point of the optical system) to the back of the eye (Figure 15.1A, right). From these measurements, we can express the relative enlargement by dividing the radius at each angle by the corresponding radius on the untreated fellow eye. From this we can see that, when only the nasal or temporal part of the retina is deprived, the corresponding region of the eye is enlarged (Figure 15.1B).

These results suggest that local retinal regions control the growth of the eye, although other explanations exist: Birds might conceivably be able to accommodate asymmetrically by tilting the lens (as first suggested by Hodos and Kuenzel 1984). Alternatively, the bird might tend to turn the eye in the direction of the opening in the occluder. Either of these behaviors might affect eye growth. Furthermore, the mechanical properties of the cornea or sclera might be altered by the raised temperature or humidity surrounding the sutured or occluded eye, either because of the direct effect of the closed eye or because of an inflammatory effect (Hodos et al. 1987). These possibilities are ruled out by three additional experiments:

1. The same effects are shown in eyes that were blind because the optic nerve had been severed before the deprivation began (partial deprivation: Troilo et al. 1987, total deprivation: Wildsoet and Pettigrew 1988).
2. Partial or total deprivation does not affect eye shape when the animals are raised in darkness (Gottlieb et al. 1987).
3. When only part of the visual field is deprived, the local enlargement and myopia occurs in the deprived region not only when the one side (nasal or temporal) of the eye is deprived (Figure 15.1), but also when it is the central or peripheral visual field that had been deprived (Figure 15.2).

The rate of growth of local regions of the posterior globe can be manipulated in both directions: Not only can the rate of growth be increased in a region by visual deprivation, but it can be decreased subsequently by removing the plastic occluders that produced the deprivation. In the latter situation, the growth rate is subnormal until the eye returns to its normal proportions and refraction (Wallman and Adams 1987). This decreased growth, like the increased growth during deprivation, can occur in local regions of the eye, while other regions are growing normally. Thus, if half the eye is deprived for two weeks, making that half enlarged

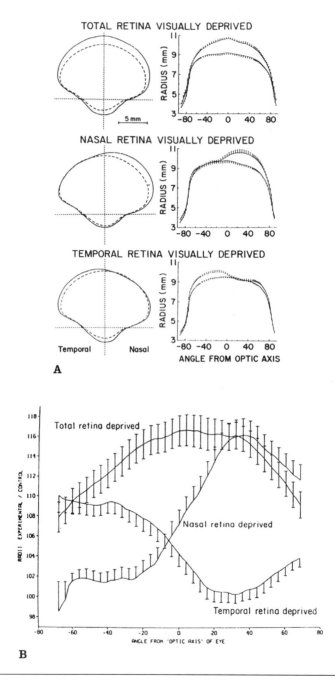

Figure 15.1. Effects of visual deprivation on the shape of the chick eye when either the entire retina was deprived, or when nasal or temporal halves were deprived. **(A)** Eyes photographed from above, traced, aligned and

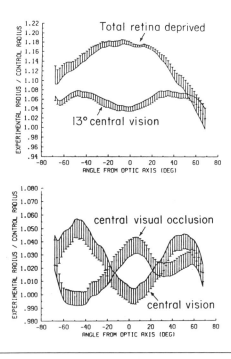

Figure 15.2. Effect of central or peripheral retinal deprivation on the shape of the chick eye. Methods are as in Figure 15.2. (Top) A small region of unobstructed central visual field reduces the elongation of the posterior vitreous chamber. The region of sclera affected is much larger than the visual field, in part because eye movements result in a larger area of retina having vision. (Bottom) Opposite effects of central and peripheral visual deprivation. The eyes with the central visual field (35 degrees) blocked by a partial occluder had a protrusion at the posterior pole of the eye; those with deprivation of the entire periphery except for the central 25 degrees had a central invagination, resulting in the axial length of the eye being essentially normal.

averaged, showing enlarged vitreous chambers only in visually deprived regions of the retina. Solid lines, experimental eyes; interrupted lines, fellow untreated eyes. (Center) Distance to the sclera from the midpoint of the line joining the corneal margins (origin of axes on left of figure). Upward error bars (sem) denote the experimental eyes; downward, the untreated fellow eyes. (B) Experimental eye radii as percentage of control eye radii at each angle. If the visual deprivation had no effect on eye size, the line would be at 100%. Values above 100% mean the experimental eye was larger. As in other sections of this figure, positive angles show nasal retinal loci. Note that only visually deprived regions are enlarged. (Adapted from Wallman et al. 1987.)

and myopic, removal of the occluder causes a rapid return to symmetry of the eye and to normal refractions along the different measuring axes.

These findings argue that local regions of the retina can control the growth of the underlying sclera, thereby resulting in enlargement of the deprived part of the eye. This enlargement appears to involve increased cell division and protein synthesis in the sclera. Specifically, we find biochemical evidence of increased DNA synthesis (increased uptake of tritiated thymidine) (Christensen and Wallman 1989), as well as histologic and autoradiographic evidence of an increased incidence of dividing cells, especially in the posterior sclera (Gottlieb et al. 1988, Christensen et al. 1990). In addition, there appears to be an increase in extracellular material, again shown both biochemically (increased uptake of labeled methionine into protein) and histologically (decreased density of cells, despite the higher rate of proliferation).

□ Is the Effect of Pattern Deprivation due to Decreased Retinal Activity?

The effects just discussed seem to require that local changes in the activity of retinal neurons cause a local change in the growth of the sclera. At first, it might seem that because deprivation of patterns, and not of light, is effective, the neurons affected must be pattern sensitive; but this is not necessarily the case. The activity of most retinal neurons viewing an unchanging stimulus decays with time. Thus the average level of activity under normal stimulus conditions would be determined largely by changes in the images viewed. Normally, eye movements would provide frequent change in the stimulation received. In lid-sutured or occluded eyes, the stimulation received before and after an eye movement would be nearly identical; thus eye movements presumably would do little to halt the decay of activity with time. The implication of this reasoning is that any cell that had transient responses would show lower activity with pattern deprivation. Thus, even non-neuronal cells, such as Müller cells, could be the relevant sensors.

As mentioned at the beginning of this chapter, one can envision that the aggregate neural activity of the retina might be maximal when an image is sharply focused on the retina — both because the contrast would be maximal and because neurons responding to small features (high spatial frequencies) would be especially active. This increased neural activity might be the signal to stop eye growth when emmetropia is reached. If this were true, in visual deprivation this "stop" signal might be absent and growth, therefore, would proceed unchecked.

If a factor controlling the growth of the eye is simply the overall neural activity, how are periods of high and low activity integrated? Does the total neural activity of some population of neurons accumulated over a day or a week determine the rate of elongation of the eye? If this were so, one could imagine a variety of seemingly inconsequential changes in behavior having large effects on the growth of the eye. For example, during reading, one can suppose that only neurons sensitive to the fine details (high spatial frequencies) of the text would be highly active; other neurons would experience little change in stimulation from one eye movement to the next because of the lack of large objects (low spatial frequencies) and thus the overall summed neural activity might be lower. This could account for the association of large amounts of reading with myopia (Wallman et al. 1987). Of course, to assess such an admittedly unconventional hypothesis, one would need to know more about how the neural activity was integrated over time. Could a few hours of mild deprivation per day in fact lead to myopia? At present, these questions are difficult to answer for humans.

To explore the time course of deprivation on myopia in chicks, we raised chicks with removable translucent occluders and gave them visual deprivation for part of each day and vision for the rest. The results were surprising: Even ten hours of visual deprivation each day (the lights were on for 14 hours) caused little myopia (Nickla et al. 1989). Thus it appears either that a small amount of vision can compensate for a large amount of deprivation or that the deprivation is ineffective unless it is continuous for a certain period of time. Similar results have been reported in monkeys visually deprived by wearing black contact lenses (Tigges et al. 1989).

If the level of retinal neural activity is the important determinant of eye growth and experimental myopia, one should be able to protect against the effect of visual deprivation by artificially raising the level of retinal neural activity. To test this hypothesis, we supplemented the illumination with a stroboscopic light. (Most retinal neurons respond to stroboscopic illumination to some extent.) We found that under these conditions, both partial and complete occluders caused much less severe eye enlargement and myopia, and some eyes are even driven considerably hyperopic by this illumination (Gottlieb and Wallman 1987).

These results are consistent with the view that increased gross neural activity is associated with decreased scleral growth. Gross activity, however, could not be the only factor. Stroboscopic illumination causes enormous variability in refraction and eye growth, some eyes becoming very myopic and others very hyperopic. When extreme hyperopia is seen, it generally occurs in the occluded eyes, not in the unrestricted fellow eyes, although the latter would presumably have even higher average neural activity. This implies that with vision, effective emmetropization can take place; without vision, some less precise control of growth based on the gross activity of some or all of the neurons remains.

If gross activity were the principal factor influencing eye growth, one would expect that any manipulation that lowered the retinal activity would produce ocular enlargement and myopia; however, this does not seem to be the case. Eyes without visual restriction in which the action potentials of neurons in the inner retina are blocked by tetrodotoxin do not become enlarged in either chicks (our unpublished data) or tree shrews (Norton et al. 1989). Furthermore, animals blinded with toxins that damage the photoreceptors and pigment epithelium do not develop enlarged eyes (Oishi and Lauber 1988). Thus, there might be two populations of retinal neurons involved in the control of scleral growth: a population having a growth-inhibiting effect and another having a growth-stimulating effect.

□ Which Neurons Might Mediate Visual Control of Growth?

Among the various types of neurons that might play a role in regulating eye growth, several cell types can be ruled out as the primary players. Retinal ganglion cells are unlikely to be necessary because eyes in which ganglion cells were eliminated as a result of earlier optic nerve section still develop pattern-deprivation myopia (Wildsoet and Pettigrew 1989). In addition, just after section of the optic nerve, eyes can support normal regulation of growth in a nondeprived part of the eye, while becoming enlarged in other parts of the same eye (Troilo et al. 1987). Although such eyes possess retinal ganglion cells, it seems unlikely that they are functioning normally.

Perhaps the most likely candidates for control of eye growth are the amacrine cells. Because over thirty types of amacrine cells have been identified, it is tempting to speculate that different types may have different roles. Evidence supporting this conjecture comes from the results of applying toxins that might be expected to have differential effects on different types of amacrine cells. Thus, kainic acid (a glutamate analog) produces enlargement of the vitreous chamber (Wildsoet and Pettigrew 1988, Barrington et al. 1988). In contrast, quisqualic acid, another glutamate analog that affects different receptors, reduces growth of the vitreous chamber, but increases the depth of the anterior chamber (Barrington et al. 1988). Finally, assays of retinas for a variety of neurotransmitters and peptides show a complex pattern of increases and decreases with pattern deprivation. Of particular interest is the fact that in chicks (Stone et al. 1989) and in monkeys (Iuvone et al. 1989), lid suture causes a decrease in retinal dopamine levels. In monkeys, vasoactive intestinal peptide (VIP) has been shown to be increased by lid suture (Stone et al. 1988). Of course, because pattern vision is a major retinal function, it is not surprising that its deprivation changes the levels of various neuropeptides and neurotransmitters. The problem is to identify which of these changes are functionally connected with eye elongation or its inhibition. A step in this direction has been taken with respect to dopamine, by showing that visual deprivation causes less axial elongation if the dopamine agonist apomorphine is given daily to chicks (Stone et al. 1989) or monkeys (Iuvone et al. 1990).

Even if one knew which cells were the visual sensors involved in regulating the growth of the sclera, there would remain a major obstacle to understanding how growth regulation could be accomplished: How does the retina influence the sclera? Because an intact optic nerve is not needed, the brain does not seem to be essential. Assuming that the influence is humoral, one must explain how the humoral agent penetrates the tight barrier of the pigment epithelium, and then how it traverses the extensive fenestrated vasculature of the choroid, without becoming widely distributed. These mysteries are all unplumbed.

EMMETROPIZATION

Both humans and chicks are born generally hyperopic with highly variable refractions, which quickly move toward emmetropia with less variability (Figure 15.3). The results presented up to this point argue that it is at least plausible that vision plays a role in the growth toward emmetropia. The important question is whether the role of vision is to guide the eye toward emmetropia from either direction by some kind of feedback mechanism, or whether the eye simply grows away from hyperopia until emmetropia is reached, at which point some visual cue causes it to stop. As an aid to discussion of experiments on emmetropization, consider Figure 15.4, which shows the four important factors that determine whether the image is focused behind or in front of the retina. Using the clinical convention of

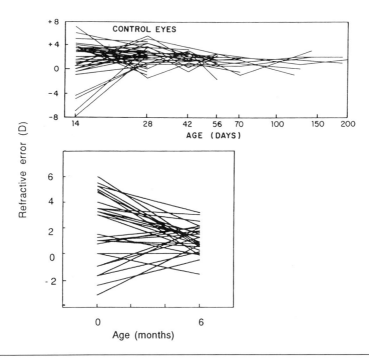

Figure 15.3. Emmetropization in chicken and human neonates. Upper: Change in distribution of spherical refractive error of chicks at different ages. Arrows point to median (From Wallman and Adams 1987). Lower: Change in cycloplegic refractive error in infants measured at birth and 6 months of age. (Data replotted from Doctoral Thesis of Dr. Caroline Thompson, Aston University.)

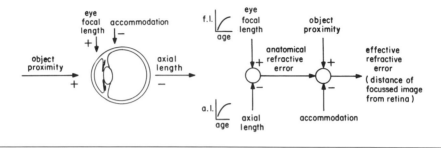

Figure 15.4. Diagrammatic representation of the effect of different factors on the refractive error of the eye. Factors with positive signs change the refractive error in the direction of hyperopia; those with negative signs change it in the direction of myopia. The diagram on the right shows a slightly more formal treatment of the same variables shown at left. In young eyes, both the focal length and the axial length of the eye grow. If they grow at the same rate, there is no anatomical refractive error. If the accommodation and object proximity are also balanced, the image will be focused on the retina.

positive signs for hyperopic refractive errors, both the resting focal length of the eye and the object proximity (relative to optical infinity) are given positive signs because an increase in either causes the image to be focused behind the retina (effective hyperopia), whereas accommodation and axial length are given negative signs because an increase in either causes the image to be focused in front of the retina (effective myopia). The anatomical refractive error is given by the difference between the resting focal length and axial length; this difference corresponds to whether the image is in front of or behind the retina (effective refractive error) only when the amount of accommodation is exactly equal to the proximity of the object viewed.

□ Experimental Studies of Emmetropization

The only adequate way to test the hypothesis that emmetropization is regulated by visual feedback would be to change the effective refractive error by varying one of the inputs shown in Figure 15.4 and to look for a compensatory change in the axial length or the resting focal length. I have already discussed the evidence that visual deprivation causes ocular elongation and myopia. This is, however, weak evidence that emmetropization is normally guided by vision. Conceivably, visual deprivation might have pathological effects on the retina or brain via mechanisms that do not normally play a role in emmetropization. For example, the visual deprivations used in the experiments discussed earlier may attenuate the amplitude of normal circadian cycles of dopamine and melatonin (Stone et al. 1989). The attenuation of these rhythms might play a role in deprivation-induced myopia, but such attenuation might never normally occur and thus would not be involved in normal emmetropization.

More relevant to the mechanism of emmetropization are experiments in which the eye is made, in effect, more hyperopic or myopic than it otherwise would be, in order to see the consequences on its subsequent growth. This can be accomplished in three general ways: One can actually change the optical power of the eye, by means of spectacles, contact lenses, or radial keratotomy; one can make the environment closer than usual to the animal, which is optically identical to making the animal hyperopic (images are focused behind the retina and accommodation is required for clear vision); or one can make the eye myopic or hyperopic by prior visual deprivation and then examine its subsequent growth. Such experiments test whether the growing animal can sense that it is hyperopic or myopic and adjust growth to compensate for it; they say nothing about what mechanism is used to sense the refractive error. This is an important caveat because several studies have assumed that since hyperopic eyes need to accommodate more, any response to an imposed hyperopia (such as by forced near viewing) must be mediated by accommodation.

The most direct test of whether induced refractive errors can be compensated for was that of Schaeffel et al. (1988), who made chicks either functionally myopic, with positive lens spectacles, or functionally hyperopic, with negative lens spectacles, and found that the refractions and axial lengths changed to compensate for the imposed refractive errors; that is, the functionally hyperopic eyes grew longer and became less hyperopic (with the spectacles), and the functionally myopic eyes stayed shorter and became less myopic. To assess whether accommodation was the cue for refractive error or the mechanism for change in axial length, Schaeffel and Howland, in collaboration with D. Troilo and myself, repeated this experiment in animals unable to accommodate because of a lesion of the Edinger-Westphal nucleus (the source of the premotor neurons driving the ciliary muscle); the same compensation for the imposed refractive error occurred, suggesting that accommodation is not essential for this regulation of growth (Schaeffel et al. 1990).

Concomitantly, Troilo followed the eye growth of chickens made myopic by being raised with translucent occluders or hyperopic by being raised in darkness. In these cases as well, eyes grew to compensate for their refractive errors, even when they could not accommodate because of Edinger-Westphal lesions (Troilo 1989). Even more surprisingly, eyes in which the optic nerve had been severed grew in the correct direction to compensate for their refractive errors, although they did not stop at emmetropia. This result suggests that the eye by itself can sense both the magnitude and direction of its refractive error and direct its growth toward emmetropia. This seems to rule out the simplest mechanism introduced at the start of this chapter — that eyes grow longer when blurred images are present and cease growth when sharp images are present. Rather, the eye seems able to discern the difference between myopic and hyperopic images and to modulate growth appropriately to compensate for either type of refractive error.

Even local regions of the retina may be able to provoke local growth to compensate for effective hyperopia imposed on part of the retina. F.A. Miles did an experiment in our laboratory in which he raised chicks in large enclosures with a patterned cloth ceiling just over their heads, so that the ventral part of the retina viewed only nearby objects. As mentioned earlier, the presence of nearby objects caused the part of the retina viewing them (in this case, the ventral retina) to be functionally hyperopic. In these eyes, the ventral halves became longer and more myopic than the ventral halves of the eyes of birds reared identically except that the cloth ceiling was 9 feet over their heads (Miles and Wallman 1990). This result suggests that local regions of retina can sense their refractive error and direct growth of the subjacent regions of sclera to correct the functional ametropia. Our laboratory has further evidence that emmetropization can take place within local retinal regions in that we find that when locally myopic eyes have the occluders removed early in life, the myopic portions return to emmetropia, and the shape of the eye changes from having a protuberance in the deprived region.

The four experiments just discussed form two complementary pairs. In the experiments in which the eye is recovering from myopia and hyperopia, visual factors cause an abnormally shaped eye to return to its normal proportions, whereas in the spectacle experiments, visual factors cause an eye of normal proportions to become more or less elongated than it would otherwise be. These results argue that refractive error can be sensed and can determine the spatial pattern of eye growth. Similarly, the recovery from local deprivation involves growth toward normal shape, whereas the low-ceiling experiment involves local growth away from normal. These results argue that refractive error might be sensed and direct growth, even in arbitrary regions of the eye. Such local emmetropization could account for the fact that in flounders and skates (Sivak 1982), pigeons (Fitzke et al. 1985), and other birds (Erichsen and Hodos 1989), the ventral visual field is myopic, which may be an adaptation to the effective hyperopia caused by the proximity of the ground.

Visual factors, however, may not be the only influences on growth in these circumstances. A curious finding in these four experiments is that growth toward the normal condition occurred very rapidly, by tens of diopters per week, whereas growth away from the normal condition in the lens or low-ceiling condition was much slower. In addition, in the birds recovering from hyperopia, the shape of the cornea and of the posterior globe continued to change in the direction of those of normal eyes, even after emmetropia was attained. Thus, a nonvisual growth mechanism may be present, which adjusts the shape of the eye and which is also disabled by visual deprivation. In the recovery experiments, this mechanism might add together with the visual one to cause rapid recovery to normal eye-proportions, but, when the experimental conditions require that the eye grow away from normal proportions to attain emmetropia, the two mechanisms might be opposed, resulting in slower growth.

□ What Error Signal Might Guide Emmetropization?

The results discussed here show that eyes experimentally manipulated so that images are focused in front of the retina seem to grow differently from eyes in which images are focused in back of the retina in such a way as to compensate for the altered effective refractive error. This permits us to redraw Figure 15.4 as Figure 15.5, showing that any change that causes the image to be formed behind the retina (effective hyperopia or positive effective refractive error) leads to two different forms of compensation: change in accommodative output and change in rate of ocular elongation. Let us first consider the accommodative loop (upper part of the figure). Near objects make the eye effectively hyperopic. This effective hyperopia induces an accommodative response, which tends to correct the refractive error. However, negative feedback systems do not completely nullify the error signal (that is, the difference between input — in this case, proximity — and output — in this case, accommodation). For example, if an object at 0.25 m dis-

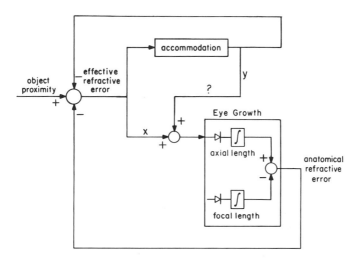

Figure 15.5.   A highly simplified diagram of the two feedback loops that control where images are focused in relation to the retina. The upper loop is a simplified version of the accommodation controller. The bottom is the hypothesized eye growth controller. Conventions as in Figure 15.4. Within the eye growth box, the focal length is assumed to increase relatively independently of the refractive status of the eye, whereas the axial length is modulated by the refractive error. The rectifying element represents the fact that growth can only go in one direction; the integrating element represents the fact that the dimensions of the eye constitute its accumulated growth.

tance (a 4.0 D stimulus) results in 3.8 D of accommodation, there will be an error of 0.2 D, which is the steady-state effective hyperopia. Thus, the 3.8 D of accommodative output is driven by the 0.2 D error signal.* Consequently, on a shorter time scale, when effective hyperopia is present, the eye increases its accommodation, which reduces the effective hyperopia by making the lens more powerful (decreased focal length), thereby moving the images forward toward the retina. On a longer time scale, the eye increases in length (lower loop), which reduces the effective hyperopia by moving the retina back toward the image.

For the error signal that is the input to the eye elongation loop, Figure 15.5 shows the three possibilities: a signal related to the effective refractive error itself (x), the output of the accommodation system (y), or both could signal the effective refractive error. The experiments described earlier show that accommodation is not necessary for emmetropization; therefore, y cannot be the only input. No definitive experiments show that a change in accommodation by itself causes a change in eye elongation; therefore, I have marked the y input with a question mark.

Viewed this way, both the accommodation system and the emmetropization system are similar in that they act to alter the relation of the optical power of the eye to its length, thereby minimizing effective refractive error and, as a result, optimizing image sharpness. In this sense, they differ only in time scale; the accommodation system acts in tenths of a second, but the emmetropization system acts over days, weeks, or years. Might they both use the same optical attribute of effective refractive error as an error signal? It is well established that the principal error signal used by the accommodation system is blur, although accommodation is aided by the presence of the spectral cues furnished by the chromatic aberration of the eye (different patterns of color occur for opposite signs of defocus), as well as by perceptual factors such as change in object size, which inform the brain that the object viewed is more likely to be getting nearer or farther. Blur by itself presents a difficulty as an error signal for either the accommodation or the emmetropization systems: It is not obvious how the eye or brain could tell whether the image is blurred because the eye is focused too close (myopic) or too far (hyperopic). The signals provided by chromatic aberration could provide the needed directional signal.

If the accommodation and emmetropization systems do use the same error sig-

---

*The diagram in Figure 15.5 is an oversimplification in that it shows the accommodation system as a proportional controller, whereas it probably is closer to an integrating controller (Schor et al. 1986). This probably does not affect the basic arguments made here, as the integration is not perfect and an error signal is continuously present. Consequently, the main effect of the integrator, as far as the present argument goes, is that the accommodation error signal would be smaller than that shown.

nal, it might seem that the emmetropization system would need to be more sensitive to this error signal than the accommodation system because otherwise the accommodation system, being more rapid, would focus the eye so accurately that the error signal would be eliminated as far as the emmetropization system is concerned. However, this is not entirely true. If a given error signal is adequate to maintain accommodative output, it would also be adequate to maintain an eye growth output. Alternatively, if the emmetropization system used an error signal other than blur, it could make use of the fact that the accommodation system cannot focus the eye perfectly because the nonzero depth of focus of the eye means that a certain amount of blur cannot be distinguished from a sharp image. For this reason, the eye tends to be slightly hyperopic for near objects and slightly myopic for distant ones. Perhaps this slight refractive error left uncorrected by the accommodation system furnishes the emmetropization system with the sign of the ametropia.

Although the scheme shown in Figure 15.5 may be correct in general, it fails to account for two important aspects of emmetropization. First, because most objects that we view are closer than infinity, it would seem that the retina would always tend to be at least slightly effectively hyperopic, which ought to lead to growth toward slight myopia, rather than emmetropia.

Second, Figure 15.5 does not take account of tonic accommodation. The accommodation controller does not produce zero output for zero input. Rather, with no input there is a moderate amount of tonic accommodation. Only when objects are at the distance corresponding to an individual's level of tonic accommodation is there no blur (zero error signal). At nearer distances, the accommodation controller produces somewhat less accommodation than required (lag of accommodation), whereas at farther distances, it produces somewhat more accommodation than required (lead of accommodation). These lags and leads occur because of an imperfect accommodation system, which always leaves an error signal that increases as a function of how far the input signal is from the zero point, that is, the tonic accommodation. It is not clear how the eye growth system avoids growing toward this refraction (moderate myopia) rather than emmetropia.

One possible solution to both problems is for the eye growth controller to use both the visual error signal (x) and the accommodation output (y) to compute the actual proximity of objects, regardless of the amount of accommodation. In this way, it would be using the accommodation output as an efference-copy signal, analogous to the mechanism by which we can infer the speed of a moving visual target when our eyes are also moving by adding together the visual speed on our retina to the known speed of the eye. Another solution, suggested by M. Bullimore of the University of California at Berkeley, would be for the eye-growth controller to somehow offset its setpoint by the level of tonic accommodation. If tonic accommodation tended to match the average proximity of objects in our environment, accurate emmetropization would result. How this might be accomplished is obscure.

■

CONCLUSIONS

This chapter has discussed two mysteries of eye growth: how lack of form vision can increase the growth of particular regions of the eye, leading to myopia, and how the normal eye can assess its refractive error and grow to correct it. It is unclear at this point what the relation of the mechanism of deprivation myopia is to that of emmetropization. It is tempting to think that the highly variable growth seen in deprived eyes, especially those under stroboscopic illumination, represents the aberrant stimulation of different classes of retinal neurons, which normally direct the growth of the eye toward myopia or hyperopia to achieve emmetropia.

On the basis of available evidence, the eye appears able to discern whether it is myopic or hyperopic. The mystery of what error signal is used to do this is deepened by the facts that this discrimination can be accomplished by the eye disconnected from the brain by optic nerve section and that it can be accomplished within local regions of the retina. These facts place additional constraints on the possible mechanism, which must rely not on the uncharted powers of the brain but on the more limited processing available within a local region of retina.

■

REFERENCES

Barrington M, Sattayasai J, Zappia J, Ehrlich D. Excitatory amino acids interfere with normal eye growth in posthatch chick. Curr Eye Res 1989;8:781–792.

Bercovitz AB, Harrison PC, Leary GA. Light induced alterations in growth pattern of the avian eye. Vis Res 1972;1:1253–1259.

Chiu PSL, Lauber JK, Kinnear A. Dimensional and physiological lesions in the chick eye as influenced by the light environment. Proc Soc Exp Biol Med 1975;148:1223–1228.

Christensen AM, Wallman J. Increased DNA and protein synthesis in scleras of eyes with visual-deprivation myopia. Invest Ophthalmol Vis Sci (ARVO Suppl) 1989;30:402.

Christensen AM, Nickla DL, Gottlieb MD, et al. Asymmetric regional growth in the chick sclera: a comparison of normal and form-deprived eyes. Invest Ophthalmol Vis Sci (ARVO Suppl) 1990;31:253.

Erichsen JT, Hodos W. Lower-field myopia in birds: an adaptation that keeps the ground in focus. Invest Ophthalmol Vis Sci (ARVO Suppl) 1989;30:31.

Ferree CE, Rand G, Hardy C. Refractive asymmetry in the temporal and nasal halves of the visual field. Am J Ophthalmol 1932;15:513–522.

Fitzke FW, Hayes BP, Hodos W, et al. Refractive sectors in the visual field of the pigeon eye. J Physiol 1985;369:33–45.

Gottlieb MD, Joshi HB, Wallman J. Local changes in the sclera of chick eyes made myopic by form deprivation. Invest Ophthalmol Vis Sci (ARVO Suppl) 1988;29:32.

Gottlieb MD, Wallman J. Retinal activity modulates eye growth: evidence from rearing in stroboscopic illumination. Soc Neurosci Abstr 1987;13:1297.

Gottlieb MD, Wentzek LA, Wallman J. Different visual restrictions produce different ametropias and different eye shapes. Invest Ophthalmol Vis Sci 1987;28:1225–1235.

Hayes BP, Fitzke FW, Hodos W, Holden AL. A morphological analysis of experimental myopia in young chickens. Invest Ophthalmol Vis Sci 1986;27:981–991.

Hodos W, Kuenzel WJ. Retinal-image degradation produces ocular enlargement in chicks. Invest Ophthalmol Vis Sci 1984;25:652–659.

Hodos W, Revzin AM, Kuenzel WJ. Thermal gradients in the chick eye: a contributing factor in experimental myopia. Invest Ophthalmol Vis Sci 1987;28:1859–1866.

Iuvone PM, Tigges M, Fernandes A, Tigges J. Dopamine synthesis and metabolism in rhesus monkey retina: development, aging, and the effects of monocular visual deprivation. Vis Neurosci 1989;2:465–472.

Iuvone PM, Tigges M, Stone RA, et al. Apomorphine inhibits development of myopia in visually-deprived infant rhesus monkeys. Invest Ophthalmol Vis Sci (ARVO Suppl) 1990; 31:254.

Lauber JK, Oishi T. Lid suture myopia in chicks. Invest Ophthalmol Vis Sci 1987;28:1851–1858.

Miles FA, Wallman J. Local ocular compensation for imposed local refractive error. Vis Res 1990;30:339–349.

Millodot M. Effect of ametropia on peripheral refraction. Am J Optom Physiol Opt 1985; 58:691–695.

Nickla DL, Panos SN, Fugate-Wentzek LA, et al. What attributes of visual stimulation determine whether chick eyes develop deprivation myopia? Invest Ophthalmol Vis Sci (Suppl) 1989;30:31.

Norton TT, Essinger JA, McBrien NA. Lid-suture myopia in tree shrew despite blockade of ganglion cell action potentials. Invest Ophthalmol Vis Sci (ARVO Suppl) 1989;30:31.

Oishi T, Lauber JK. Chicks blinded with formoguanamine do not develop lid suture myopia. Curr Eye Res 1988;7:69–73.

Oishi T, Lauber JK, Vriend J. Experimental myopia and glaucoma in chicks. Zoo Sci 1987; 4:455–464.

Pickett-Seltner RL, Sivak JG, Pasternak JJ. Experimentally induced myopia in chicks: morphometric and biochemical analysis during the first 14 days after hatching. Vis Res 1988; 28:2:323–328.

Raviola E, Wiesel TN. Effect of dark-rearing on experimental myopia in monkeys. Invest Ophthalmol Vis Sci 1978;17:485–488.

Regal DM, Boothe R, Teller DY, Sackett GP. Visual acuity and visual responsiveness in dark-reared monkeys (*Macaca nemestrina*). Vis Res 1976;16:523–530.

Schaeffel F, Troilo D, Wallman J, Howland HC. Developing eyes that lack accommodation grow to compensate for imposed defocus. Vis Neurosci 1990;4:177–183.

Schaeffel F, Glasser A, Howland HC. Accommodation, refractive error, and eye growth in chickens. Vis Res 1988;28:639–657.

Schor CM, Kotulak JC, Tsuetaki T. Adaptation of tonic accommodation reduces accommodative lag and is masked in darkness. Invest Ophthalmol Vis Sci 1986;27:820–827.

Sivak JG. Optical characteristics of the eye of the flounder. J Comp Physiol 1982;146:345–349.

Stone R, Laties AM, Raviola E, Wiesel TN. Increase in retinal vasoactive intestinal polypeptide after eyelid fusion in primates. Proc Natl Acad Sci USA 1988;85:257–260.

Stone RA, Lin T, Laties AM, Iuvone PM. Retinal dopamine and form-deprivation myopia. Proc Natl Acad Sci USA 1989;86:704–706.

Tigges M, Tigges J, Fernandes A, et al. Axial eye growth of normal and visually deprived infant monkeys. Invest Ophthalmol Vis Sci (ARVO Suppl) 1989;30:301.

Troilo D. The visual control of eye growth in chicks. Doctoral Thesis, City Univ. of New York, 1989.

Troilo D, Gottlieb MD, Wallman J. Visual deprivation causes myopia in chicks with optic nerve section. Curr Eye Res 1987;6:993–999.

Van Alphen GWHM. On Emmetropia and Ametropia. Ophthalmologica (Suppl) 1961; 142:1–92.

Wallman J, Adams JI. Developmental aspects of experimental myopia in chicks: susceptibility, recovery and relation to emmetropization. Vis Res 1987;27:1139–1163.

Wallman J, Adams JI, Trachtman JN. The eyes of young chickens grow toward emmetropia. Invest Ophthalmol Vis Sci 1981;20:557–561.

Wallman J, Gottlieb MD, Rajaram V, Fugate-Wentzek LA. Local retinal regions control local eye growth and myopia. Science 1987;237:73–77.

Wallman J, Turkel J, Trachtman J. Extreme myopia produced by modest changes in early visual experience. Science 1978;201:1249–1251.

Wildsoet CF, Pettigrew JD. Experimental myopia and anomalous eye growth patterns unaffected by optic nerve section in chickens: evidence for local control of eye growth. Clin Vis Sci 1988;3:99–107.

Wildsoet CF, Pettigrew JD. Kainic acid-induced eye enlargement in chickens; differential effects on anterior and posterior segments. Invest Ophthalmol Vis Sci 1988;29:311–319.

Wildsoet CF, Pettigrew JD. Lid-sutured induced myopia in chickens is not dependent on ganglion cell activity. Invest Ophthalmol Vis Sci (ARVO Suppl) 1989;30:31.

Yinon U, Koslowe KC. Eyelid closure effects on the refractive error of the eye in dark- and in light-reared kittens. Am J Optom Physiol Opt 1984;61:271–273.

Yinon U, Koslowe KC. Hypermetropia in dark-reared chicks and the effect of lid suture. Vis Res 1986;26:999–1005.

Yinon U, Koslowe KC, Lobel D, et al. Lid suture myopia in developing chicks: optical and structural considerations. Curr Eye Res 1983;2:877–882.

_16

Mechanical Considerations in Myopia

Peter R. Greene

☐

■

THEORETICAL ISSUES

The fundamental problem in myopia research is that only the back of the eyeball is distorted. The forward portion of the corneoscleral shell remains normal. The eye starts out being approximately spherical in a young person but slowly and steadily, typically over the 10-year period from age 8 to 18, the posterior sclera appears to creep into the shape of a prolate spheroid. If this circumstance is to be explained in mechanical terms there are only two possibilities: (1) Either the back of the myope's ocular shell is _mechanically weak_ in some sense (that is, has a lower yield stress, or a greater propensity to creep), or (2) _concentrated forces_ are some-how exerted in this area and not elsewhere. A third possibility is that both of these mechanisms occur together. To date, our research has been concerned exclusively with the first possibility, namely, examining factors that can influence the _creep rate_ of the ocular shell. We have found that the temperature and pressure are important parameters in determining the rate at which the sclera creeps (Greene and McMahon 1979).

The classical picture of the corneoscleral shell of an axially myopic eye is shown in Figure 16.1. The degree of scleral distortion shown here represents about 18.00 D of myopia. Note that the geometry is that of a prolate spheroid, and the posterior sclera is thinned. A schematic sketch of the fundus of the pathologically myopic eye is shown in Figure 16.2. This left eye shows an elliptical region, which

This was supported in part by the National Institutes of Health Grant 5-RO1-EY-01907-02 and by the Division of Applied Sciences, Harvard University, Cambridge, Massachusetts. Special thanks go to William R. Baldwin, Carter C. Collins, Brian J. Curtin, David L. Guyton, Thomas A. McMahon, and Francis A. Young for their review and comments about this manuscript. The author would also like to thank B. Budiansky and J.J. Connor for some very helpful discussions.

Figure 16.1.
Geometry of the axially
myopic globe
superimposed on the
normal emmetropic
globe. Sketch shows the
prolate geometry and
scleral thinning
characteristic of the
posterior half of the
axially myopic eye. Also
note that the degree of
implied stretching is
greater on the temporal
side. This sketch
represents a horizontal
section through the left
globe, viewed from
above. (Modified after
Southall 1961.)

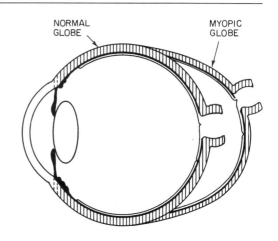

Figure 16.2. Fundus
sketch of the posterior
staphyloma from an eye
with pathologic myopia.
Fundus of the left eye,
viewed from the front,
is shown. Shaded area
represents the localized
herniation or out-
pouching characteristic
of this problem. The
staphyloma varies
among individuals in
size, shape, depth,
abruptness of the
margin, and associated
changes in the optic
nerve and retinal
vessels. (Modified after
Curtin 1977.)

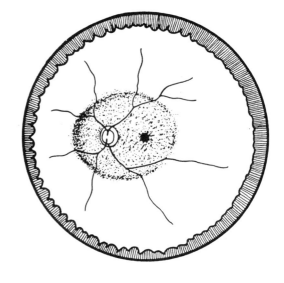

envelopes both the optic nerve head and the fovea. The shaded region represents the extent of the posterior staphyloma and can be thought of as a localized bulge in the posterior sclera. The staphyloma varies in geometry and location from one individual to the next, occasionally occurring nasally, but usually occurring temporally as shown in Figure 16.2.

Other important considerations suggest that mechanical concentrations can occur in the back of the ocular shell, particularly near and around the optic nerve entrance. To begin with, the attachment lines of both the inferior and superior oblique muscle insertions are located in the back half of the shell, the inferior oblique often being close to the optic nerve entrance. Figure 16.3 shows different artists' portrayals of the situation for the human eye (Sobotta 1957, Hogan et al. 1971). In addition, the entrance of the optic nerve into the back of the ocular shell creates a problem similar to the problem in applied mechanics of a stress-free hole in an infinite plate. (The lamina cribrosa partially reinforces the hole, but we have no mechanical data about the strength of the reinforcement.) Such a hole in a plate or shell-like structure inevitably gives rise to an augmentation of mechanical stress at the edge of the hole; for this reason, rivet holes in airplane wings and in the hulls of ships are often a source of mechanical failure (Timoshenko and Goodier 1934).

In engineering, mechanical stress is an important concept (Crandall et al. 1972). For a solid body subjected to external forces, the mechanical stress varies from point to point within the solid, and the forces are said to give rise to a "stress field" or a "stress distribution" within the solid. Stress is specified in units of force per unit area, and can be *tensile, compressive,* or *shear.* When one pulls on a rubber band, the forces produce uniaxial tensile stress; that is, the rubber band is under tension. In the case of an inflated spherical shell, such as the eye, the material is under biaxial stress, being pulled equally in all directions in the plane of the shell. The magnitude of the stress, s, is given by Laplace's law (Kraus 1967):

$$s = \frac{(p_i - p_o)R}{2h} \tag{1}$$

where s = stress (g/mm^2)
  p_i = internal pressure of the sphere (g/mm^2)
  p_o = outside pressure of the sphere (g/mm^2)
  R = radius of the sphere (mm)
  h = thickness of the spherical shell (mm)

In Equation 16.1, the difference $(p_i - p_o)$ is referred to as the *transmural pressure drop*, literally, the pressure drop "across the wall," and is the difference between the internal and external pressures on the spherical shell. The wall stress is directly proportional to this transmural pressure. In the context of the posterior sclera, the external pressure, p_o, refers to the pressure of the orbital contents

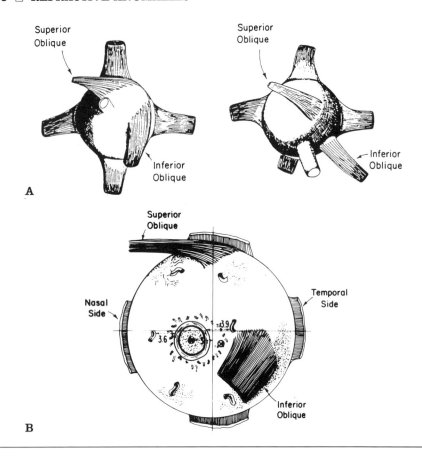

Figure 16.3. **(A)** Two slightly different views of the posterior aspect of the normal human globe showing the attachment locations of the superior and inferior oblique muscles. Note that the attachment widths and locations with respect to the optic nerve can vary (Modified after Sobotta 1957). **(B)** Another view of the posterior aspect of the normal human eye showing the inferior oblique attaching very close to the optic nerve entrance port. Dimensions quoted are in millimeters. Circle with X represents the location of the fovea. (Modified after Hogan et al. 1971.)

(Moller 1955), and the internal pressure, p_i, refers to the pressure of the supra-choroidal space (which is only slightly different from the vitreous pressure). Assuming a transmural pressure of 15 mm Hg, a globe radius of 12 mm and a shell thickness of 1 mm, one finds that the wall stress imposed by this pressure is 1.2 g/mm^2. This is an important reference number, which will be compared (in the next section) to the stress imposed by the oblique muscles.

Two additional classic results from the field of applied mechanics should be mentioned to appreciate the distribution of tensile stress in the posterior sclera. The first concerns a point force exerted parallel to the surface of a flat plate, and the second concerns the effects of a circular hole in a flat plate under tension.

Figure 16.4 shows the idealized notion of a point force acting parallel to a plate. This example is presented as a first approximation to the situation where an extra-ocular muscle pulls tangentially to the ocular shell. In the next section, this point of force solution will be integrated numerically to include the case of line of force, analogous to the line of attachment of the oblique muscle insertions on the posterior sclera. The analytical solution of the point force problem is (Timoshenko and Goodier 1934):

$$s_x = \frac{P \cos \Theta}{4 \ rh} \left[- (3 + v) + 2(1 + v) \sin^2 \Theta \right] \qquad (2)$$

where s_x = tensile (or compressive) stress in the x direction (g/mm²)
     P = force (g)
     r = radial distance from (x,y) to the point of force of P (mm)
     h = plate thickness (mm)
     v = Poisson's ratio (0< v <0.5)
     Θ = angle as shown in Figure 16.4A

Figure 16.4. (A) Tensile and compressive stress distribution caused by an in-plane point source of force. Ahead of the force P the stresses are compressive, whereas behind the force they are tensile. (B) Perspective view of a plate showing the idealized mathematical notion of an in-plane point source of force.

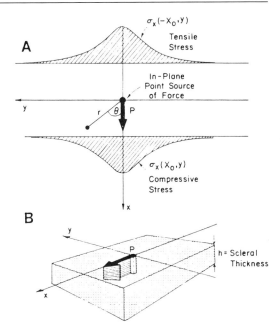

For the sclera, Poisson's ratio is 0.5 (Woo et al. 1972). Under these circumstances, Equation 16.2 becomes:

$$S_x = \frac{P \cos \Theta}{4 \, rh} [3 \sin^2 \Theta - 3.5] \qquad (3)$$

The x-direction stresses are the largest in the problem. The complete solution also involves shear stresses and stresses in the y-direction, but they are not presented here because they are smaller.

The importance of the point force solution, as given in Equation 16.3, is that the stress becomes distributed in the plane of the plate. To some extent, the effects of the force P are felt everywhere in the plate, but they are greatest near the point of application and diffuse out as one moves away from this point. As shown in Figure 16.4A, the stress distribution is symmetric in shape about the line x = 0, but of opposite sign on either side of this line. In other words, the plate supports the load P, half by compressive stresses ahead of the force, and half by tensile stresses behind the force. The situation is exactly symmetric. Also, as indicated in Figure 16.4A, it is important to note that the stress diffuses laterally away from the line of the force (that is, is not concentrated along the line y = 0).

Finally, there is the problem of the circular hole in the plate under tension, which is similar to the mechanical situation in the vicinity of the ocular shell where the optic nerve enters. The solution to this problem is too complex to present here, so only the results are shown in Figure 16.5 (Timoshenko and Goodier 1934). Tension is applied uniformly at the upper and lower borders of the plate. The stress is smoothly distributed about the hole and is amplified by a factor of 3.0 at the edge of the hole. This phenomenon is referred to as a "stress concen-

---

Figure 16.5.
Distribution of tensile stress in the x-direction around a hole in a flat plate. The plate is under a uniform state of tension applied far away from the hole. The stress is augmented by a factor of 3.0 at the edge of the hole. The claim is that a similar phenomenon occurs around the optic nerve.

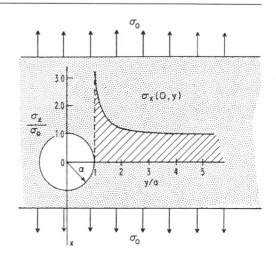

tration," and this particular problem is said to have a "stress concentration factor" of 3.0. It is well known that mechanical failure (that is, crack growth, fatigue, creep, etc.) always occurs first at the edge of such holes, as predicted by the theoretical solution shown in Figure 16.5 (Timoshenko and Goodier 1934).

STRESSES ON THE POSTERIOR SCLERA

The engineering concepts presented in the foregoing section will now be extended to the case of the back of the human eyeball. First, the isolated point force solution for a plate will be used to calculate the stress field produced by the two oblique muscles when pulling simultaneously in antagonistic directions. The problem is considerably more difficult when shell curvature is included, but this is beyond the scope of this chapter (Kraus 1967). The primary change caused by including shell curvature is the addition of localized bending stresses near sites of applied force, in addition to the in-plate tensile, compressive, and shear stresses already discussed.

The range of forces to be expected from either oblique muscle is from 10 to 40 g. These values are well within the range expected for the extraocular muscles, the lower value representing the resting tension. Robinson (1964) shows that the extraocular muscles can generate 150 g (peak) and routinely produce 40 g during large amplitude saccades. It would be valuable to have direct measurements of the force developed in all six of the extraocular muscles during convergence, and other ocular maneuvers as well; however, this is a very difficult experimental task. Electromyogram records do exist, but Davson (1969) cautions that electromyography is not an indicator of force of a muscle, but only of electrical activity. A muscle can easily withstand force, that is, by being stretched, without producing a change in the electromyographic signal.

We are now in a position to calculate the distribution of tensile and compressive stresses imposed on the posterior sclera by the pull of the oblique muscles. As mentioned in the discussion of a point force applied in the plane of a plate, one half of the load is carried by compressive stresses on the trailing edge of the attachment line, and one half of the load is carried by tensile stresses at the leading edge of the attachment line (see Figure 16.4A). The magnitude of these stresses is given by:

$$s = \frac{P}{2\,Ah} \tag{4}$$

where P = muscle force (g)
    h = thickness of the scleral shell (mm)
    A = width of the line of attachment (mm)

Neglecting shear stress, Equation 16.4 can be derived by drawing a control volume enclosing the oblique attachment line and then shrinking this volume to the attachment. The width of the oblique muscle attachments can be anywhere from 5 to 14 mm, a considerable variation from one subject to the next (Hogan et al. 1971). Finally, the posterior sclera is usually about 1 mm thick, but can be as thin as 0.1 mm in advanced cases of pathologic myopia (Friedman 1966). Table 16.1 shows the results of plugging various forces P and muscle widths A into Equation 16.4 for a scleral thickness fixed at 1.0 mm. These numbers represent the mechanical stress in a plate due to the pull of one muscle attached along a line. For two muscles attached close to each other pulling in opposite directions, these numbers all double. For a thinner sclera, these stresses all increase: For instance, for a 0.1 mm thick sclera, the stresses in Table 16.1 all become greater by a factor of 10.

The values for mechanical stress quoted in Table 16.1 are meaningful when referred to the stress imposed on the ocular shell by the vitreous pressure. As already shown, a transmural stress of 15 mm Hg produces a scleral stress of 1.2 g/mm. Thus, the oblique muscles can exert stresses locally that are of the same order of magnitude or greater than the wall stress produced by the vitreous pressure. This muscle-induced stress depends strongly on oblique tension, the width of the attachment line, and the thickness of the posterior sclera. The worst case would be realized with narrow muscle attachment lines only 5 mm wide, the superior and inferior oblique muscles attached very close together, an oblique muscle tension of 40 g, and a sclera only 0.1 mm thick. Under these circumstances, the tensile stress in the region between the oblique muscles is 80 g/mm².

Because the problem is linear, the actual stress experienced by the posterior sclera is the sum of the stress induced by the intraocular pressure and that induced by the oblique muscles. Thus, the compressive stresses produced on the trailing

Table 16.1. **Mechanical Stress in Sclera Near Oblique Muscle Attachments (g/mm²) as a Function of Muscle Force and Attachment Width**[a]

Muscle attachment width, A (mm)	Muscle force, P (g)			
	10	20	30	40
5	1.0	2.0	3.0	4.0
7	0.71	1.43	2.13	2.84
9	0.56	1.12	1.68	2.24
11	0.45	0.90	1.35	1.80
14	0.36	0.71	1.08	1.44

[a]This table assumes a scleral thickness of 1.0 mm.

edge of the oblique attachment are partially cancelled by the Laplace stress, whereas the tensile stresses produced on the leading edge of the oblique attachment are augmented by the Laplace stress.

The stress diffuses laterally away from the line of the applied force in a plate with two muscles attached and pulling in opposite directions. Because the problem is linear and superposable (Timoshenko and Goodier 1934), a large number of point sources of force can be located along a line on a plate as shown in Figure 16.6. For the sake of this particular calculation, 200 points of force were used along each muscle attachment. Figure 16.7 shows the results of the calculation. Traverses are made across the plane of the plate along various lines as indicated, and the distribution of the stress, s, is plotted with the traverse line as 0 reference. As expected, the region between the oblique muscle attachments is under tensile stress. As Figure 16.7A shows, the tensile stress diffuses laterally to a considerable extent, and for the geometry shown in Figure 16.3A, the optic nerve will encounter a considerable amount of tensile stress, even though it is off the center line. When the stress concentration factor of 3.0 is taken into account, the mechanical stress at the temporal border of the optic nerve entrance hole could easily be the greatest stress in the problem. This seems consistent with the fact that the posterior staphyloma in pathologic myopia always envelopes the optic nerve and is usually most pronounced on the temporal side of the globe (Curtin 1977).

Fibers in general are best at withstanding *tensile* stress; therefore, it would make good sense to align all fibers parallel to the direction of the tensile stresses and perpendicular to the direction of the compressive stresses. It would seem that

---

Figure 16.6.
Coordinate system for the computer program, which models plate stretching due to the antagonistic pull of the superior and inferior oblique muscles. A line of N point sources, each of equal strength, is used to model the pull of each oblique muscle on the sclera. A separate (r, θ) coordinate system is attached to each point source of force, in order to calculate its contribution at the point (x, y) in the plane.

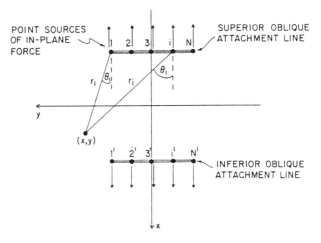

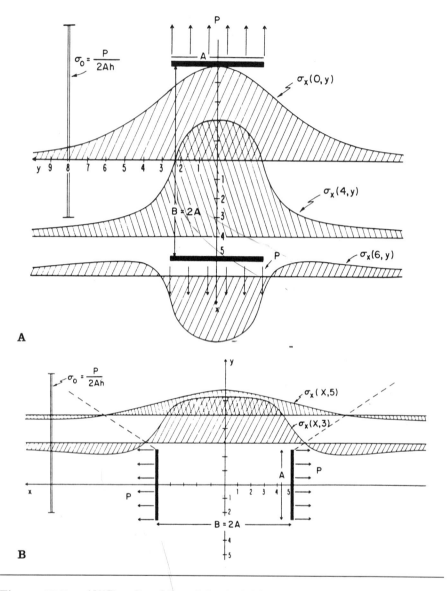

Figure 16.7. **(A)** Results of the plate-stretching computer program showing the distribution of stress at three different traverse locations with respect to the oblique muscles. For this particular case, the muscles are separated by a distance equal to twice their width. Note that in all cases, the stress field diffuses considerably off the center line. Also note that in some regions, the stress field changes sign from tensile to compressive stress. **(B)** Same as A, except that the traverses are made in a perpendicular direction. Note that the zero-crossing, where the stress changes from tensile to compressive, radiates away from the corners of the oblique attachment along the dashed line, as indicated for the 2 cases shown. Optimally, the optic nerve entrance hole should be located on this line to minimize stress concentration at the edge of the hole.

Figure 16.8. **(A)** Schematic diagram showing primary fibril bundle orientation in the posterior sclera. Note that the sclera seems to have responded to the structural demands placed on it by the antagonistic pull of the superior and inferior oblique muscles. **(B)** Fibril bundle directions as viewed from the top of the right eye. To a certain limited extent, the same effect of altered fiber directions can be detected near and around the superior rectus, but the effect is less pronounced than with the superior oblique. (Modified after Hogan et al. 1971.)

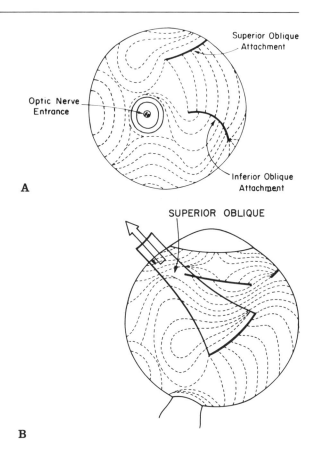

this is exactly what nature has arranged in the sclera. In Figure 16.8A and B, note that the fibers near the trailing edge of the attachment line of the superior oblique muscle run perpendicular to the compressive stress, s, in this area. The preferential orientation of the collagen fibrils seems to be clear proof that the oblique muscles exert significant stresses on the ocular shell.

MECHANICAL EFFECTS OF ACCOMMODATION AND CONVERGENCE COMPARED

The mechanical effects of accommodation are limited by the physical strength of the ciliary muscle, just as the mechanical effects of convergence are limited by the strength of the medial rectus muscle. The peak force exerted by the ciliary muscle is 0.6 g (Van Alphen 1961), whereas the peak force capability of the medial rectus muscle is 150 g (Robinson 1964). On this basis alone, it simply must be true that convergence mechanically dominates accommodation. The fundamental question now is, "How could the pull of the medial rectus muscle, being attached anteriorly and nasally, possibly have an effect on the stress distribution in the back of the scleral shell?" Several investigators have published experimental evidence that clearly indicates the effect is the result of an increase in *vitreous pressure*.

Coleman and Trokel (1969), in an unusual study in which intraocular pressure was measured directly in a human subject, recorded pressure increases of 5 to 10 mm Hg when the subject diverted his eyes from the straight-ahead position. Young (1975) reported an increase in vitreous pressure of 7 mm Hg in monkeys when accommodating and converging at close range. The effect lasts as long as the monkey's attention is held on the target. Finally, Collins et al. (1967) reported a vitreous pressure increase of 14 mm Hg in cats when the force developed by the extraocular muscles was increased by 11.6 g. This report very clearly shows that the mechanism by which the rectus muscles increase the vitreous pressure is *local indentation of the sclera*, thereby decreasing intraocular volume. The pressure remains elevated for 3 minutes of chemically induced muscle contraction. These three studies report experiments in which vitreous pressure rises from 5 to 14 mm Hg as a result of the pull of the extraocular muscles. These increases are considerably greater than those created by the choroid during accommodation.

Van Alphen found maximum choroid tension during accommodation to be 0.6 g for a strip of choroid 6.0 mm wide. This corresponds to an increase in vitreous pressure of less than 2 mm (Greene 1978). Furthermore, Van Alphen (1961) pointed out that a vitreous pressure increase generated by the choroid actually shields the sclera; in fact, he measured a pressure *drop* in the suprachoroidal space of 1.0 mm Hg.

Because the problem is linear, the total stress experienced by the posterior sclera is the sum of the stress induced by the vitreous pressure and that induced by the oblique muscles. During convergence, the region of the sclera between the two oblique muscle attachments will be subjected to tensile stresses higher than those at any other locale on the globe. Consequently, if the material properties of the sclera cause it to yield and creep for stresses above a certain magnitude (Greene and McMahon 1979), then this locale is the most likely to yield first.

■

CONCLUDING REMARKS

This chapter presents a review of the mechanical phenomena most likely to cause myopia. The calculations indicate that the oblique muscles can exert significant amounts of localized tensile stress on the posterior sclera, and with the increase in vitreous pressure associated with convergence, this concentrated stress may be sufficient to stretch the sclera permanently out of shape (Greene and McMahon 1979). The important mechanical and geometric parameters are the following:

1. Width of the oblique muscle attachment lines
2. Tension in the oblique muscles, both statically and during convergence
3. Location of the attachment lines with respect to the optic nerve entrance port (Figure 16.8C)
4. Thickness of the posterior sclera
5. Intrinsic mechanical properties of the posterior sclera
6. Vitreous pressure, both statically and during convergence.

A knowledge of all these parameters allows one to calculate the local mechanical stress (g/mm^2) experienced by the posterior sclera at both the leading and trailing edges of the attachment lines of the oblique muscles, before and during convergence, and to estimate the likelihood of permanent scleral distortion. The worst case is realized by narrow attachment lines, high tension in the oblique muscles, oblique attachments close to the optic nerve, a thin posterior sclera, a sclera with a high propensity to creep, and, finally, high vitreous pressure.

SUMMARY

In conclusion, it seems plausible that human myopia and experimental myopia in animals may have as a common denominator the mechanical stress imposed on the posterior sclera by the combined influence of the extraocular muscles and the vitreous pressure.

REFERENCES

Coleman DJ, Trokel S. Direct-recorded intraocular pressure variations in a human subject. Arch Ophthalmol 1969;82:637–640.

Collins CC, Bach-y-Rita P, Loeb DR. Intraocular pressure variation with oculo-rotary muscle tension. Am J Physiol 1967;213:1039–1043.

Crandall SH, Dahl NC, Lardner YJ. Introduction to the Mechanics of Solids. New York: McGraw-Hill Book Co, 1972.

Curtin BJ. The posterior staphyloma of pathological myopia. Trans Am Ophthalmol Soc 1977;75:67–84.

Davson H. Muscular Mechanisms, in the Eye, 2nd ed., vol. 3. New York: Academic Press, Inc, 1969.

Friedman B. Stress upon the ocular coats: effects of scleral curvature, scleral thickness, and intraocular pressure. Eye Ear Nose Throat Mon 1966;45:59–66.

Greene PR. Mechanical aspects of myopia. PhD Thesis. Division of Applied Sciences, Harvard University, 1978.

Greene PR, McMahon TA. Scleral creep vs temperature and pressure in vitro. Exp Eye Res 1979;29:527–537.

Hogan MJ, Alvarado JA, Weddell JE. Histology of the Human Eye, an Atlas and Textbook. Philadelphia: WB Saunders Co, 1971.

Kraus H. Thin Elastic Shells: An Introduction to the Theoretical Foundations and the Analysis of their Static and Dynamic Behavior. New York: John Wiley and Sons, 1967.

Moller PM. The Pressure in the Orbit. Copenhagen: Munksgaard, 1955.

Robinson DA. The mechanics of human saccadic eye movement. J Physiol 1964;174:245–264.

Sobotta J. Atlas of Descriptive Human Anatomy, ed. and trans. Uhlenhuth, 7th English ed., New York: Publishing Co., 1957.

Southall JPC. Introduction to Physiological Optics. New York: Dover, 1961.

Timoshenko SP, Goodier JN. Theory of Elasticity. New York: McGraw-Hill Book Co, 1934.

Van Alphen GWHM. On emmetropia and ametropia. Acta Opthalmologica (suppl) 1961. p. 1–92.

Woo SLY, Kobayashi AS, Schlegel WA, Lawrence C. Nonlinear material properties of intact cornea and sclera. Exp Eye Res 1972;14:29–39.

Young FA. The development and control of myopia in human and subhuman primates. Contacto 1975;19(6):16–31.

__17__

Accommodation and Vitreous Chamber Pressure: A Proposed Mechanism for Myopia

Francis A. Young and George A. Leary

☐

Although myopia has existed for centuries, its prevalence remained at a relatively low level of approximately 13% until the middle 1950s when it began to increase so rapidly that it was referred to as an "epidemic" of myopia (Roberts and Rowland 1978). The view of Steiger (1913) was that the refractive state of the eye results from a randomly distributed relationship between the power of the cornea and the axial length of the eye and, therefore, was a genetically determined condition. He based his conclusion on a study of the corneal power measurements, which seemed to fit a normal curve. He made no measurements of axial length, as no technique was available to do this during his lifetime. His assumption of the random distribution of axial length was later disproved in a paper published by Stenström (1948), who used x-rays to measure the axial length of the eye and found that axial length was not distributed normally and was the major cause of myopia, correlating -0.76 with refractive error.

■
STRUCTURAL CHANGES DURING ACCOMMODATION

Hess (1904) and Heine (1905) pressed a needle through the sclera and choroid of a live monkey and found that the exposed part of the needle moved toward the back of the eye when accommodation was induced and moved back to its original position when accommodation was relaxed. They reasoned that the backward movement of the needle must have been due to the choroid moving forward during accommodation. When accommodation is relaxed, the choroid moved back to the original position, moving the needle back to its original position.

This procedure was repeated by Van Alphen (1961) with the same results. Van Alphen then trephined a small hole in the sclera of the live monkey eye and observed that the choroid bulged out through the hole when the eye was not accommodated and disappeared and pulled away from the hole in the sclera when the eye was accommodated. He also measured the pressure at the hole and found that the pressure increases when accommodation is relaxed and decreases when accommodation is stimulated.

These studies suggest that the choroid must be involved in the process of accommodation. To determine the relationship, Young and Leary (1987) applied Leary's (1981) ocular component analysis approach to the accommodated monkey eye. This procedure permits the calculation of the relative contribution of each optical component to the back vertex power of the anterior segment of the eye. Corneal refracting power is determined by keratometry; anterior chamber depth, lens thickness, and vitreous chamber depth are determined by the use of ultrasound; and the power of the two lens surfaces is measured by photographic phakometry. After these values are obtained, it is possible to determine what percentage each contributes to the back vertex power of the anterior segment of the eye (the distance of the focal point behind the posterior lens surface). Typical values for human eyes under cycloplegia are cornea, 53%; anterior chamber, 7%; front lens surface, 10%; lens thickness, 13%; and rear lens surface, 17%. Thus, under cycloplegia, the rear lens surface is the second-most powerful refracting component of the eye.

Ocular component analysis was applied to the right eyes of twelve female *Maccaca nemestrina* (pigtail) monkeys with the following ages: 13 years (2), 7 years (3) and 3 years (7). An iridectomy was performed on each animal by cutting the iris at the 6 and 12 o'clock positions so that the iris drops out of sight. Atropine was used twice a day for 7 days to achieve a high level of cycloplegia; and eserine was used to induce accommodation.

Under cycloplegia, mean results were similar to those for humans (in parentheses): cornea 52.4% (53.0%); anterior chamber 7.6% (7.0%); front lens surface 9.7% (10%); lens thickness 13.5% (13.0%); and rear lens surface 16.7% (17.0%). For both humans and monkeys, the lens provides 40% of the total vergence, and the cornea and anterior chamber provide 60%. Under eserine, which brought about an average of 10.00 D of accommodation, the results show a greatly different picture: The contribution of the cornea and anterior chamber drops to 47.7%, and the contribution of the lens increases to 52.3%. It was found that the rear lens surface remains fixed (within the experimental error of 0.3 mm, for ultrasound), and the front surface of the lens moves forward an average of 0.75 mm causing the mean thickness of the lens to increase from 3.63 to 4.38 mm. This forward movement of the front lens surface reduces the anterior chamber depth by about 0.80 mm. Neither atropine nor eserine brought about a change in the monkey's vitreous chamber depth. This finding was in contrast to the results of Coleman et al. (1969) who, working with humans, reported that one-third showed no change in vitreous depth, one-third showed an increase in vitreous depth, and one-third showed a decrease in depth.

Using phakometry with a human subject able to change accommodation at the request of the investigator, it is possible to photograph the changes in the appearance of the lens surface under different amounts of accommodation. The resulting photograph (Figure 17.1) demonstrates that three changes occur in the lens during accommodation: The front surface moves forward, the front surface increases in convexity, and the rear surface also increases in convexity. However, whereas the front surface change is a simple decrease in radius of curvature, the rear surface assumes a more complicated, wavelike form (Figure 17.1C).

Fincham (1937) suggested that the difference in the front and rear lens surfaces under accommodation may be due to the attachment ring of the hyaloid membrane on the rear surface of the lens capsule. This ring results in much thicker capsule walls that surround a circle of much thinner capsule wall within the center

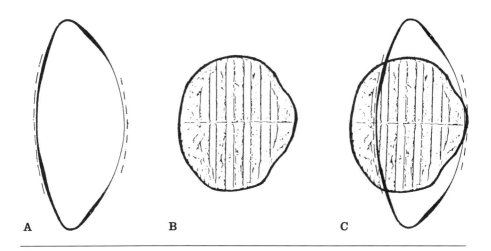

Figure 17.1.   **(A)** Fincham's idealized human lens capsule magnified for comparison purposes about 10× larger than an average human eye. The dashed lines represent the actually measured front lens and rear lens surface curvatures, and the separation between the two sets of lines is the depth of the lens under atropine for the mean of twelve monkey eyes. **(B)** Clay model of the same volume as the Fincham eye modeled to the actual surface curvatures and depth of the average lens size for the same twelve monkey eyes under eserine. **(C)** Overlay of the Fincham capsule and the accommodated eye with the rear lens surfaces aligned, as there was no change in the back surface position of the accommodated and unaccommodated eyes. (All monkeys eyes are under 10× magnification, and the front lens surface of all eyes is to the left and the rear surface to the right.)

of the rear lens surface. This thinner center of the rear lens capsule would allow the lens to bulge in the center, creating the wavelike appearance of the rear lens surface under accommodation. This mechanism would work in a manner similar to that of the pressure concept of accommodation proposed by Colemen (1970).

PRESSURE CHANGES
DURING ACCOMMODATION

A number of investigators have studied the changes in intraocular pressure during accommodation (Armaly et al. 1958, 1961, 1962). These studies have shown that intraocular pressure decreases as much as 4 mm Hg in young adults and 2.5 mm Hg in 65-year-olds during accommodation. Furthermore, the pressure remains low as long as accommodation is maintained. Recently, Perkins and Young (1987) have followed the pressure changes that occur with rapidly increasing accommodation and have found that the pressure drop follows the increase in accommodation immediately, with no measureable lag.

Young (1975) implanted the radiosonde pressure transducer invented by Collins (1967) in one eye of each of two sexually mature *Macaca nemestrina* (pigtail) males, and determined the direction of the pressure changes associated with eye-contact controlled accommodation. These male animals will maintain eye contact with a human as long as the human does not break eye contact. The results demonstrated that there is an increase in pressure in the vitreous chamber when a person walks toward the monkey (sitting in a restraining chair) as long as eye contact is maintained. If the person stares at the monkey at a distance of approximately 1 foot, the pressure remains constant as long as eye contact is maintained. If the person walks backward from the monkey while maintaining eye contact, the pressure in the vitreous chamber decreases in a monotonic manner, as the fixation distance decreases. Unfortunately, at the time of the experiment, we had no equipment for calibrating the pressure transducer, so numerical values of the pressure changes could not be maintained.

A cylindrical pressure chamber, with an inside diameter of 33 cm and an inside length of 66 cm, is now available for use in calibrating the radiosonde transducer. The top is removable, having ten locking screws and gaskets to provide an airtight seal. The monkey with the transducer implanted in the vitreous chamber is anesthetized with ketamine hydrochloride and strapped to the board with tape. The transmitter and receiver are also mounted on the board with the monkey. The board, with the monkey and the equipment, is inserted into the calibration chamber, which is held in a horizontal position by a cradle. The chamber is sealed, and the air pressure is raised from 0 to 20 mm Hg in 5 mm steps as measured by a manometer. The output is recorded on a Beckman R511 recorder. The pressure increase in the vitreous chamber was found to reach 12 mm Hg when the viewing distance was 20 cm. The pressure increase occurred within a fraction of a second, and the pressure decrease was a mirror image of the pressure increase. When accommodation is elicited by eserine, the pressure increase again reaches 12 mm Hg but requires 30 minutes to reach this level. There is no drop in pressure as long as the eserine is working; the pressure decreases only with a reduction in accommodation.

□ Fluid Movement within the Eye

Suzuki (1973) studied the movement of radio-opaque dyes injected into the vitreous chamber of cat eyes by means of fluoroscopy. When an oil soluble dye was injected, the dye did not dissipate or move; when a water soluble dye was injected, the dye started to dissipate and moved forward around the lens, between the lens and the iris, through the pupil into the anterior chamber, and out of the eye. Wesner (1985) used fluorescein injected into the vitreous chamber of monkey eyes to determine the effects of a variety of drugs that affect accommodation, such as eserine and cyclopentolate hydrochloride. The fluorescein was injected into the center of the vitreous chamber, where it dissipated throughout the chamber and was visible in the anterior chamber as a curling, twisting stream in the upper portion of the pupil, approximately 15 minutes after injection.

It appears, therefore, that there is a continuous movement of fluid from the vitreous chamber into the anterior chamber. The nature and speed of this movement is constant enough to ensure maintenance of intraocular pressure in spite of the changes that occur in the eye with accommodation. Any concept of the mechanism of accommodation must deal with the following changes that take place during accommodation: (1) the drop in anterior chamber pressure, (2) the increase in vitreous chamber pressure, (3) the change in the position of the choroid, and (4) the changes in the geometry of the lens.

□ Differential Chamber Pressures

If the anterior chamber pressure drops while the vitreous chamber pressure increases during accommodation, as has been demonstrated, there must be two separate pressures in the eye, which means that a membrane must separate the two chambers. The hyaloid membrane, which is attached to the rear lens capsule and covers the front surface of the vitreous body, could serve to separate the vitreous chamber from the posterior and anterior chambers. At the present time, little is known about this membrane. The rigidity imparted to the rear lens capsule by the attachment of this membrane suggests that the membrane should be investigated more closely.

The radiosonde pressure measurements of vitreous chamber pressure indicate that there is a direct and linear relationship between the amount of accommodation achieved and the amount of pressure exerted. What causes this pressure increase? It is possible that the ciliary muscle puts tension on the choroid, tightening it around the vitreous body. This would explain the forward movement of the choroid, as well as the pulling away from the hole in the sclera as described by Van Alphen. As the ciliary muscle increases its pull on the choroid, the muscle itself may be displaced toward the back of the eye, which would bring about an increase in the volume of the anterior chamber, causing the anterior chamber pressure to drop. Thus, both the drop in anterior chamber pressure and the increase in vitreous chamber pressure may be caused by the tension of the ciliary muscle on the choroid.

The attachment ring on the rear lens capsule would move forward under pressure, causing the front lens surface to move forward also. The lens may increase in its anterioposterior thickness by as much as 1 mm under strong accommodation. With this increase in thickness, the equatorial diameter of the lens decreases, while the radius of the front surface decreases to increase the power of this surface. The ringlike pressure on the rear lens surface would cause the center within the ring to bulge backward with a smaller radius of curvature, increasing the rear surface power and giving rise to the more complicated shape of this surface.

Another study that bears on the relationship of myopia and increased pressure in the vitreous chamber was reported by Deller, O'Connor, and Sorsby (1947). In this study, the x-ray method was used to measure the anteroposterior diameter and the vertical and horizontal equatorial diameters of nineteen emmetropic, eleven hypermetropic, and fifteen myopic eyes. The correlations between all three axes over all subjects averaged 0.73, which suggests that as the eye enlarges there is an overall increase in size before the typical elongation of the anteroposterior axis occurs in higher levels of myopia.

PROPOSED MECHANISM FOR THE DEVELOPMENT OF MYOPIA

In a series of studies dealing with the development of myopia in monkeys (Young 1961, 1962, 1963, 1965), monkeys developed myopia when placed in a near-visual environment in a manner similar to that of humans, but more rapidly because the monkeys were in the near-visual environment intermittently and randomly. Young monkeys (12 to 24 months of age) resisted the development of myopia for 4 to 6 months in the near-visual situation, but when they started to develop myopia, they developed it more rapidly and became more myopic than the adolescent (3- to 4-year-old) monkeys who had resisted for 2 to 3 months, and the adults, who had resisted from 1 to 2 months. Consistently, 70 to 86% of the monkeys developed myopia.

If accommodation produces an increase in vitreous chamber pressure, how does that result in the development of myopia? If the increase in pressure is brought about by the tension of the choroid on the vitreous body, resulting in less pressure on the sclera (as indicated by Van Alphen 1961), we may conclude that the tension of the choroid around the vitreous body reduces the blood supply to both choroid and retina. Over time, the choroid and retina will weaken and begin to thin and stretch. Because the volume in the vitreous chamber will increase as a result of the compression thinning of the choroid and retina, more fluid will enter the vitreous chamber to maintain normal intraocular pressure when accommodation is relaxed.

Accommodation is assumed to be a reflex mechanism, which is activated when the image on the retina is blurred. Thus, the development of myopia is an adjustment mechanism that permits the eye to see clearly in near vision without the need to accommodate. When this adjustment has been reached, the eye will assume a steady state, which will be maintained as long as the person is satisfied with the status quo. As Sato (1976) pointed out, Japanese students could tolerate 1 or 2 D of myopia as long as there was no car to drive or television to watch. After the war, however, when both the automobile and television became accessible, no amount of accommodation improved the situation; and students were fitted with minus lenses and instructed to wear them during all their waking hours. This meant that the earlier process of accommodation had to be repeated because they were now effectively emmetropes instead of myopes.

During the development of the first phase of myopia, the pressure against the sclera is reduced (Van Alphen 1961) as a result of the tension on the choroid exerted by the ciliary muscle. As the need for accommodation to see at near was reduced by the thinning of the retina and sclera (between 0.41 and 0.70 mm), the tension of the ciliary muscle relaxed and the pressure against the sclera increased and continuously remained increased, in contrast to the premyopic state, in which the pressure against the sclera was intermittent rather than continuous.

Because the sclera is plastic rather than elastic (Ku and Greene 1981), the continuous pressure would eventually result in stretching of the sclera. Once the sclera is stretched, it is more easily stretched. Thus, the alternative accommodation and reduction of accommodation elicited by the yearly change in minus lenses will increase the amount of myopia that is developed. Oakley and Young (1975) showed that this yearly increase in myopia can be prevented by substituting for single-vision minus lenses a highly-placed + 1.50 D bifocal add. However, bifocals have not been found to be satisfactory by other investigators (Mandell 1959, Roberts and Banford 1967). Atropine will also prevent the progression of myopia, as Bedrossian (1966), Gostin (1963), Kelly et al. (1975) have demonstrated; others have shown that some children immediately begin to progress into myopia as soon as the atropine treatment is discontinued.

■

REFERENCES

Armaly MF, Burian HM. Changes in the tonogram during accommodation. Arch Ophthalmol 1958;69:60–69.

Armaly MF, Rubin ML. Accommodation and applanation tonometry. Arch Ophthalmol 1961;65:415–423.

Armaly MF, Jepson NC. Accommodation and the dynamics of the steady state intraocular pressure. Invest Ophthalmol 1962;1:480–483.

Bedrossian R. Treatment of progressive myopia with atropine. Proceedings of the XX International Congress of Ophthalmology, Munich, 1966;612–617.

Coleman DJ. Unified model for accommodative mechanism. Am J Ophthalmol 1970; 69:1063–1079.

Coleman DJ, Wuchinich D, Carlin B. Accommodative changes in the axial dimension of the human eye. In: Gitter KA, Keeney AH, Sarinand LK, Meyer D, eds. Ophthalmic Ultrasound. St Louis: CV Mosby Co, 1969;134–141.

Collins CC. Miniature passive pressure transensor for implanting in the eye. IEEE Trans Biomedical Engineering 1967;14:74–83.

Deller JFP, O'Connor AD, Sorsby A. X-ray measurements of the diameters of the living eye. Proc R Soc Lond 1947;134:456–467.

Fincham E. The mechanism of accommodation. Br J Ophthalmol 1937;8:1–9.

Gostin SB. Prophylactic management of progressive myopia. Guildcraft 1963;37:5–13.

Heine L. Ein versuch über akkommodation und intraokularen druck am uberlebenden kinderauge. Graefes Arch Ophthalmol 1905;60:448–451.

Hess C. Beobachtungen üeber den akkommodations vorgang. Klin Monatsbl Augenheilkd 1904;42:309–315.

Kelly TS-B, Chatfield C, Tustin G. Clinical assessment of the arrest of myopia. Br J Ophthalmol 1975;59:529–538.

Ku D, Greene P. Scleral creep in vitro resulting from cyclic pressure pulses. Am J Optom Physiol Opt 1981;58:528–535.

Kupfer C. The promise of eye research. Sightsaving Rev 1979;49:21–29.

Leary GA. Ocular component analysis by vergence contribution to the back vertex power of the anterior segment. Am J Optom Physiol Opt 1981;58:899–909.

Mandell RB. Myopia control with bifocal correction. Am J Optom Arch Am Acad Optom 1959;36:652–658.

Oakley KH, Young FA. Bifocal control of myopia. Am J Optom Physiol Opt 1975;52: 758–764.

Perkins ES. Morbidity from myopia. Sightsaving Rev 1979;49:11–19.

Perkins ES, Young FA. Unpublished data, 1987.

Roberts J, Rowland M. Refractive status and mobility defects of persons 4–74 years United States 1971–1972. Hyattsville, MD: US Department of Health Education & Welfare. HEW Publication No. (PHS) 78-1654, 1978.

Roberts WL, Banford RD. Evaluation of bifocal correction techniques in juvenile myopia. Optom Weekly 1967;58(38):25–31, (39):21–30, (49):23–28, (41):27–34, (43):19–26.

Sato T. Personal communication, 1976.

Steiger A. Die entstehung der sphärischen refraktionen des menschlichen auges. Berlin: S Karger, 1913.

Stenström S. Variations in the size and shape of the eye. Acta Ophthalmol 1948;26:559–567.

Suzuki H. Observations on the intraocular changes associated with accommodation; an experimental study using radiographic technique. Exp Eye Res 1973;17:119–128.

Van Alphen GWHM. On emmetropia and ametropia. Ophthalmologica (Suppl 142) 1961.

Wesner MF. The influence of cycloplegic, mydriatic and miotic drugs on intraocular fluid movement in pigtailed monkeys. PhD Thesis, Washington State University, 1985.

Young FA. The effect of restricted visual space on the primate eye. Am J Ophthalmol 1961;52:799–806.

Young FA. The effect of nearwork illumination level on monkey refraction. Am J Optom Arch Am Acad Optom 1962;39:60–67.

Young FA. The effect of restricted visual space on the refractive error of the young monkey eye. Invest Ophthalmol 1963;2:571–577.

Young FA. The effect of atropine on the development of myopia in monkeys. Am J Optom Arch Am Acad Optom 1965;42:439–449.

Young FA. The development and control of myopia in human and subhuman primates. Contacto 1975;19:16–31.

Young FA. Vision and the autonomic nervous system. In: Goss DA, Edmondson, LL, Bezan DJ. Proceedings 1986 NE Okla State Un Symposium on Theoretical and Clinical Optometry. Tahlequah, OK, Northeastern State Un, 1986.

Young FA, Leary GA. Unpublished data, 1987.

_18_

Effects on the Resting States of Accommodation and Convergence

Clifton Schor

☐

■

POSITIONS OF REST FOR ACCOMMODATION AND VERGENCE

In a normal visual environment, both accommodation and vergence operate as closed-loop systems. Accommodation responds to target distance by sensing the discrepancy — error signal — between the eye's accommodative state and the accommodation required by the target, whereas convergence responds by sensing the discrepancy between the vergence of the eyes and the vergence required by the target. When the error signal for accommodation is removed by placing a pinhole pupil before the eye and the error signal for vergence is removed by occluding one eye, the feedback loops for accommodation and convergence are no longer closed. Each of the motor systems, therefore, no longer responds to target distance but assumes a default, or open-loop position known as the _position of rest_. Maddox (1893) believed that the position of rest for vergence was determined by intrinsic tonic innervation; Heath (1956) proposed a similar explanation for the position of rest for accommodation. More recently, Liebowitz and Owens (1975) proposed that the intrinsic innervation for accommodation consisted of the balance between the sympathetic and parasympathetic branches of the autonomic nervous system.

Tonic innervation for accommodation is demonstrated by the difference between the position of rest of accommodation — which ranges from about 2 m to

I thank John Kotulak, Tracy Tseutaki, and Leon MacLin for their assistance in data collection, analysis, and thoughtful discussions. The project was supported by a grant (RO1 - EY - 03432) from the National Eye Institute.

67 cm (0.5 to 1.5 D) — and the far point of the eye under full cycloplegia. Similarly, the position of rest for vergence, which is normally divergent by about 1 degree, is much less divergent than the anatomical position of rest. One of the questions to be explored in this chapter is the following: Do these positions of rest place demands on the visual system and potentially contribute to refractive error?

□ Accommodation Resting States: Instrument, Space, and Night Myopia

The magnitude and direction of the positions of rest for both accommodation and vergence depend on how their respective feedback loops are opened. Three classical procedures for opening the accommodative loop make use of (1) the pinhole pupil, (2) the optically empty field, and (3) darkness. The position of rest when a pinhole pupil is used has been referred to as *instrument myopia* (Schober et al. 1970); the position of rest in an optically empty field is known as *space myopia* or *empty field myopia* (Whiteside 1952); and the position of rest in darkness is known as *night myopia* (Campbell 1953).

Night myopia is generally greater in amount than instrument myopia or space myopia, due to changes in the eye's optical system and in the spectral luminance sensitivity in darkness (Heath 1956). These changes include (1) the dilation of the pupil in darkness, which introduces 0.75 D of spherical aberration; and (2) the Purkinje shift of the eye's sensitivity toward longer wavelengths, which accounts for an additional 0.50 D of night myopia.

□ Vergence Resting States: Phoria and Dark Vergence

The position of rest for vergence, which requires a target that minimizes the accommodative response, is the well-known *distance phoria*. When one eye is occluded and the open eye views a distant target, the normal eye diverges approximately 1 degree (Morgan 1944); however, when both eyes are occluded or an observer is placed in darkness, the eyes converge approximately 5 degrees (Levy 1969). This convergence of the eyes (dark vergence) is not correlated with the resting state of accommodation because (1) the time courses for reaching the resting postures of accommodation and vergence in darkness are unequal, and (2) the accommodative and vergence postures are sometimes found to occur in opposite directions (Kotulak and Schor 1986, Bohman and Saladin 1980, Owens and Leibowitz 1980).

These differences in resting states for accommodation and vergence can be illustrated as follows: When an observer views a target binocularly through base-out prisms (inducing increased vergence) while wearing plus lenses (including decreased accommodation) and is subsequently placed in darkness, the eyes diverge and accommodate (Kotulak and Schor 1986). The immediately preceding closed-loop situation influences direction of vergence and accommodation in their open-loop states.

―――■――――――――――――――――――――――――――

DIRECT ADAPTATION OF VERGENCE AND ACCOMMODATION TO PRISMS AND LENSES

☐ Vergence Adaptation

Vergence adaptation is an aftereffect; it refers to the changes in the phoria that occur after vergence responses to prisms. The eyes become more esophoric after wearing base-out prisms and more exophoric after wearing base-in prisms, the effect due to base-out prisms being the larger of the two (Schor 1979). Vergence adaptation is thought to underlie the process of *orthophorization* — the process by means of which the distance phoria tends to become orthophoric or nearly orthophoric. Vergence adaptation is also thought to underlie the rapid adjustments to optical distortions produced by prismatic components in spectacle corrections (Schor 1983). Vergence adaptation appears after only 15 seconds of disparity vergence, and its amplitude often reaches 80 to 90% of that of the vergence stimulus (Schor 1979a, Henson and North 1980).

☐ Accommodation Adaptation

Unlike vergence adaptation, accommodative adaptation measured in the dark is less than 10% of the accommodative stimulus, even after strenuous and prolonged monocular stimulation of accommodation (Ebenholtz 1983, Baker et al. 1983, Schor et al. 1984). However, Schor et al. (1986) measured large accommodative aftereffects in the light with a pinhole pupil or an optically empty field (Ganzfeld), but not in darkness. Aftereffects of 50 to 90% of the accommodative stimulus amplitude were produced after accommodating monocularly for only 15 to 30 seconds. The duration of the aftereffects increased exponentially with the stimulus duration: a 1-minute stimulus resulted in an aftereffect that lasted only 1 minute, but a 5-minute stimulus resulted in an aftereffect that lasted for an hour. The magnitude and duration of the accommodative adaptation, manifested only in the light, rivals the aftereffect of the vergence system (Schor 1980).

Given the preceding results, it seems appropriate to ask, "Can accommodation adapt to a *vergence response,* and can vergence adapt to a monocular *accommo-*

dative response?" In other words, does the resting state of accommodation adapt after vergence accommodation, and does the phoria adapt after accommodative vergence? This question of cross-linked adaptation has an important bearing on the possible roles of excessive accommodation and convergence in the etiology of myopia.

CROSS-LINKED ADAPTATION OF VERGENCE AND ACCOMMODATION TO PRISMS AND LENSES

Adaptation of the resting states of vergence and accommodation to responses of the other system was investigated by providing one system (vergence or accommodation) with a step stimulus (8 Δ base-out or −2.00 D) while the other system (vergence or accommodation) was placed in an open-loop state to allow it to adapt. When vergence was stimulated, the eyes viewed a fusion target through pinhole pupils that increased the eye's depth of focus to ±4.00 D. When accommodation was stimulated, the fellow eye was occluded to permit a vergence response to take place. Stimulus periods of 5 seconds and 2 minutes were used; the feedback loop of the stimulated system was opened after each stimulus period. In other words, right after stimulating accommodation with the −2.00 D lens, a pinhole was added to open the accommodation loop. Similarly, after stimulating vergence with the base-out prisms, one eye was occluded to open the vergence loop. Both accommodation and vergence were objectively measured during and after the stimulus period.

□ Adaptation of Vergence Accommodation

During a 5-second stimulus by base-out prism, one subject's convergence response increased 8 prism diopters and his accommodative response increased 0.75 D. When the left eye was then occluded after this short wearing period (opening the vergence loop), there was a rapid decay within 5 seconds of both the immediate esophoria and the increased (vergence) accommodation. However, when the left eye was occluded after wearing the same prism for 2 minutes, the immediate esophoria and accommodation decayed approximately equally and slowly, taking 1 to 1.5 minutes.

This latter result can be explained in one of two ways. First, vergence and accommodation adapt separately in response to the prism-induced vergence. Alternatively, vergence adapts and the vergence aftereffect then stimulates vergence accommodation. The first explanation is supported by the results obtained from three subjects whose vergence and accommodation adapted unequally. For these subjects, the 8 Δ base-out prism induced an esophoria, which decayed within 5 seconds after occluding one eye, and an accommodation, which persisted for more than 1 minute. In some subjects, accommodation and vergence adapt separately to a prism stimulus. For these subjects, the aftereffect of vergence accommodation is not the result of accommodation being stimulated by tonic vergence.

In investigating the influence of darkness on the aftereffects of vergence accommodation, it was found that accommodation adapted (decayed slowly) when the accommodative loop was opened by a pinhole pupil or by an optically empty field, but the accommodation aftereffect decayed rapidly in darkness. (The effect of prism-induced vergence on accommodation reappeared in the light when the visual stimulus, viewed through a pinhole pupil, was switched on again.) The phoria in darkness (dark vergence) was more esophoric than the phoria in light. An increaed convergence and decreased accommodation in darkness illustrates independence of accommodation and vergence in darkness (Kotulak and Schor 1986).

The reduction of vergence accommodation aftereffects to baseline resting focus in darkness suggests that the same monocular adaptive mechanism is responding to lenses and prisms, since aftereffects to both stimuli are masked in darkness.

□ Adaptation of Accommodative Vergence

A −2.00 D lens was added to the right eye for 5 seconds and later for 2 minutes. After each stimulus period, the accommodative loop was opened by using the pinhole pupils; both accommodation and vergence were objectively measured. One subject accommodated 1.5 D and had an accommodative vergence response of 7.5 prism diopters. When the accommodative loop was opened after 5 seconds of stimulation, there was a rapid decay of both accommodation and accommodative vergence. When the accommodative loop was opened after 2 minutes of stimulation, there was more accommodation and convergence than occurred with 5 seconds of stimulation; both aftereffects decayed slowly to their resting levels in 1 to 1.5 minutes.

For another subject, however, vergence adaptation was exhibited after only 5 seconds of prism stimulation, whereas demonstrated accommodation adaptation required 40 to 80 seconds of minus lens stimulation. This same subject showed greater aftereffects of vergence than of accommodation for both prism and lens stimulation. This dissociation in the time courses indicates that vergence and accommodation are adapting separately to reflex accommodation and that the aftereffect of accommodative vergence is not the result of vergence being stimulated by tonic accommodation.

□ Influence of Adaptation Aftereffects on Clinical Measures of Refractive Error

The results of this study illustrate that (1) not only does tonic vergence adapt to disparity vergence, but also it adapts to accommodative vergence; and (2) not only does tonic accommodation adapt to accommodative stimulation, but also it adapts to vergence accommodation (Schor et al. 1986). Prior studies have not revealed aftereffects of accommodative vergence on the phoria or aftereffects of vergence accommodation on the resting state of accommodation. Previous measures of accommodative-vergence aftereffects differed from those reported here by using shorter adaptation periods and by objectively monitoring accommodative vergence but not accommodation (Schor 1979b). Previous measures of vergence-accommodation aftereffects were made in darkness after adapting to combined prism and lens stimuli (Owens and Leibowitz 1980). No aftereffect would be expected for accommodation under these conditions because tonic aftereffects of accommodation are masked in darkness (Schor et al. 1986). In addition, it would be difficult to separate the effects due to the lens from those due to the prism.

The results clearly illustrate that the accommodative system is adaptable and responds both to direct stimulation with lenses and to indirect (cross-linked) stimulation with prisms via vergence accommodation. Thus an exophoric observer with convergence insufficiency may experience an accommodative spasm by overexerting either accommodative or convergence effort. The question is: "What is the influence of such accommodative spasm on refractive error?"

The spasm is likely to have a neurological basis rather than a muscular basis, since it is readily switched off in darkness and reappears suddenly when the retina is stimulated by either an optically empty field (Ganzfeld) or a pattern viewed through a pinhole pupil. Owens reports (Chapter 19) that longer adaptation stimulus periods (days or months) produce changes in the resting state of accommodation in darkness. It is possible that these long-term aftereffects have a different underlying basis than the short-term aftereffects reported here.

Clearly the short-term aftereffects have no immediate influence on refractive state other than to distort its measurement. If a patient accommodates strongly (as in reading or responding to clinical tests of accommodation), then measures of the refractive error are susceptible to being biased in the myopic direction, with an overestimation of the degree of myopia. Such short-term accommodative stimuli are not expected to have long-term or permanent influence on the actual refractive state. However, if the accommodative system is stimulated over a long period of time (days or years), the neurologic mechanism could have a secondary effect on the ciliary muscle controlling the power of the lens, or perhaps even on the axial length of the eye as a result of traction placed on the eye's choroidal tissue. One could discriminate between these two hypotheses by performing cycloplegic refractions on the subjects undergoing long-term nearpoint stimulation of accommodation. If the aftereffects disappeared under cycloplegia, then changes in axial length could be ruled out.

An important experiment needs to be performed in which the refractive state in the light is compared with the refractive state in the dark after long-term adaptation in the open-loop state. A true refractive error should exhibit itself in both the light and dark. If the resting focus of the eye is found to be more myopic when measured in the light than in the dark, as occurs after short-term adaptation, then the adaptive accommodation is unlikely to account for a myopic refractive change. If, on the other hand, the resting focus is found to be equally myopic in light and dark, then accommodative adaptation would be clearly implicated in a myopic shift in refraction.

REFERENCES

Baker R, Brown B, Garner L. Time course and variability of dark focus. Invest Ophthalmol Vis Sci 1983;24:1528–1531.

Bohman CE, Saladin JJ. The relationship between night myopia and accommodative convergence. Am J Optom Physiol Opt 1980;57:551–558.

Campbell FW. Twilight myopia. J Opt Soc Am 1953;43:925–926.

Ebenholtz SM. Accommodative hysteresis: a precursor for induced myopia. Invest Ophthalmol Vis Sci 1983;24:513–515.

Garner L, Brown B, Baker R, Cogan M. The effects of phenylepherine hydrochloride on the resting focus of accommodation. Invest Ophthalmol Vis Sci 1983;24:393–395.

Heath GG. Components of accommodation. Am J Optom 1956;33:569–579.

Henson DB, North R. Adaptation to prism-induced heterophoria. Am J Optom Physiol Opt 1980;57:129–137.

Kotulak JC, Schor CM. The dissociability of accommodation from vergence in the dark. Invest Ophthalmol Vis Sci 1986;27:94–101.

Krishnan VV, Shirachi D, Stark L. Dynamic measurements of vergence accommodation. Am J Optom Physiol Opt 1977;54:470–473.

Leibowitz HW, Owens DA. Anomalous myopias and the intermediate dark focus of accommodation. Science 1975;189:646–648.

Levy J. Physiological position of rest and phoria. Am J Ophthalmol 1969;68:706–713.

Maddox EE. The Clinical Use of Prisms, 2nd ed. Bristol, England: John Wright and Co, 1893.

Morgan MM. Accommodation and its relationship to convergence. Am J Optom 1944; 21:183–195.

Owens DA, Leibowitz HW. Accommodation, convergence, and distance perception in low illumination. Am J Optom Physiol Opt 1980;57:540–550.

Owens DA, Leibowitz HW. Perceptual and motor consequences of tonic vergence. In: Schor C, Ciuffreda K, eds. Vergence Eye Movements: Basic and Clinical Aspects. Boston: Butterworths, 1983;25–74.

Schober HA, Dehler WH, Kassel R. Accommodation during observations with optical instruments. J Opt Soc Am 1970;60:103–107.

Schor CM. The influence of rapid prism adaptation upon fixation disparity. Vis Res 1979a; 19:757–765.

Schor CM. The relationship between fusional vergence eye movements and fixation disparity. Vis Res 1979b;19:1359–1367.

Schor CM. Fixation disparity and vergence adaptation. In: Schor C, Ciuffreda K, eds. Vergence Eye Movements: Basic and Clinical Aspects. Boston: Butterworths, 1983; 465–516.

Schor CM. Adaptive regulation of accommodative vergence and vergence accommodation. Am J Optom Physiol Opt 1986;63:587–609.

Schor CM, Johnson CA, Post RB. Adaptation of tonic accommodation. Ophthalmol Physiol Opt 1984;4:133–137.

Schor CM, Kotulak J, Tsuetaki T. Adaptation of tonic accommodation reduces accommodative lag and is masked in darkness. Invest Ophthalmol Vis Sci 1986;27:186–193.

Whiteside TCD. Accommodation of the human eye in a bright and empty field. J Physiol Lond 1952;118:65.

__19__

Near Work, Accommodative Tonus, and Myopia

D. Alfred Owens

☐

Understanding the basis of myopia has posed a tantalizing problem to vision prac-titioners and scientists for centuries. Among visual disorders, myopia appears to be the hallmark of civilization. It appears to be rare in hunter-gatherer societies, more prevalent in agricultural societies, and commonplace in industrialized soci-eties that place a premium on prolonged near tasks (Post 1962). Although long considered to arise from genetic, as well as environmental, factors, myopia is widely regarded as a "disease" of eyestrain and near work. This view undoubtedly springs from the recurrent and widespread observation that myopia is most prev-alent among such groups as artisans, scholars, and others whose activities are dom-inated by near work. Almost 300 years ago, Ramazzini (1713) offered the following account in his treatise on *The Diseases of Workers*:

> In our list of workers are some who are employed in craftsmanship of the utmost delicacy, e.g., goldsmiths, makers of automatic machines, I mean timepieces, painters of pictures on gems, and such writers as he must have been who wrote out the Iliad of Homer on a piece of parchment that would go into a nutshell, that is if we may believe Cicero. Over and above the evil effects of a sedentary life, *the affliction in store for such workman as a result of their craft is myopia*, a well known affliction of the eyes which obligates one to bring objects closer and closer to the eyes in order to see them clearly; hence we may see nearly all such workers using spectacles when they are elaborating the details of their handwork. (P. 323, emphasis added)

The author gratefully acknowledges the assistance of Deborah Harris in collating and annotating literature for this chapter. He would also like to express appreciation for constructive comments on an earlier draft of this chapter that were offered by Michael Barris, Kenneth Ciuffreda, Sheldon Ebenholtz, Bernard Gilmartin, Herschel Leibowitz, Neville McBrien, Michel Millodot, and Mark Rosenfield. Preparation of this work was supported by Franklin & Marshall College and Grant # EY 03898 from the National Eye Institute.

Ramazzini went on to suggest that the reason such craftsmen "hardly ever escape the weakness of vision called myopia" is that the continuous "muscular tension" required for near tasks causes the eyes to "contract a certain habit, the retiform tunic becomes firmly set in the same position and persists in it thereafter; nor can it any longer be moved at will for the purposes of seeing clearly things more remote" (P. 325).

Similar views were advanced by numerous later theorists including Helmholtz (1909), who states: "Nearsightedness is usually the result of occupation or habits requiring the close and minute examination of small objects" (P. 129). When considering how near visual activities produce such effects, however, he was less confident than Ramazzini. Anticipating contemporary views, Helmholtz suggested that myopia depends on genetic as well as environmental factors: "The original cause is known to be a disposition, either constitutional or acquired by weakness of some kind, and the effect of over-exertion with close work. . . . As to how and why over-exertion with close work is injurious, there has come to be a wide diversity of opinion" (P. 379).

Although a consensus about the theoretical basis of myopia has yet to emerge, many investigators agree that accommodation plays a role, at least in the type of myopia associated with habitual close work and appearing relatively late in life (Goldschmidt 1968, McBrien and Barnes 1984, Grosvenor 1987, Rosner and Belkin 1987). Young (1981) has proposed that the development of such myopia is a two-phase process. The first stage, which is a direct outcome of prolonged near fixation, "is an induced tonic change in the ciliary muscle which keeps the lens in a more or less continuously accommodated posture" (P. 564). This phase fits the subjective experience often reported by individuals who have tried to read a distant target after a prolonged close task. Clinically, such excessive accommodative tonus is commonly referred to as *pseudo*myopia. According to Young, the increased ciliary tonus has an important secondary effect — it mechanically increases the pressure in the vitreous chamber. Thus, in the second phase, increased vitreal pressure induced by accommodative tonus slowly enlarges the globe, producing greater axial length and, thus, true myopia. Van Alphen (1986; 1961, 1961 as cited by McBrien and Barnes 1984) has advanced a similar theory of the role of accommodative tonus, and others have proposed that variations of accommodative tonus may be precursors to the development of myopia (Charman 1982, Ebenholtz 1983). It is interesting to note that the accounts offered by Young and van Alphen are reminiscent of a comment by Ramazzini, who claimed that the afflictions of near work are due to weakening of "the tonus of membranes and filaments of the eye" (P. 417). Lacking an understanding of the mechanism of accommodation, however, Ramazzini assumed the pupil to be the key mechanism.

A major difficulty for theories linking the development of myopia to close work is the fact that a substantial number of individuals, who spend much of their life doing exactly the sort of work that is supposed to cause myopia, never become myopic. Beyond reference to presumed genetic dispositions, such individual differences remain to be explained. Even if genetic factors do contribute to near-work myopia, the mechanism by which this predisposition is expressed must be identified. Recent investigations of the resting state of accommodation have provided new insights that may well help to clarify the basis of near-work myopia. Similar to skeletal muscle, the ciliary muscle continues to receive innervation in the absence of (visual) stimulation. This tonic innervation produces a refractive state that is intermediate in the normal range of accommodation, corresponding on the average to about 1.5 D (Leibowitz and Owens 1978). Since no stimulation or effort is involved, some investigators have referred to this state as the *physiological resting position* or *Akkommodationsrühelage* (for example, Schober 1954). Others prefer to emphasize its presumed physiological basis by referring to the state as *tonic accommodation*. In an effort to avoid theoretical presumptions, Leibowitz and his colleagues introduced the term *dark focus* as an operational definition, which emphasizes the conditions of measurement.

This chapter summarizes new evidence about the tonic, or resting, state of accommodation and considers its implications for understanding the development of myopia. A key concept throughout the discussion will be that individual differences in the resting state may represent a key for unlocking the mystery of myopia.

—■———————————————————————————

INTERMEDIATE RESTING STATE OF THE EYES

Popular theory and textbook accounts notwithstanding, the emmetropic eye does *not* relax at optical infinity. Rather, both accommodation and binocular vergence, the eyes' adjustments for the third dimension, rest at an intermediate distance (Owens 1984).

☐ Rival Views and Anomalous Myopias

The notion that the eyes relax at their far point has been widely accepted since Helmholtz's influential contributions in the late nineteenth century. According to this theory, accommodation is a one-way response. Increasing activity brings the eye's focus to a proportionately nearer distance, and decreasing activity passively "relaxes" the eye's focus toward the far point. This theory was based primarily on anatomical evidence gained from examination of cadavers, with little or no consideration of physiological or behavioral evidence. Thus, the resting state was conceptualized in terms of mechanical factors, such as elasticity of the lens capsule and supporting fibers, while the role of tonic innervation to the ciliary muscle was neglected.

At about the same time as Helmholtz's early work, Th. Weber proposed that the eyes relax at an intermediate distance (Cornelius 1861). This view holds that, similar to skeletal muscle systems, accommodation is a two-way response, involving opposite actions for adjustment to near and to far distances. Accordingly, the resting state was conceptualized as depending on physiological rather than anatomical factors. In the absence of adequate stimulation, accommodation was thought to maintain an intermediate resting posture, which reflected the balance point of tonic innervation from the near and far subsystems.

The intermediate resting state hypothesis gained little credence for more than a century, although it was advocated by several highly respected theorists, including Cogan (1937), Morgan (1946, 1957), and Schober (1954). Perhaps their arguments were overshadowed by Helmholtz's powerful influence. More likely, they were discounted because of technical difficulties that made direct measurement of the resting state problematic, and because the rest-at-infinity hypothesis provided a simple framework for defining and correcting refractive errors. Standard refraction techniques use a fixation target that stimulates the observer's accommodation and, therefore, does not assess the resting state, which would be obtained in the absence of visual stimulation. Moreover, from a functional standpoint, the individual's far point is of primary concern, and it serves as the index by which refractive error is defined. Thus, the assumption that the eye's far point and its resting state are identical provided a simple and parsimonious rationale for clinical practice.

The rest-at-infinity theory was not without problems, however. Most notable were the anomalous myopias. Beginning with the British astronomer, Nevil Maskelyne (1789, Levene 1965), it has often been observed that many individuals become myopic under low-visibility conditions. According to the rest-at-infinity theory, these refractive errors are due to maladaptive accommodative activity, which is puzzling given the usual efficiency of accommodation. The intermediate resting state theory suggested a more plausible explanation, that accommodation simply relaxes to its natural, relatively myopic resting posture when stimulation is degraded. Although plausible, confirmation of this account awaited development of new techniques for measuring the eye's resting focus.

In retrospect, it appears that both theories of the resting state were partly correct. The resting focus of cadavers is determined entirely by anatomical factors and, if the cadaver were emmetropic, this final resting focus is likely to correspond to infinity or beyond. Recent research, however, has established that the resting focus of living, alert persons rarely falls at infinity. Rather, it almost always lies at a point intermediate in the eye's focus range. Although the physiological basis of the resting focus is still uncertain, the available evidence supports the notion that this physiological resting posture is determined by tonic activity of opposing parasympathetic and sympathetic mechanisms (Cogan 1937, Morgan 1946, Siebeck 1953, Toates 1972, Gilmartin 1986).

□ Dark Focus: Individual Differences

A new opportunity to study the resting state of accommodation came in the early 1970s with the advent of the laser optometer (Hennessy and Leibowitz 1972, Charman 1974). Unlike conventional refraction techniques, the laser optometer allows precise measurement of the eye's focus without stimulating accommodation because the speckled test pattern, which is created by optical interference, remains sharply imaged regardless of the eye's refractive state. Because the test pattern cannot be blurred, it provides no feedback to stimulate an accommodative response and, in the popular jargon of control theory, accommodation remains "open-loop," or unstimulated. Thus, the laser optometer offered an accurate means to measure accommodation at rest. Further, by virtue of its simple design, the laser optometer could be used in a variety of viewing conditions, including total darkness, naturalistic situations, and with optical instruments.

The unique advantages of the laser optometer were first exploited by Herschel Leibowitz and his students at the Pennsylvania State University. Motivated by problems of visual performance that arise under challenging conditions, Leibowitz's group used the laser optometer initially to investigate accommodative behavior in optical instruments and in low-visibility situations such as darkness and inclement weather. Consistent with the intermediate resting state theory, first advanced by Th. Weber more than a century earlier, they found that accommodation consistently adjusts to an intermediate distance whenever the stimulus is either degraded or immune to blur. In addition, they discovered a basic aspect of the resting focus that had previously gone undetected: The refractive state of accommodation at rest varies widely among individuals who have normal vision.

Figure 19.1 illustrates the distribution of resting focus values obtained in dark-

Figure 19.1.
Distribution of dark focus values of 220 college students. All measures were taken with a laser optometer with the subjects' normal refractive correction in place. (From Leibowitz and Owens 1978.)

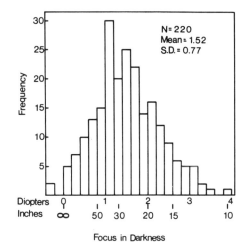

N= 220
Mean= 1.52
S.D. = 0.77

Focus in Darkness

ness from 220 college students. All subjects were either emmetropic or wearing their normal spectacle correction, and they were instructed to "relax" their eyes while observing the test pattern of a laser optometer that was flashed intermittently in darkness. The average measure, referred to as the dark focus, clearly corresponded to an intermediate value, equal to 1.5 D of "myopia." What is more, the data also revealed substantial individual differences, with a few subjects focusing to optical infinity as claimed by Helmholtz, while others focused as near as 25 cm, corresponding to 4.00 D of "myopia" (Leibowitz and Owens 1975a, 1978).

Research from other laboratories has generally confirmed these findings, although there is growing evidence that the average resting focus of the general population may be somewhat less myopic than that of college students (Epstein et al. 1981, Simonelli 1983). Although the dark focus exhibits considerable fluctuations over short periods of time (Johnson et al. 1984), several studies have also shown that individual dark focus values are relatively stable over extended time periods of up to a year (Miller 1978, Mershon and Amerson 1980, Heron et al. 1981, Owens and Higgins 1983, Post et al. 1984), suggesting that an individual's resting focus is a rather enduring visual characteristic.

□ Dark Focus: A Measure of Resting Accommodation

It seems reasonable to assume that the dark focus corresponds to the physiological resting state of accommodation. Not only is it the posture obtained in total darkness, but also it is highly correlated with, and often equivalent to, measures of accommodation taken under a wide variety of conditions, including dim natural scenes; bright, empty fields; interference patterns; small pupils; and optical instruments (Hennessy et al. 1976, Leibowitz and Owens 1978, Ward and Charman 1985). Furthermore, these studies have shown that whenever stimulation is gradually degraded, as with reduced luminance or contrast, accommodative responses are progressively biased toward the individual's dark focus posture.

This change in focusing behavior, illustrated in Figure 19.2, is functionally similar to the onset of presbyopia. As stimulation is degraded, the eye's focusing range gradually diminishes. The growing "lead" and "lag" of accommodation, which result from the dark-focus bias, produce increasing "hyperopia" for stimuli nearer than the individual's dark focus, just as they produce increasing "myopia" for stimuli farther than the dark focus. It is interesting to note, however, that unlike presbyopia, this loss of accommodative facility generally goes unnoticed. Surprisingly few individuals spontaneously recognize they have night myopia before they observe the enhancement afforded by the appropriate optical correction.

The dark-focus bias also helps to explain another interesting phenomenon, known as the Mandelbaum effect. As originally reported by the ophthalmologist, Joseph Mandelbaum (1960), when one views a distant scene through an intervening surface, such as a fence or a window screen, accommodation may become

Figure 19.2. When stimulus conditions deteriorate, as with reduced illumination or contrast, accommodative responses are progressively biased toward the observer's dark focus. The result is functionally similar to presbyopia, with increasing accomodative "myopia" for stimuli farther than the dark focus, and increasing accommodative "hyperopia" for stimuli nearer than the dark focus distance. Under severely degraded conditions, accommodation remains near the dark focus regardless of stimulus distance, producing a flat response function. Note that accommodation is always accurate for stimuli located at the observer's dark focus distance. (From Owens 1984.)

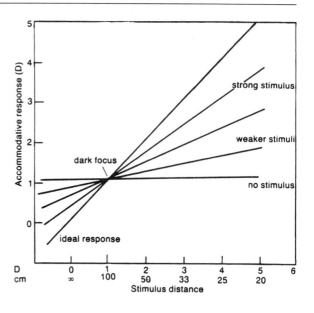

trapped by the intervening structure. This effect is most troublesome when the unattended surface lies near the distance of the observer's dark focus (Owens 1979). As noted by Roscoe (1980, Roscoe and Hull 1982), the Mandelbaum effect is potentially hazardous to drivers or pilots who are attempting to see weak distant stimuli through a dirty or scratched windshield.

Thus, the "anomalous myopias," discovered by investigators ranging from Maskelyne (1789) to Mandelbaum (1960), can all be seen as a consequence of normal variations in the behavior of accommodation. Whenever the mechanisms controlling accommodation are deprived of necessary feedback, or they are offered their choice of focusing planes, responses are involuntarily biased toward the dark focus, which is usually somewhat myopic. Following this interpretation, several studies have found that the problems of "night myopia" and "empty-field myopia" can be predicted and corrected on the basis of the individual's dark focus (Owens and Leibowitz 1976, Post et al. 1979, Luria 1980, Hope and Rubin 1984).

On the theoretical side, a growing body of evidence indicates that the ciliary muscle receives sympathetic as well as parasympathetic innervation (Siebeck 1953, Toates 1972, Gilmartin 1986). According to Gilmartin and Bullimore (1987), sympathetic innervation is (1) inhibitory and probably mediated by β-adrenergic receptors, (2) slow, (3) small in magnitude relative to parasympathetic input, and (4) augmented by increased background parasympathetic tone. Although the central mechanisms of accommodative control are still obscure, these data provide a physiological foundation for the intermediate-resting-state theory. In this context, the dark focus may be considered to reflect the balance of tonic parasympathetic and sympathetic innervation to the ciliary muscle.

DARK FOCUS AND REFRACTIVE ERROR

At this stage, one may be willing to accept the intermediate-resting-state theory of accommodation, but still be justified in asking what all this has to do with understanding true myopia. Indeed, the issue of tonic accommodation may seem irrelevant when one considers that good vision depends on "working" rather than on "resting" eyes. The concept of resting state is fundamental, however. It dictates one's conception of how the accommodative system operates and thus sets an important component of the theoretical foundation for clinical assessment and management of many visual disorders, including refractive errors. But this assertion begs the question, for it fails to identify exactly what, if anything, the resting focus has to do with true myopia.

□ Myopia Associated with Near Work

Before looking at evidence concerning the possible connection of tonic accommodation (dark focus) and refractive error, it may be helpful to recall general insights about the development of myopia. From all accounts, there appears to be more than one form of myopia (Goldschmidt 1968, McBrien and Barnes 1984, Grosvenor 1987). Of particular interest here is a class of myopia referred to as *early-adult-onset* (Grosvenor 1987) or *late-onset* myopia (McBrien and Millodot 1986, 1987a; Bullimore and Gilmartin 1987a). Unlike youth- or early-onset myopia, which ceases progression by the mid-teenage years (Goss and Winkler 1983), this class of myopia appears first during the teens or later. It is commonly associated with close work, as illustrated by studies of cadets at military academies (for example, O'Neal and Connon 1987), submariners (Kinney et al. 1980), and military personnel assigned to duty in missile silos (Greene 1970).

Although genetic disposition may be important (Goldschmidt 1968), many theorists, from the time of Ramazzini to the present, have concurred that prolonged accommodation is likely to be a precipitating factor. In particular, Young (1981) and Van Alphen (1986) have pointed toward changes in ciliary tonus as the first stage in development of myopia from near work. Although specific predictions were not made, this view suggests two hypotheses: (1) The tonic accommodation of myopes may be different from that of emmetropes and hyperopes, and (2) changes of tonic accommodation, which are proported to contribute to the development of myopia, should be observed during or after strenuous near visual tasks. These implications gained special significance when the great individual differences of dark focus were recognized and, during the past few years, they have become a topic of increased research interest.

□ Dark Focus and Refractive Error Compared

Attempts to uncover a simple correlation between individual differences in dark focus and refractive errors have yielded inconsistent results, except for the general finding that there is not a very strong relationship. Two early investigations reported evidence that the dark focus is negatively correlated with ametropia. That is, when their far points are equated optically, hyperopes tend to have a nearer (more myopic) dark focus than myopes (Maddock et al. 1981, Epstein et al. 1981). A third investigation reported the opposite relation — that relative to the far point, myopes tend to have a nearer dark focus than hyperopes (Simonelli 1983). The basis for this discrepancy is not clear, but it may be related to sampling or methodological differences.

More recent studies, which used objective infrared measures of dark focus and refractive error, tend to support the negative correlation, but only after distinguishing between early-onset (before age 14) and late-onset (age 15 or older) myopes. McBrien and Millodot (1987a) reported that the mean dark focus of fifteen hyperopes corresponded to 1.3 D of myopia, whereas those of seventeen emmetropes and fourteen early-onset myopes corresponded to 0.89 and 0.92 D, respectively, and that of late-onset myopes corresponded to 0.49 D. A similar difference was reported by Bullimore and Gilmartin (1987a), who found the mean dark focus of emmetropes to be 1.14 D and that of late-onset myopes to be 0.81 D of myopia. Thus, although conclusions must be tentative due to limited data, there may be significant differences between the tonic accommodation of late-onset myopes as compared with other refractive groupings. If the preliminary findings survive further investigation, we may conclude that late-onset myopes have signifcantly lower dark focus values than early-onset myopes, emmetropes, and hyperopes.

Viewed in the context of dual-innervation theory, this outcome suggests that late-onset myopes are characterized by an imbalance of the opposing sympathetic and parasympathetic innervations that determine the individual's dark focus. One interpretation, which assumes that sympathetic innervation to the ciliary muscle is excitatory, would be that the late-onset myopes' dark focus is less myopic because their sympathetic innervation and, therefore, their negative accommodation are relatively weak (Charman 1982). There is evidence, however, that the sympathetic innervation to the ciliary muscle is largely inhibitory, and that it varies in proportion to parasympathetic activity (Gilmartin 1986). Moreover, recent evidence from pharmacological studies indicates that individual differences in dark focus may be due primarily to variations of parasympathetic rather than sympathetic innervation (Gilmartin et al. 1984, Gilmartin and Hogan 1985a, 1985b). This suggests that it may be more accurate to describe the late-onset myope as exhibiting relatively weak parasympathetic tonus, which would shift the level of tonic accommodation at rest toward the individual's far point (Gilmartin and Bullimore 1987).

□ Change in Dark Focus with Near Work

In recent years, several laboratories have reported that the resting focus of many subjects is readily modified by strenuous visual tasks. Most notably, brief periods of near fixation can produce a myopic shift of the dark focus, which persists for some time after the task is finished. This shift presumably reflects a change in tonic innervation to the ciliary muscle. It may serve the adaptive function of enabling a worker to stay on task longer with minimal loss of performance. In the long run, however, such shifts of accommodative tonus may be detrimental. If persistent and cumulative over time, increasingly myopic tonic accommodation is likely to reduce one's ability to focus distant targets and, consistent with theories discussed earlier, this increased tonus could induce more permanent myopic refractive error. Growing evidence seems to bear out these predictions, suggesting that adaptive variations of tonic accommodation may provide a key for understanding the basis of late-onset myopia.

The first evidence for task-related variations of the dark focus was reported by Ostberg (1980), a Swedish researcher investigating the vision of air-traffic controllers and office workers. He found a significant myopic shift of the dark focus of air-traffic controllers, from 0.94 to 1.62 D, after 2 hours at a radar scope. In addition, after duty the controllers exhibited decreased accommodative responsiveness for targets nearer and farther than their dark focus distance. This reduced focusing ability appears to represent fatigue of the accommodative system, a phenomenon that has been difficult to reproduce in laboratory settings. Ostberg also found that clerical workers and switchboard operators exhibit changes of dark focus after a day's work, thus demonstrating that air-traffic controllers are not the only workers subject to task-related changes of accommodation.

Similar findings soon emerged from several laboratory investigations. Ebenholtz (1983) found that as little as 8 minutes of continuous fixation at the near point produced a significant myopic shift of the dark focus, whereas fixation at the far point produced a smaller hyperopic shift, and fixation at the observer's dark focus distance produced no change in the dark focus. Referring to these changes as accommodative hysteresis, Ebenholtz proposed that the near shift of dark focus is a precursor of myopia. At about the same time, Brown et al. (1982) reported that reading can induce esophoric shifts in dark vergence posture, as well as myopic shifts of dark focus, thus adding evidence that ordinary tasks can modify the resting (or tonic) state of oculomotor mechanisms. Another study, by Miller et al. (1983) reported that accommodation was not affected by a prolonged and stressful visual task that was located at the dark focus distance. And still another, by Schor et al. (1984), found that reading newsprint for 30 minutes at a near distance (6 D, equivalent to 16.6 cm) produced inconsistent results for different subjects. Although the combined data from nine subjects showed a significant shift in the dark focus averaging 0.5 D, individual measures showed myopic shifts for six subjects, no change for two, and a hyperopic shift for one.

These findings comprised the first experimental evidence on humans supporting the long-standing hypothesis that near visual tasks affect tonic accommodation. Typical of such advances, they raised a number of new and important questions: Why did some subjects exhibit the expected myopic change of dark focus, while others showed no change or even a hyperopic shift? Are these changes related to symptoms of visual fatigue associated with near work? And, more pertinent to the present volume, can repeated exposure to close work induce a sustained change of the resting focus that, in turn, produces clinically significant myopia?

□ Resting State and Susceptibility to Symptoms of Visual Fatigue

In hopes of gaining insight to these questions, Karen Wolf and I conducted a series of experiments on the effects of reading on oculomotor tonus. One of our primary goals was to investigate the basis of individual differences in visual problems associated with near work. It was noted earlier that a major difficulty for theories linking myopia to near work is the fact that not all craftsmen, students, and submariners become myopic. In a similar vein, a report from the National Research Council (1983) confirmed observations that not all clerical workers experience asthenopia from prolonged work at a computer station. Perhaps one's susceptibility to asthenopia from near work is related to the resting (tonus) state of the individual's accommodative and vergence systems.

One study was designed to assess both the effects of display system and the role of individual differences in resting state on refractive and subjective symptoms of visual fatigue (Owens and Wolf 1983, Owens and Wolf-Kelly 1987). Two groups of college students were required to read text material for 1 hour, either from the original paper copy or from a video-display terminal (VDT). Headrests were used to assure that both kinds of material were viewed from a distance of 20 cm. The procedure was straightforward. Immediately before and after the 1-hour reading period, we administered five vision tests: (1) tonic accommodation (dark focus), (2) tonic vergence (dark vergence), (3) accommodative responses for a matrix of optotypes presented monocularly over a range of optical distances (infinity to 4 D), (4) visual acuity for a distant wall chart, and (5) lateral heterophoria. Measures of accommodation and dark focus were obtained with a polarized vernier optometer; measures of dark vergence were obtained with a nonius alignment technique. In addition, after the reading period, the subjects were asked to rate their subjective feeling of visual fatigue on a scale of 1 to 7, where a rating of 1 meant no fatigue and 7 meant extreme fatigue.

The results confirmed our hypothesis that the resting or tonus states of accommodation and vergence are related to an individual's susceptibility to problems of near work. What is more, they provided evidence for an unexpected dissociation of the roles of tonic accommodation and tonic vergence. They also indicated that, at least when reading distance, posture, and textual material are held constant, there is no difference between the effects of reading from paper and a VDT.

The accommodation data are summarized in Figure 19.3. Consistent with Ostberg's study (1980) our reading task produced a significant myopic shift of dark

Figure 19.3. Mean dark focus and accommodative response functions before (solid lines) and after (dashed lines) subjects read for 1 hour at a distance of 20 cm. Both the dark focus and accommodative responses exhibited significant shifts in the myopic direction. Vertical bars indicate two standard errors of the means. (From Owens and Wolf-Kelly 1987.)

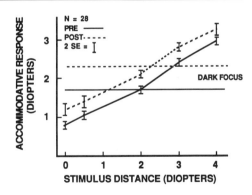

focus, which averaged 0.6 D. This change of the resting focus, indicated by the horizontal lines, was accompanied by a significant tendency for accommodative responses for the monocular array of optotypes to shift toward increased myopia. This means that, parallel to changes in dark focus, the far point of accommodation shifted in the myopic direction, while accommodation for targets nearer than the dark focus improved. These changes were most dramatic for subjects whose dark focus initially corresponded to a relatively far distance. As shown in Figure 19.4A those whose initial dark focus was less than or equal to 1.0 D exhibited an average myopic shift of nearly 1 D, whereas those whose initial dark focus was more than 1 D showed an average shift about half as large. This outcome is consistent with the hypothesized relation of tonic accommodation and late-onset myopia (Gilmartin and Bullimore 1987).

A similar pattern of results, illustrated in Figure 19.4B, was obtained for measures of dark vergence. It is important to note, however, that neither the initial resting posture nor the magnitude of changes of dark vergence was closely correlated with those of dark focus.

The similarities and differences between dark vergence and dark focus are significant for practical as well as theoretical reasons. Consistent with earlier research (Owens and Leibowitz 1983, Owens 1984, 1987a), this study showed that the resting states of accommodation and vergence are broadly similar. Both generally correspond to an intermediate distance, and both can be modified by visual tasks such as near work. In addition, our reading experiment showed that adaptive changes of both tonic vergence and tonic accommodation, which are produced by near work, are greatest for individuals whose initial resting postures correspond to a far distance.

Although the parallels are impressive, they reveal only part of the story, for there are important differences between the resting states of accommodation and vergence. Several studies had reported that measures of dark focus and dark vergence are only weakly correlated (Fincham 1962, Owens and Leibowitz 1980). In contrast to measures taken when either response is activated by an effective stimulus, this low correlation suggests that there is little interaction between the accommodative and vergence systems at rest. Our study of the effects of reading showed that adaptive changes of resting vergence and accommodation induced by a near task are not even weakly correlated ($r = 0.06$). In short, although they appear similar in function, accommodative and vergence tonus may be determined largely by separate mechanisms.

This distinction between the resting states of accommodation and vergence has an interesting practical connection to problems of visual fatigue. Not surprisingly, many of the subjects in our study experienced symptoms of fatigue after an hour of near reading. About half of the subjects (fifteen of twenty-eight) reported feeling visual fatigue at levels of 5 or greater on the scale of 1 to 7, and one third of a larger sample (seventeen of fifty-two) exhibited reduced visual acuity for a distant chart after reading. Comparison of these symptoms with changes of dark vergence and dark focus revealed an unexpected dissociation. Subjective ratings of fatigue were significantly correlated with changes of dark vergence (rho $= 0.58$), but they

Figure 19.4.
Histograms illustrating the change in resting (tonic) positions of accommodation and vergence. Vertical bars indicate two standard errors of the means. For both accommodation and vergence, the changes induced by reading were greatest for subjects whose resting posture initially corresponded to a far distance. Correlational analyses indicated that myopic shifts of the dark focus were associated with reduced distance acuity, while esophoric shifts of dark vergence were associated with subjective ratings of fatigue. (From Owens and Wolf-Kelly 1987.)

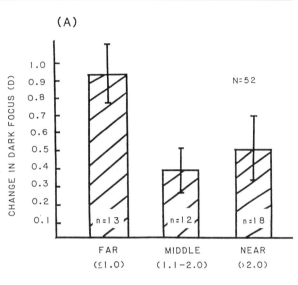

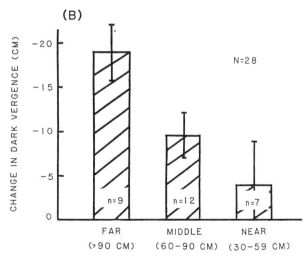

showed no relationship to changes of dark focus (rho = 0.13). The opposite was true for losses of visual acuity, which were significantly correlated with changes of dark focus (r = 0.35) but unrelated to changes of dark vergence (r = −0.12).

Researchers in other laboratories have also continued to examine the effects of visual tasks on the resting state of accommodation, yielding mixed results. In general, average dark focus values consistently tend to shift toward the distance of the visual task, but this effect is not exhibited by all subjects. Consistent with our results, Ebenholtz (1985) found that adaptive changes in tonic accommodation depended largely on the difference between the visual task and the individual's initial dark focus level. Also similar to our findings, Wolf et al. (1987) found no difference in the effects of reading from paper as compared with video displays; both produced progressive near shifts of tonic accommodation and tonic vergence, which were not closely correlated in magnitude or time course. Other studies have found that changes of dark focus are often, but not always, accompanied by parallel changes of accommodation for adequate stimuli. Similar to our findings, Pigion and Miller (1985) report that reading *Pride and Prejudice* for 1 hour produced a myopic shift of the dark focus when the reading distance was 30 cm, but no change when the reading distance was 6 m. Unlike our findings however, there were no consistent changes of accommodative responses for adequate stimuli. Ebenholtz and Zander (1987) found that brief periods of fixation (8 minutes) at the subject's near point or far point produced significant shifts of dark focus toward the distance of fixation. These changes of dark focus were accompanied by parallel changes of the near point, but no change of far point. A similar study by Fisher et al. (1987) examined the effects of 10 minutes of near fixation on tonic accommodation and accommodative responses for near and distant targets. Again, the results showed a highly significant myopic shift of the dark focus (mean = 1.1 D). In this case, the change in dark focus was accompanied by parallel myopic shifts of both the near point and the far point of accommodation, although the latter (far-point) change was relatively small.

The apparent discrepancies in the results among these studies might be due to several methodological differences, such as the duration and distance of the visual tasks, techniques for assessing accommodation, and the samples and classification of subjects. The last possibility, classification of subjects, is of particular interest for two reasons. First, as illustrated in Figure 19.4, we found that subjects with a relatively far resting state exhibit greater adaptive changes after near work than those with a relatively near resting state. As noted earlier, Ebenholtz (1985) found similar results with brief visual tasks. Thus, changes in accommodative function might be rather small if subjects are not grouped separately according to their initial levels of tonic accommodation, particularly if the overall sample includes a large proportion of subjects who begin with a relatively near resting focus. Second, as mentioned earlier, recent evidence indicates that late-onset myopes may characteristically exhibit lower dark focus values than those of other refractive groupings (for example, Bullimore and Gilmartin 1987a, McBrien and Millodot 1986, 1987a). This suggests that individual differences in susceptibility to adaptive changes of resting tonus may be related to refractive grouping as well as dark focus (Gilmartin and Bullimore 1987). I shall return to this interesting possibility in the next section.

ADAPTIVE CHANGES OF DARK FOCUS AND REFRACTIVE ERROR

Returning now to the central question for this chapter: What is the relationship between tonic accommodation and myopia? The evidence so far appears to be consistent with theories that attribute early stages of the development of some forms of myopia to changes in ciliary tonus. One class of myopes, those with late (early adult) onset, are reported to exhibit less ciliary tonus than other refractive groupings; that is, their dark focus lies closer than average to their far point. Moreover, we have found that such individuals (those with a "far" dark focus) are most likely to show a substantial myopic shift of the dark focus and far point of accommodation after close work. This effect, referred to as *transient accommodative myopia*, is probably analogous to accommodative spasms frequently observed in the examining room. Are these adaptive variations of tonic accommodation, or accommodative spasms, a step toward the development of true myopia? Two lines of evidence, which suggest the answer is yes, are just beginning to emerge.

□ Comparison of Different Refractive Types

Recent reports from researchers in the United Kingdom indicate that late-onset myopes are more likely to exhibit changes of tonic accommodation than subjects of other refractive categories. As noted in an earlier section, Bullimore and Gilmartin (1987a, 1987b) have found that late-onset myopes have lower dark focus values than emmetropes. In addition, they report that late-onset myopes are significantly more likely to show myopic changes of dark focus due to cognitive factors (backward counting by 7s in darkness). Perhaps more pertinent to the present discussion is recent evidence that late-onset myopes are most susceptible to adaptive changes of accommodation after near work. McBrien and Millodot (1986, 1987a) also reported that late-onset myopes (i.e., onset at age 15 or later) have lower dark focus values than early-onset myopes, emmetropes, or hyperopes. Further, they found that the late-onset myopes exhibited significantly greater myopic shifts of the dark focus after 15 minutes of near fixation. More recently, McBrien and Millodot (1988) have replicated and extended these findings, showing that late-onset myopes exhibit greater myopic shifts of the dark focus after tasks performed at a distance of 37 cm as well as 20 cm, and that the magnitude of such adaptive changes is negatively correlated with the subjects' initial resting state. In other words, consistent with the data illustrated in Figure 19.4, they found that individuals with relatively low initial dark focus values show greater "myopic" adaptation after near work. Moreover, McBrien and Millodot (1988) also obtained the converse finding: Fixation of a distant target (6 m) induced a negative or "hyperopic" shift of dark focus in subjects of all refractive groupings except late-onset myopes. Again, a significant negative correlation was found, indicating that subjects with a relatively near resting focus, who must exert the greatest accommodative effort to focus a distant target, are most likely to show an adaptive reduction of dark focus level after distant fixation.

These studies provide new and intriguing support for the notion that late-onset myopes have low dark focus values because of reduced sympathetic innervation to the ciliary muscle. As a consequence, the parasympathetic activity required for a near task is not effectively counteracted by inhibitory sympathetic activity, and tonic accommodation shifts toward a more myopic posture (Gilmartin and Hogan 1985a, 1985b; Gilmartin and Bullimore 1987; McBrien and Millodot 1988). Distant fixation, on the other hand, may stimulate relatively little sympathetic activity in the late-onset myope, producing relatively little "hyperopic" shift of the resting posture. If cumulative, both of these effects could contribute to a gradual progression of accommodative myopia in the late-onset myope.

☐ A Longitudinal Study of Dark Focus and Myopia

A second line of evidence for a relationship between changes in tonic accommodation and the development of late-onset (early-adult) myopia comes from our laboratory at Franklin & Marshall College. We have recently conducted a longitudinal study of college students (Owens and Harris 1986), which suggests that adaptive changes of tonic accommodation are cumulative and persistent over time. The study began by recruiting at freshman orientation a group of twenty-two entering students, who were willing to participate in a series of vision tests during the academic year. Optometric refractions were obtained for all subjects in early September, late January, and late April. Refractions of sixteen of the subjects were also obtained after summer break in September of their sophomore year. In parallel with these optometric tests, laboratory measures of the dark focus and accommodative responses for monocular targets presented over a range of distances were collected on five occasions during the freshman year and in September of the sophomore year for the sixteen students who continued to participate in the study. To minimize measurement bias, the data from optometric and laboratory measures were filed separately so that the optometrist and experimenters would not be aware of concurrent measures from the other component of the study.

The results, illustrated in Figure 19.5, revealed progressive increases both in myopic refractive error and in the dark focus throughout the academic year. Mean refractive error increased significantly, from -0.13 D to -0.39 D from September to April; but for the sixteen subjects who returned after September, refractive errors had regressed to a value approximately half-way between the levels at the beginning and end of the previous academic year. Although the data are more

Figure 19.5. Mean refractive error and dark focus values of twenty-two college freshmen measured on different occasions during the academic year. Both refraction and dark focus exhibited significant myopic shifts over the duration of the 8-month study, and both variables regressed toward original levels in sixteen subjects who were tested again after summer vacation, in September of their sophomore year. (Owens and Harris 1986.)

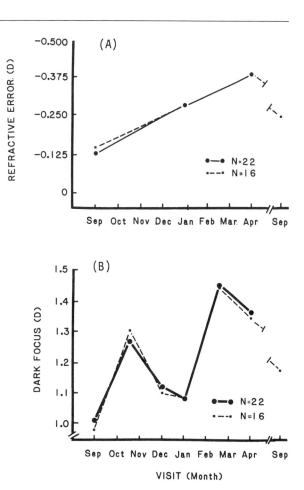

variable, a similar outcome is seen for the dark focus. Mean dark focus increased significantly, from 1.08 D to 1.37 D from September to April of the freshman year. Also similar to changes of refractive error, the mean dark focus of students who returned in September of their sophomore year was found to decrease by approximately half of the progression during the previous academic year. Preliminary analyses of data from a smaller group of subjects who continued to participate in our study through their senior year indicate that, at least for some individuals, both the dark focus and refractive errors continued to shift toward increased myopia throughout their college education.

These results appear to be exactly what is predicted by the theory that changes of ciliary tonus are reflected in concomitant changes of refractive error. On closer scrutiny, however, the findings are not so clear-cut. Consistent with our predictions, correlational analyses of individual data revealed a significant relationship between the subject's initial dark focus and magnitude of changes in dark focus over time ($r = -0.66$), indicating that subjects with lower dark focus values generally exhibited greater "myopic" changes in the dark focus over the academic year. However, correlational analyses did not find significant correlations between the subjects' initial dark focus values and changes in refractive error ($r = -0.12$), nor between the changes in dark focus and changes in refractive error ($r = 0.22$). Theory would predict strong correlations in both cases: Initial dark focus values should have been negatively correlated with changes of refractive error because individuals with low dark focus values are supposed to be most susceptible to development of late-onset myopia. And changes of dark focus should have been directly reflected in changes of refractive error, as our earlier work indicated that changes in far point occur in parallel with changes in resting focus (Figure 19.3). Thus, although data from the group as a whole appear fully consistent with the theory, those of individual subjects do not follow theoretical predictions so closely.

Two methodological limitations might account for the failure of individual data to confirm theoretical predictions. First, due to the small sample ($N = 22$) and the restricted range of refractive errors, which ranged from -2.0 to $+1.0$ D at the outset, correlational analyses would have limited statistical power. It is possible that a relationship existed that was not detected by our analyses. Second, and perhaps more likely, the results from individual subjects may have been clouded by another factor, the fact that the dark focus, as measured by a subjective (polarized-vernier) optometer, is a rather noisy variable (Johnson et al. 1984, Post et al. 1984, 1985). Evaluations of test-retest reliability showed that the dark focus measures in this study were substantially less reliable ($r = 0.46$ to 0.74) than assessments of refractive error ($r = 0.90$ to 0.94).

This unwelcome variance, which would weaken statistical correlations, might have arisen from two sources. As discussed earlier, the dark focus is readily modified by visual activities such as close work. Although we asked subjects not to read for at least 1 hour before each test session, this request was not strictly enforced and, in accord with the rhythms of academic life, it is possible that activities before testing varied widely during the course of the year. Even if we assume that the students conscientiously observed the 1-hour restriction, it is possible that dark focus measures after several days of "cramming" for examinations differ from those after a more relaxed period. In addition to transient variations of dark focus due to adaptation or "hysteresis," recent evidence indicates that measures of the dark focus can be biased by subjective measurement techniques, particularly with naive subjects (Post et al. 1985). Such task-related biases would be most troublesome for measurements obtained at the first test session, in September of the freshman year, which are the very measures one would want to use for predicting subsequent changes of refractive error. The loss of statistical power could be reduced or avoided by limiting analyses to data collected later in the year, after the students were more familiar with the laboratory situation and tasks. The problem with this strategy is that it restricts the time period over which accommodative and refractive changes can be studied. Nonetheless, comparison of the changes of dark focus and refractive error occurring over the 3-month period from mid-January to mid-April of the freshman year yielded a significant correlation (r = 0.42).

While firm conclusions are not justified, the results of our longitudinal study are encouraging. They provide the first empirical evidence for parallel myopic changes of tonic accommodation and refractive error in young adults who engage in near work on a routine basis. Moreover, they indicate that these myopic changes tend to regress when time spent on near tasks decreases, as during summer break; however, these data do not establish a causal connection. Even if we had succeeded in finding a strong statistical correlation between changes in individuals' dark focus and refractive errors, which we did not, much work would remain, for we would have yet to uncover the mechanism that links tonic accommodation and refractive error. Perhaps a longitudinal study of the future, which includes a larger subject sample and uses objective measures of dark focus, or possibly an extensive clinical assessment project, will bring us closer to a definitive answer.

CONCLUSIONS, SPECULATIONS, AND CLINICAL RELEVANCE

We have learned a great deal about tonic accommodation during the past 15 years. Much of this new evidence seems to support the hypothesis that changes in ciliary tonus play an important role in the development of some types of myopia. The view presented here is that major insights have built on the fundamental observation that tonic accommodation, as reflected in the dark focus, varies widely among people with normal vision.

Contrary to traditional views, the physiological resting state of accommodation does not lie at optical infinity. Rather, it typically corresponds to an intermediate "myopic" position which, although usually not assessed by conventional clinical tests, has important implications for many visual functions. We have seen that whenever stimulation is degraded or the need for accurate accommodation is reduced, focusing responses are passively biased toward the observer's characteristic dark focus. This effect is responsible for anomalous refractive errors, such as night myopia and empty-field myopia, which long eluded explanation. Recognition of individual differences of the dark focus provided a basis for understanding and correcting this class of situation-specific myopias.

Individual differences in the resting state of accommodation were also found to be useful for predicting one's susceptibility to asthenopic symptoms associated with near work. For many individuals, strenuous near tasks induce adaptive changes of tonic vergence as well as tonic accommodation. These changes are most striking for individuals whose resting state(s) initially lie at a relatively far distance, suggesting that the adaptation is induced by oculomotor effort. In the case of binocular vergence, adaptive changes induced by near work appear to be related to subjective symptoms of visual fatigue. In the case of accommodation, adaptive changes were accompanied by a myopic shift of the far point, thus producing a temporary refractive error similar to the clinical phenomenon of accommodative spasm, but here referred to as transient accommodative myopia.

Beyond these situational myopias, the relation of tonic accommodation and clinical myopia remains somewhat obscure, but new evidence is accumulating rapidly. Recent studies have reported that late-onset (early-adult) myopes tend to have low dark-focus values, which are more susceptible to adaptive changes from near work or cognitive factors. The Franklin & Marshall longitudinal study, which tracked changes in refractive error and oculomotor functions in college students, found parallel myopic changes of both the dark focus and refractive error. Although this may reflect a link between work-related changes on tonic accommodation and the development of late-onset myopia, a clear correlation has not yet been demonstrated at the individual level.

Although available evidence appears to be broadly consistent with the notion that increased ciliary tonus is a precursor of late-onset myopia, a causal connection remains to be established. Resolution of this issue may hinge ultimately on empirical demonstration that ciliary tonus can modify axial length. Vision science has long recognized that the primary structural correlate of refractive error is axial length of the globe. In general, myopic eyes tend to be long eyes. A key finding was recently reported by McBrien and Millodot (1987b), who reported that late-onset myopia, in particular, is also associated with axial elongation. Thus, demonstrating that ciliary tonus can influence globe length, as hypothesized by Young (1981) and Van Alphen (1961, 1986), could establish the causal link and close the argument.

It seems appropriate, however, to consider the possibility of an alternate outcome. It may be that not all clinically significant myopia can be attributed to abnormal axial length. Avoiding for now discussion of the correlation among refractive components of the eye, we should consider data recently summarized in a review by Grosvenor (1987). Drawing on data from a massive study by the U.S. Department of Health, Education, and Welfare (now Health and Human Services) along with several of the most extensive clinical optometric investigations, Grosvenor distinguishes four classes of myopia on the basis of age-related prevalence. Of special interest to the present discussion, he reports that, over the human life span, the prevalence of myopia peaks sometime between the ages of 20 and 40, and thereafter declines. This late peak is surprising in view of reports from other studies claiming that the "age of cessation" of progression of myopia is the mid-teenage years (Goss 1983, Goss and Winkler 1983). Most likely, the difference reflects characteristics of the populations under consideration. Rural, agricultural populations, which were dominant in early investigations and Goss and Winkler's

(1983) database, may well exhibit lower incidence and earlier age of cessation of myopia progression than the current population at large. Indeed, Grosvenor's review indicates that the age of cessation is much later for a significant segment of the population, that segment in which myopia appears in early adulthood. Grosvenor also notes that in many cases, the myopia that appears in early adulthood does not progress to high levels and may regress or disappear in later life. Although this later regression may be due to tissue changes that modify the structure of the lens or globe, the possibility of a physiological basis seems tenable as well. Perhaps the appearance of late-onset myopia and its subsequent regression are the result of sustained variations of ciliary tonus. If so, then it seems inappropriate to limit the rubric of myopia to cases that involve changes in axial length.

We have all heard of cases where substantial myopia developed during school or college years and then miraculously disappeared when the patient went on to view broader horizons. My mentor and colleague, Herschel Leibowitz, once commented that he was becoming increasingly myopic as a 17-year-old college student, but the trend reversed as he abruptly changed occupations during military service in the infantry. Another close colleague, Robert L. Owens, who practices optometry in Amish country, has observed that the myopia of his "plain" patients generally ceases to progress and often regresses when they leave school after the eighth grade. Although this second example comes close to the "age of cessation" found by Goss and Winkler (1983) in clinical records of a predominantly rural sample, the observed regression of myopia may be less typical.

Of course, anecdotes and isolated cases cannot be taken as adequate foundation for scientific theory. But neither should they be neglected, for they represent the front line of empirical observation. The point of introducing these observations is not to draw conclusions, but rather to raise a basic question. Given the fact that a large portion of the population develops significant levels of myopia relatively late in life (early adulthood), and then subsequently loses this myopia, should we assume that variations of true refraction are necessarily caused by fluctuations of axial length? Are there any longitudinal data documenting such variations of axial length over the life span of individuals who exhibit late-onset myopia? If not, then the possibility that this class of myopia is primarily accommodative remains open.

In the next few years, we may gain a much fuller account of the extent to which tonic accommodation contributes to clinically significant myopia. With this progress will come a clearer view of the mechanisms controlling accommodation, as well as their role in the etiology of refractive error. Achieving these goals could be greatly enhanced by contributions from clinical investigators. Presently a small but growing number of clinicians measure the dark focus routinely. Research indicates that these measures can be valuable for treating difficulties of night vision and asthenopia. Potential benefits for treating presbyopia, assessing the consequences of visual training, and perhaps general prescription of ocular refractive corrections seem likely but are largely unexplored (Weisz 1980a, 1980b). Clinical practitioners are more likely than laboratory investigators to recognize such applications, and they may be in a better position to evaluate potential benefits. As more practitioners become familiar with the dark focus concept and with the fact that it can be measured with ordinary clinical equipment using a technique known as dark retinoscopy (Owens et al. 1980, Bullimore et al. 1986), we may see a groundswell of new information about the role of tonic accommodation for visual functions. Through the cooperative efforts of clinical and laboratory investigators, we may solve the puzzle of myopia and near work in time for the tricentennial of Ramazzini's classical speculations.

■

REFERENCES

Brown K, Wolf K, Owens DA. Effects of reading on accommodation and vergence. Presentation at the Annual Meeting of the American Academy of Optometry, Philadelphia, 1982.

Bullimore MA, Gilmartin B, Hogan RE. Objective and subjective measurement of tonic accommodation. Ophthalmic Physiol Opt 1986;6:57–62.

Bullimore M, Gilmartin B. Aspects of tonic accommodation and emmetropia and late-onset myopia. Am J Optom Physiol Opt 1987a;64:499–503.

Bullimore MA, Gilmartin B. Tonic accommodation, cognitive demand, and ciliary muscle innervation. Am J Optom Physiol Opt 1987b;64:45–50.

Charman WN. On the position of the plane of stationarity in laser refraction. Am J Optom Physiol Opt 1974;51:832–838.

Charman WN. The accommodative resting point and refractive error. The Ophthalmic Optician 1982;22:469–473.

Cline D, Hofstetter HW, Griffin JR. Dictionary of Visual Science, 3rd ed., Radnor, PA: Chilton, 1980;505.

Cogan DG. Accommodation and the autonomic nervous system. Arch Ophthalmol 1937; 18:739–766.

Cornelius CS. Die Theorie des Sehens und räumlichen Vorstellens. Halle: H. W. Schmidt, 1861;283–285.

Ebenholtz SM. Accommodative hysteresis: a precursor for induced myopia? Invest Ophthalmol Vis Sci 1983;24:513–515.

Ebenholtz SM. Hysteresis magnitude and decay rate as a function of fixation target distance from the dark focus. Invest Ophthalmol Vis Sci (Suppl) 1984;26:269.

Ebenholtz SM. Accommodative hysteresis: relationship to resting focus. Am J Optom Physiol Opt 1985;62:755–762.

Ebenholtz SM, Zander PAL. Accommodative hysteresis: influence on closed loop measures of far point and near point. Invest Ophthalmol Vis Sci 1987;28:1246–1249.

Epstein D, Ingelstam E, Jansson K, Tengroth B. Low-luminance myopia as measured with a laser optometer. Acta Ophthalmol 1981;59:928–943.

Fincham EF. Accommodation and convergence in the absence of retinal images. Vis Res 1962;1:425–440.

Fisher SK, Ciuffredda KJ, Levine S. Tonic accommodation, accommodative hysteresis and refractive error. Am J Optom Physiol Opt 1987;64:799–809.

Fisher SK, Ciuffreda KJ, Levine S, Wolf-Kelly KS. Tonic adaptation in symptomatic and asymptomatic subjects. Am J Optom Physiol Opt 1987;64:333–343.

Garner LF, Kinnear RF, McKellar M, Klinger J, Hovander MS, Grosvenor T. Refraction and its components in Melanesian schoolchildren in Vanuatu. Am J Optom Physiol Opt 1988;65:182–189.

Gilmartin B. A review of the role of sympathetic innervation of the ciliary muscle in ocular accommodation. Ophthalmol Physiol Opt 1986;6:23–37.

Gilmartin B, Bullimore MA. Sustained near-vision augments inhibitory sympathetic innervation of the ciliary muscle. Clin Vis Sci 1987;1:197–208.

Gilmartin B, Hogan RE. The role of the sympathetic nervous system in ocular accommodation and ametropia. Ophthalmic Physiol Opt 1985a;5:91–93.

Gilmartin B, Hogan RE. The relationship between tonic accommodation and ciliary muscle innervation. Invest Ophthalmol Vis Sci 1985b;26:1024–1029.

Gilmartin B, Hogan RE, Thompson SM. The effect of timolol maleate on tonic accommodation, tonic vergence, and pupil diameter. Invest Ophthalmol Vis Sci 1984; 25:763–770.

Goldschmidt E. On the Etiology of Myopia: An Epidemiological Study. Munksgaard: Copenhagen, 1968.

Goss DA. Parameters of the change in clinical refractive error in young myopes. In: Breinin GM, Siegel IM, eds. Advances in Diagnostic Visual Optics. Springer: New York, 1983.

Goss DA, Winkler RL. Progression of myopia in youth: age of cessation. Am J Optom Physiol Opt 1983;60:651–658.

Greene MR. Submarine myopia in the Minuteman launch control facility. J Am Optom Assoc 1970;41:1012–1013.

Grosvenor T. A review and a suggested classification system for myopia on the basis of age-related prevalence and age of onset. Am J Optom Physiol Opt 1987;64:545–554.

Helmholtz H. Handbook of Physiological Optics, 3rd ed., vol. 1. Hamburg: Voss, 1909. English trans by Southall JPC. Dover Publications, 1962.

Hennessy RT. Instrument myopia. J Opt Soc Am 1975;65:1114–1120.

Hennessy RT, Iida T, Shiina K, Leibowitz HW. The effect of pupil size on accommodation. Vis Res 1976;16:587–589.

Hennessy RT, Leibowitz HW. Laser optometer incorporating the Badal principle. Behav Res Methods Instrumentation 1972;4:237–239.

Heron G, Smith AC, Winn B. The influence of method on the stability of dark focus position of accommodation. Ophthalmic Physiol Opt 1981;1:79–90.

Hope GM, Rubin ML. Night myopia. Surv Ophthalmol 1984;29:129–136.

Hung GK, Semmlow JL. Static behavior of accommodation and vergence: computer simulation of an interactive dual-feedback system. IEEE Trans Biomed Eng 1980;BME-27:439–447.

Johnson CA, Post RB, Tsuetaki TK. Short-term variability of the resting focus of accommodation. Ophthalmic Physiol Opt 1984;4:319–325.

Kinney JAS, Luria SM, Ryan AP, Schlicting CL, Paulson HM. The vision of submariners and national guardsmen: a longitudinal study. Am J Optom Physiol Opt 1980;57: 469–478.

Leibowitz HW, Owens DA. Anomalous myopias and the intermediate dark focus of accommodation. Science 1975a;189:646–648.

Leibowitz HW, Owens DA. Night myopia and the intermediate dark focus of accommodation. J Opt Soc Am 1975b;65:1121–1128.

Leibowitz HW, Owens DA. New evidence for the intermediate position of relaxed accommodation. Doc Ophthalmol 1978;46:133–147.

Leibowitz HW, Sheehy JB, Gish KW. Correction of night myopia: the role of vergence accommodation. In Night Vision: Current Research and Future Directions, Symposium Proceedings. Washington, DC: National Academy Press, 1987.

Levene JR. Nevil Maskelyne, F.R.S., and the discovery of night myopia. Royal Society of London Notes and Reports, 1965;20:100–108.

Luria SM. Target size and correction for empty-field myopia. J Opt Soc Am 1980;70: 1153–1154.

Maddock RJ, Millodot M, Leat S, Johnson CA. Accommodation responses and refractive error. Invest Ophthalmol Vis Sci 1981;20:387–391.

Mandelbaum J. An accommodation phenomenon. Arch Ophthalmol 1960;63:923–926.

Maskelyne N. An attempt to explain a difficulty in the theory of vision, depending on the different refrangibility of light. Philosophical Transactions of the Royal Society, 1789; 19:256–264.

McBrien NA, Barnes DA. A review and evaluation of theories of refractive error development. Ophthalmol Physiol Opt 1984;4:201–213.

McBrien NA, Millodot M. Amplitude of accommodation and refractive error. Invest Ophthalmol Vis Sci 1986;27:1187–1190.

McBrien NA, Millodot M. The relationship between tonic accommodation and refractive error. Invest Ophthalmol Vis Sci 1987a;28:997–1004.

McBrien NA, Millodot M. A biometric investigation of late-onset myopic eyes. Acta Ophthalmol 1987b;65:461–468.

McBrien NA, Millodot M. Differences in adaptation of tonic accommodation with refractive state. Invest Ophthalmol Vis Sci 1988;29:460–469.

Mershon DH, Amerson TL. Stability of measures of the dark focus of accommodation. Invest Ophthalmol Vis Sci 1980;19:217–221.

Miller RJ. Temporal stability of the dark focus of accommodation. Am J Optom Physiol Opt 1978;55:447–450.

Miller RJ, Pigion MF, Wesner MF, Patterson JG. Accommodation fatigue and dark focus: the effects of accommodation-free visual work as assessed by two psychophysical methods. Percept Psychophysics 1983;34:532.

Morgan MW. A new theory for the control of accommodation. Am J Optom 1946;23: 99–110.

Morgan MW. The resting state of accommodation. Am J Optom 1957;34:347–353.

National Research Council. Video Displays, Work, and Vision. Washington, DC: National Academy Press, 1983.

National Research Council. Emergent Techniques for Assessment of Visual Performance. Washington, DC: National Academy Press, 1985.

O'Neal MR, Connon TR. Refractive error change at the U.S.A.F.A. — class of 1985. Am J Optom Physiol Opt 1987;64:344–354.

Ostberg O. Accommodation and visual fatigue in display work. In: Grandjean E, Vigliani E, eds. Ergonomic Aspects of Visual Display Terminals. London: Taylor and Francis, 1980.

Owens DA. The Mandelbaum effect: an accommodative bias toward intermediate distances. J Opt Soc Am 1979;69:646–652.

Owens DA. The resting state of the eyes. Am Scientist 1984;72:378–387.

Owens DA. Normal variations of accommodation and binocular vergence: some implications for night vision. In: Night Vision: Current Research and Future Directions. Washington, DC: National Academy Press, 1987a.

Owens DA. Oculomotor tonus and visual adaptation. Acta Psychol 1987b;63:213–231.

Owens DA, Harris D. Oculomotor adaptation and the development of myopia. Invest Ophthalmol Vis Sci (Suppl) 1986;27:80.

Owens DA, Leibowitz HW. Night myopia: cause and a possible basis for amelioration. Am J Optom Physiol Opt 1976;53:709–717.

Owens DA, Leibowitz HW. Accommodation, convergence, and distance perception in low illumination. Am J Optom Physiol Opt 1980;57:540–550.

Owens DA, Leibowitz HW. Perceptual and motor consequences of tonic vergence. In: Schor C, Ciuffreda KJ, eds. Basic and Clinical Aspects of Binocular Vergence Eye Movements. Boston: Butterworths, 1983.

Owens DA, Mohindra I, Held R. Near retinoscopy and the effectiveness of a retinoscope beam as an accommodative stimulus. Invest Ophthalmol Vis Sci 1980;18:942–949.

Owens DA, Wolf KS. Accommodation, binocular vergence, and visual fatigue. Invest Ophthalmol Vis Sci (Suppl) 1983;19:23.

Owens DA, Wolf KS. Dissociation of dark focus and tonic vergence by near work. Invest Ophthalmol Vis Sci (Suppl) 1984;25:183.

Owens DA, Wolf-Kelly K. Near work, visual fatigue, and variation of oculomotor tonus. Invest Ophthalmol Vis Sci 1987;28:743–749.

Owens RL, Higgins KE. Long-term stability of the dark focus of accommodation. Am J Optom Physiol Opt 1983;60:32–38.

Pigion RG, Miller RJ. Fatigue of accommodation: changes in accommodation after visual work. Am J Optom Physiol Opt 1985;62:853–863.

Post RH. Population differences in vision acuity: a review with speculative notes on selection relaxation. Eugenics Q 1962;9:189–192.

Post RB, Johnson CA, Tsuetaki TK. Comparison of laser and infrared techniques for measurement of the resting focus of accommodation: mean differences and long-term variability. Ophthalmic Physiol Opt 1984;4:327–332.

Post RB, Johnson CA, Owens DA. Does performance of tasks affect the resting focus of accommodation? Am J Optom Physiol Opt 1985;62:533–537.

Post RB, Owens RL, Owens DA, Leibowitz HW. Correction of empty field myopia on the basis of the dark focus of accommodation. J Opt Soc Am 1979;69:89–92.

Ramazzini B. Diseases of Workers. 1713. Trans. by Wilmer Cave Wright, Chicago: The University of Chicago Press, 1940.

Roscoe SN. Aviation Psychology. Iowa State University Press, 1980.

Roscoe SN, Hull JC. Cockpit visibility and contrail detection. Hum Factors 1982;24: 659–672.

Rosner M, Belkin M. Intelligence, education, and myopia in males. Arch Ophthalmol 1987; 105:1508–1511.

Schober H. Uber die Akkommodationsrühelage. Optik 1954;6:282–290.

Schor CM. The relationship between fusional vergence eye movements and fixation disparity. Vis Res 1979;19:1359–1367.

Schor CM. Fixation disparity and vergence adaptation. In: Schor C, Ciuffreda KJ, eds. Basic and Clinical Aspects of Binocular Vergence Eye Movements. Boston: Butterworths, 1983.

Schor CM, Johnson CA, Post RB. Adaption of tonic accommodation. Ophthalmic Physiol Opt 1984;4:133–137.

Semmlow JL, Hung GK. The near response: theories of control. In: Schor C, Ciuffreda KJ, eds. Basic and Clinical Aspects of Binocular Vergence Eye Movements. Boston: Butterworths, 1983.

Siebeck R. The antagonistic innervation of the ciliary muscle and the rest position of accommodation. Optician December 11, 1953, 535–540.

Simonelli NM. The dark focus of the human eye and its relation to age and visual defect. Hum Factors 1983;25:85–92.

Tan RKT. The effect of accommodation response on the dark focus. Clin Exp Optom 1986; 69:156–159.

Toates FM. Accommodation function of the human eye. Physiol Rev 1972;52:828–863.

Van Alphen GWHM. On emmetropia and ametropia. Ophthalmologica (Suppl) 1961; 142:1–92.

Van Alphen GWHM. Choroidal stress and emmetropization. Vis Res 1986;26:723–734.

Ward PA, Charman WN. Effect of pupil size on steady state accommodation. Vis Res 1985; 25:1317–1326.

Weisz CL. The accommodative resting state: theoretical implications of lens prescriptions. Rev Optom 1980a;117(7):60–70.

Weisz CL. The accommodative resting state. Rev Optom 1980b;117(8):62–74.

Wolf KS, Ciuffreda KJ, Jacobs SE. Time course and decay of effects of near work on tonic accommodation and tonic vergence. Ophthalmic Physiol Opt 1987;7:131–135.

Young FA. Primate myopia. Symposium paper. Am J Optom Physiol Opt 1981;58: 560–566.

Management of Myopia: Functional Methods

Theodore Grosvenor

☐

Although the experience of most vision practitioners suggests that juvenile myopia tends to progress no matter what is done, many methods have been advocated for its control. These include the use of eye exercises or visual training, undercorrecting or overcorrecting the myopia, wearing of bifocal lenses, use of minus lenses for distance vision only, wearing of contact lenses, and daily instillation of pharmaceutical agents. In this chapter, the progress that has been made with each of these methods will be assessed, with the exception of the use of pharmaceutical agents, which will be covered in the next chapter.

THE BATES SYSTEM OF EYE EXERCISES

One of the earliest advocates of the use of eye exercises in an attempt to control myopia was William H. Bates, an ophthalmologist. After having examined 1,500 schoolchildren in Grand Forks, Iowa, in 1903, Bates found that some of the children failed the visual acuity test on the first trial but passed on the second or third trial. One of the teachers was so impressed by the improvement in visual acuity on repeated testing that she asked Bates to allow her to place a Snellen chart permanently in her class room. The children were instructed to read, at least once every day, the smallest row of letters that they could see from their seats. The Snellen chart was subsequently used in all of the public schools in Grand Forks for a period of 8 years, after which Bates (1920) reported that during this period myopia was reduced from 6 to 1%. Unfortunately, he failed to report his criterion for myopia, either in terms of refractive error or visual acuity.

The Bates methods were popularized by a number of his disciples, including Peppard, Corbett, and the author Aldous Huxley, each adding touches of his or her own. Peppard (1936) supplemented the Bates procedures with practice in blinking and the "long swing." Corbett (1953) suggested the use of a commercial calendar, having a "large month" at the top and two "small months" at the bottom, rather than a Snellen chart. Huxley (1942) went one step further, suggesting the use of a large wall calendar for distance vision and a small pocket calendar for near vision and recommending what sounds very much like the near-far accommodative facility training commonly used by many optometrists.

These methods of training were based on the erroneous conclusion that accommodation was brought about by the extraocular muscles rather than the ciliary muscle. Bates (1920) argued that his experiments with cats, dogs, rabbits, and other animals seemed to leave no room for doubt that neither the lens nor any muscle inside the eyeball has anything to do with accommodation, but that the process whereby the eye adjusts itself for vision at different distances is entirely controlled by the action of the muscles on the outside of the globe. Not surprisingly, there has never been any scientific evidence that these methods were of any help in controlling the presence of myopia.

□ Flashes of Clear Vision

Many followers of the Bates methods reported seeing "flashes of clear vision"; apparently it was these flashes that motivated them to continue the training procedures. By advertising in a newspaper and contacting Bates training schools, Marg (1952) was able to find five people who could obtain flashes of clear vision. Uncorrected visual acuity for these subjects ranged from 6/60 (20/200) to 6/120 (20/400), but during flashes of clear vision, acuity improved to a range of 6/15 (20/50) to 6/24 (20/80). Neither retinoscopy nor refraction with a coincidence optometer, performed during the flashes of clear vision, showed a change in refraction for any of the five subjects. Marg concluded that the increase in visual acuity obtained by these individuals must be central to the retinal image (that is, in the physiological or perceptual image). An interesting point made by Marg was that even though visual acuity during a flash was no better than 6/15 (20/50), the subjective experience was seeing more clearly than he had ever seen with glasses, even though the glasses corrected the acuity to 6/4.5 (20/15).

Giglio (1952) examined four myopes who reported "clearing" of vision and demonstrated that, for these patients, the episodes of clear vision occurred as a result of a flattening of the tear layer. The first patient described by Giglio was a 9.00 D myope, corrected to 6/7.5+ (20/25+), who wore his glasses principally for reading, saying that he didn't need them for outdoor activities such as baseball or tennis. On the third visit, he was able to demonstrate that he could read the 6/7.5+ (20/25) line on the distance chart without glasses.

Thinking that the cornea may be responsible for these episodes of clear vision, Giglio mounted a plate of glass on a keratometer, at a 45-degree angle, so that the patient was able to view a distance chart with the eye aligned on the axis of the keratometer. Four myopes were tested with this apparatus. Giglio reported that for all four myopes, the mire showed a section defect, which could occur in any quadrant, presenting itself as a flattening of the circle as though caused by a drop of liquid. The effect was not static, and the circle continued to shimmer until the effect disappeared. The effect was sometimes fleeting, but sometimes lasted for 20 to 30 seconds, after which the shimmering ring returned to its normal shape and the patient concurrently reported a loss of clear vision.

■
CONVENTIONAL VISUAL TRAINING

Many vision practitioners have advocated the use of various visual training procedures, usually designed to relax accommodation, for the control of myopia. The pressure on optometrists to provide this form of therapy was at its greatest during the Second World War, when large numbers of young men requested visual training in order to be accepted by (or to remain in) one of the armed services. The stated aim of these procedures was myopia reduction; however, in almost all cases, the criterion for success was an improvement in unaided visual acuity rather than a reduction in the objectively or subjectively measured amount of myopia.

When improvement in unaided visual acuity is the only criterion, one may conclude that any improvement may be due, at least in part, to the fact that the patient has learned to interpret a blurred image. An additional possibility is that the patient has simply memorized the letters on the Snellen chart, as the same Snellen chart is often used for both training and testing sessions.

The use of visual training for the control of myopia was evaluated in a prospective study conducted in 1944, known as the Baltimore Myopia Project. The Curtis Publishing Company financed the study, recruiting 111 subjects who were trained by optometrists and technicians under the sponsorship of the American Optometric Association. Subjects for the study were unselected, ranging in age from 9 to 32 years and having from 0.50 D to 9.00 D of myopia. The average number of training sessions was twenty-five, during a 13-week period. The results of the study were evaluated by staff ophthalmologists at the Wilmer Eye Institute.

The official ophthalmological report for the study was written by Woods (1945), and the official optometric report was written by Ewalt (1946). Additional reports were written by Shepard (1946), Eberl (1946), Betts (1947), and Hackman (1947). These reports analyzed the results of the study in some detail, but none of the reports described the training procedures. Although neither of the official reports provided data on the reduction in the measured amount of myopia as a result of the training, Ewalt published acuity graphs indicating (on visual inspection) an average improvement of about two lines of letters. In summarizing both the Woods and Ewalt reports, Shepard (1946) concluded that "as a demonstration of control of myopia, in face of the data reported by the Wilmer Institute, but not by the A.O.A. bureau, it must be admitted to be a complete failure. It has shown that optometry cannot control myopia" (P. 135).

BIOFEEDBACK TRAINING

More recently, a number of reports have appeared in the literature describing the use of biofeedback in connection with training designed to reduce the amount of myopia by relaxing accommodation. In such procedures, a signal (usually auditory) is used to indicate to the patient when accommodation is being relaxed. An optometer system, using infrared light, is used to monitor the amount of accommodation in play.

A biofeedback study involving seventeen subjects between the ages of 20 and 46 years was reported by Balliet et al. (1982). The subjects were given biofeedback training, with buzzers indicating the correct accommodative responses. The mean improvement in visual acuity, after thirty-eight training sessions, was 3.4 lines on the Snellen chart. No data concerning refractive error were reported.

The Accommotrac Vision Trainer, developed by Trachtman for biofeedback training, was used in a study reported by Berman et al. (1985). Using as subjects sixteen myopic patients between the ages of 9 and 37 years, binocular visual acuity was measured, both at the beginning and at the end of each training session. Seven training sessions were given, each consisting of 10 minutes of training, 10 minutes of rest, and an additional 10 minutes of training. Mean improvement in visual acuity was from 6/27 (20/90) to 6/11 (20/35). Data concerning change in refraction were not given. In a review of biofeedback studies, Trachtman (1987) made the following points:

1. His basic hypothesis was that people who are myopic learn to overaccommodate in response to blur, whereas those who are hyperopic learn to underaccommodate.
2. This inappropriate learning begins as a result of the absence of an odd-error retinal signal (that is, there is no error signal to indicate that overaccommodation is occurring).
3. The reduction in myopia due to training occurs as a result of a reduction in parasympathetic muscle tone and an increase in sympathetic muscle tone (that is, negative accommodation).

One of the best documented studies making use of the Accommotrac instrument was that of Gallaway et al. (1987). Subjects for the study were eleven myopes ranging in age from 23 to 42 years, having no more than 4.00 D of myopia and less than 1.00 D of astigmatism. Before the training was begun retinoscopy, subjective refraction, autorefraction and autokeratometry were performed on each subject. Training procedures were those outlined in the instruction manual that accompanies the instrument. Each subject was scheduled for twelve to sixteen training sessions, each session consisting of an initial visual acuity measurement followed by 10 to 15 minutes of training, a 10- to 15-minute rest period, and another 10- to 15-minute training period. At the completion of the training, retinoscopy and subjective refraction were performed by two examiners who were not connected with the study and who had no knowledge of the original refractive status of the subjects or of the training procedures; autorefraction and autokeratometry were then repeated.

Nine of the original eleven subjects completed the biofeedback training. Graphs published by Gallaway et al. (1987) indicated improvements in visual acuity for the majority of these subjects, but there were no changes in refractive error. The authors questioned whether the improvements in visual acuity were the result of training, or represented learning effects in measuring visual acuity. The possibility of learning effects was reinforced by two occurrences: (1) Before the administration of the training, the visual acuity of each subject was measured several times to establish a baseline, and it was found that visual acuity for several subjects improved with repeated testing, in these pretraining sessions; (2) an increase in visual acuity was found for one of two control subjects. These subjects were not given the biofeedback training, but their visual acuity was measured repeatedly, as was the visual acuity of the experimental subjects.

■

UNDERCORRECTION AND OVERCORRECTION OF MYOPIA

Undercorrection of myopia by 0.50 to 0.75 D has been proposed as a method of controlling the progression of myopia. However, to my knowledge, no studies (or even case reports) involving undercorrection have been published.

Goss (1984) reported a study in which overcorrection was used in an attempt to control the progression of juvenile myopia. He compared the rates of progression for thirty-six young myopes who were overcorrected by 0.75 D, and thirty-six who were not overcorrected. Subjects in the two groups were matched for sex, initial age, and the initial amount of myopia. Mean rates of progression, on the basis of subjective refraction, were found not to be significantly different for the two groups, being −0.52 D per year for the experimental group (with a range of +0.21 to −1.32 D per year) and −0.47 D per year for the control group (range, +0.28 to −1.72 D per year).

___■___

THE USE OF BIFOCALS

More than 100 years ago, Donders, the Dutch ophthalmologist (1864, reprinted 1972) proposed that myopia occurred as a result of prolonged tension on the eyes during close work. He suggested that strong convergence of the visual axes caused an increase in pressure within the ocular fluids, resulting in an extension of the globe, particularly at the posterior pole.

The role of intraocular pressure in the normal development of the eye was demonstrated by Coulombre (1956), who inserted a small glass tube into the vitreous body of one eye of each of fifty-eight 4-day-old chick embryos. The glass tube allowed the vitreous to escape, causing a reduction in intraocular pressure. During the next 4 days, the intubated eyes increased only slightly in diameter while the contralateral control eyes underwent a sixfold increase in diameter (normal for this period of development). At the end of this period, the neural retina was found to be greatly folded, the cornea and lens were appreciably smaller than normal, the corneal bulge failed to appear, and the ciliary processes were lacking. Coulombre concluded that the size of the eye, at any given time after the closure of the choroidal fissure, results from the balance between the intraocular pressure and the resistance to expansion offered by the wall of the eye.

Using rabbits as subjects, Maurice and Mushin (1966) found that myopia could be induced by increasing the body temperature to 41°C while simultaneously increasing the intraocular pressure to 40 mm Hg. They noted the resemblance to the results of Rigby et al. (1959) who found that rat-tail collagen stretched when put under tension when heated to a temperature above 40°C, and concluded that the myopia occurred due to a stretching of the eye. They suggested that this effect may be related to the myopia that had been reported to develop in fibrile diseases in children. Citing the Maurice and Mushin report, Hirsch (1972) noted that coughing increases intraocular pressure and suggested that any disease that involves both coughing and an increase in body temperature may supply the mechanism for myopia. Such diseases could include measles, scarlet fever, and whooping cough.

Kelly (1981) found that young myopes have elevated applanation pressure, and described juvenile myopia as a self-inflicted condition, which he calls "juvenile expansile glaucoma." However, Young (1975) believes that anterior chamber pressure is normal in myopia, and he has proposed that accommodation causes an increase in vitreous pressure, leading to an expansion of the vitreous chamber. Young used a surgically implanted radiosonde transducer to measure change in the vitreous chamber pressure of the pigtail monkey during accommodation. On the basis of ambient pressure, the transducer (a small drum, about the size of an aspirin tablet) amplifies or depresses the signal from a radiofrequency source outside the eye. The pigtail monkey has a strong eye contact response, and will look at the eye of a human as long as the human looks at the monkey. Using the experimenter's eye as a stimulus to accommodation for the monkey (seated in a restraining chair), it was found that the vitreous chamber pressure increased in a monotonic fashion as the experimenter moved from a distance of 6 meters to a distance of 30 cm from the monkey's face. The possible role of accommodation in the development of myopia is discussed in this volume by Young and Leary (Chapter 17), Schor (Chapter 18), and Owens (Chapter 19).

□ Earlier Bifocal Studies

Many clinicians and researchers, believing that myopia occurs as a result of prolonged accommodation, have recommended the use of bifocal lenses to reduce the accommodative demand for young myopes. Although the literature on myopia contains a large number of reports about the use of bifocals for the control of myopia, only a small number of large-scale controlled clinical studies have been reported.

Mandell (1959) reported on a survey of patient records from an optometric practice in which fifty-nine myopes had been fitted with bifocals and 116 had been fitted with single-vision lenses. He concluded that bifocal lenses had not eliminated or reduced the progression of myopia beyond what might have been expected on a chance basis. However, the patients in the two groups were not matched on the basis of age: The average age for single-vision lens wearers was 17.1 years, as compared to an average age for bifocal lens wearers of only 14.3 years.

Reporting on a study in which a group of myopes who had previously been fitted with single-vision lenses were fitted with bifocals, Miles (1962) found that the average rate of progression for the subjects (from 6 to 14 years of age) while wearing single-vision lenses was 0.75 D per year; but the average rate of progression (for the same subjects, now from 8 to 16 years of age) while wearing bifocals had decreased to 0.40 D per year. Because the subjects wearing bifocals were 2 years older than they had been when they wore single-vision lenses, it is possible that the reduction in the mean rate of progression (0.35 D per year) may have been, at least in part, due to this age difference.

In a retrospective report on mean rates of progression for eighty-five bifocal wearers and 396 single-vision lens wearers who had been seen in their optometric practice on at least two occasions before age 17, Roberts and Banford (1967) found that the bifocal wearers progressed at a mean rate of 0.36 D per year as compared to 0.41 D for single-vision lens wearers. This small difference (0.05 D per year) was reported by the authors to be statistically significant. Of the children who had worn bifocals during the entire period of the study, twelve children having a stable refraction had a mean near-point phoria of 6.0 prism diopters of esophoria; whereas twelve children having the highest rates of progression had a mean near-point phoria of 1.1 prism diopters of esophoria. Roberts and Banford interpreted these results as indicating that of all the children who wore bifocal lenses, stabilization of the myopia was more effective for those who were esophoric at nearpoint.

Results of bifocals in controlling the progression of myopia were analyzed on the basis of nearpoint esophoria by Goss (1986), who reported on a survey of the records of three optometrists who regularly prescribe bifocals for the control of myopia. Records used in this retrospective study were those of all patients who had had four or more subjective refractions between the ages of 6 and 15 years and who had worn either bifocals or single-vision lenses during the entire period. Mean rates of progression were found to be −0.37 D per year for bifocal wearers and 0.44 D per year for single-vision lens wearers: The difference (0.07 D per year) was found not to be significant at the 0.95 confidence level. Suggesting that bifocals may have had a greater effect for those children having near-point esophoria, Goss tabulated the rates of progression for bifocal and single-vision subjects in terms of the near-point phoria findings and the near-point cross-cylinder nets. For children having exophoria at near point, the difference between the mean rates of progression for single vision and bifocal groups was not statistically significant; however, for children having near-point esophoria, the bifocal group had a significantly lower progression rate (−0.32 D per year) than the single-vision group (−0.54 D per year). For children having near-point cross-cylinder nets less than +0.50 D, the difference between mean rates of progression for single-vision and bifocal groups was not significant; but for chlidren having cross-cylinder nets of +0.50 D or more, the bifocal group had a significantly lower progression rate (−0.25 D per year) than the single vision group (−0.48 D per year). According to Goss, these results suggest that if bifocals are prescribed to provide comfortable vision for myopes who have esophoria or high cross-cylinder nets at near, some level of control of myopia progression may follow as a consequence.

It should be understood, however, that the occurrence of a near-point esophoria in an uncorrected or undercorrected myope is not necessarily a cause for concern. Flom and Takahashi (1962) measured the distance and near phorias of twenty-eight previously uncorrected or undercorrected myopes. Phoria findings were taken when the full correction for the myopia was first worn and after the correction had been worn for a week or longer. For fourteen of the subjects who were esophoric at near on the initial phoria measurement, the average change after wearing the correction for a week or longer was 3.01 prism diopters in the direction of decreased esophoria at near. Flom and Takahashi reasoned that when myopia is not fully corrected, the reduction in accommodative demand at the reading distance results in a relative exophoria: Bifixation is possible only with the use of positive relative vergence, which becomes conditioned through use over a long period of time. When the myopia is fully corrected, this conditioned convergence remains in play; but with continued wearing of the correction, the conditioned convergence will be extinguished, and the near-point phoria will return to the previous level.

Oakley and Young (1975) reported the results of a retrospective study in which progression rates were compared for 269 bifocal wearers and 275 single-vision lens wearers between the ages of 6 and 21 years. The subject pool included 441 Caucasians and 156 Native Americans. Subjects for the bifocal and single vision groups were matched on the basis of sex, initial age, and the initial amount of myopia. For the bifocal wearers, the distance prescription was undercorrected by about 0.50 D, and the power of the bifocal addition was +0.75 or +1.00 D for low myopes and +1.50 or +2.00 D for higher myopes. Straight-top bifocals were used, with the segment top splitting the subject's pupil when the eyes were in the primary position. Mean rates of progression for the Caucasian children, after 3 to 4 years, were 0.02 D per year for bifocal wearers and 0.50 D per year for single-vision lens wearers; for Native American children, mean rates were 0.11 D per year for bifocal wearers and 0.37 D per year for single-vision lens wearers. Oakley and Young attributed their success to the high bifocal position. However they commented that there could have been some experimenter bias, as all of the refractions were performed by the senior author.

□ The Houston Bifocal Study

In a 3-year randomized clinical trial of the use of bifocal lenses for the control of myopia recently completed at the University of Houston (Young et al. 1985, Grosvenor et al. 1987) a table of random numbers was used to place each of 207 subjects ages 6 to 15 years in one of three experimental groups: a single-vision group, a +1.00 D add group, and a +2.00 D add group. Subjects in the three groups were matched on the basis of sex, initial age, and initial amount of myopia. Two groups of investigators were involved in the study: an evaluation team, whose task was to evaluate candidates before entering the study and to reevaluate each subject on a yearly basis for the 3-year period, and a patient care team, whose task was to prescribe glasses for each subject, as well as to counsel subjects and their parents in the correct use of the glasses, and to provide follow-up examinations every 6 months for the duration of the study.

Members of the evaluation team were not permitted to know which subjects wore single-vision lenses, +1.00 D add bifocals, or +2.00 D add bifocals; nor were they permitted to see the patient care team records until the completion of the study. In the interest of responsible patient care, members of the patient care team were permitted to know to which experimental group each subject had been assigned. An additional difference between the two teams was that members of the evaluation team determined each subject's refractive state by means of retinoscopy under cyclopentolate cycloplegia, whereas members of the patient care team determined refractive state by means of manifest retinoscopy and subjective refraction.

In the report of the patient care team, Grosvenor et al. (1987) stated that for the 124 subjects who remained in the study for the entire 3-year period, mean rates of myopia progression were 0.34 D per year for single vision lens wearers, 0.36 D per year for + 1.00 D add bifocal wearers, and 0.34 D per year for + 2.00 D add bifocal wearers (Figure 20.1). The small differences in mean rates of progression were found not to be statistically significant. When male and female subjects were considered separately (see Table 20.1), differences in mean rates of progression for the members of the three treatment groups were slightly larger but were still not statistically significant.

Figure 20.1.
Frequency distributions of mean changes in spherical equivalent refraction, right eye, for subjects wearing single-vision lenses, + 1.00 D add bifocals, and + 2.00 D add bifocals. (From Grosvenor et al. 1987.)

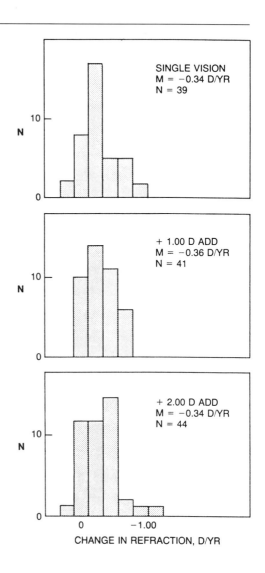

Table 20.1. Mean Change in Refraction (D/year) Based on Sex

	Single vision	+ 1.00 D Add	+ 2.00 D Add	All groups
Boys	− 0.24 (16)*	− 0.38 (20)	− 0.32 (22)	− 0.32 (58)
Girls	− 0.41 (23)	− 0.35 (21)	− 0.33 (22)	− 0.36 (66)
All subjects	− 0.34 (39)	− 0.36 (41)	− 0.34 (44)	− 0.34 (124)

(From Grosvenor et al. 1987.)
*Number of subjects in parentheses.

When rates of progression for the two sexes were considered on the basis of initial age and initial refractive error, it was found that no matter what form of treatment was used (single vision, + 1.00 D add bifocals, or + 2.00 D add bifocals), subjects who entered the study before the age of about 11 years with more than 2.00 D of myopia tended to progress rapidly, whereas subjects who entered the study beyond the age of 11 years with less than 2.00 D of myopia tended to progress slowly. This is demonstrated in the graphs in Figure 20.2 for girls wearing single-vision lenses (Figure 20.2A) and + 2.00 D add bifocals (Figure 20.2B): For the curves in the upper left quadrant of each graph (subjects having a relatively large amount of myopia at a relatively young age), the rate of progression is relatively rapid; but for those in the lower right quadrant (subjects having a smaller amount of myopia at a more advanced age), the rate of progression is relatively slow.

The authors suggested that the lack of a significant effect of the bifocals on the progression of myopia may have been due to the fact that once the eye has begun to elongate, the scleral tissue is stretched and thinned to the extent that it has lost much of its resiliency and will continue to elongate, even in the presence of lower vitreous pressure. If this is the case, bifocals would be expected to have a significant effect on the progression of myopia only if they were worn before the eye began to elongate. This would mean that bifocals would have to be worn before the onset of myopia. Since it was shown by Hirsch (1964) that the children at greatest risk for development of myopia are those with no more than 0.50 D of myopia at the age of 5 to 6 years, particularly if they also have against-the-rule astigmatism, children who fit this description could be fitted with bifocals (with plano uppers) or with reading glasses and then followed during the elementary school years. A problem with this approach, however, would be that of convincing parents (as well as children) of the need for glasses, even though no refractive error or visual problem existed.

Another possible explanation for the negative results of this study is that an increase in the length of the eye is brought about not only by excessive accommodation but also by excessive convergence. Donders (1864, reprinted 1972) sug-

Figure 20.2. (A) Graphical representation of spherical equivalent refraction, right eye, on the basis of measurements made each six months for a three-year period, for twenty-three girls wearing single-vision lenses. (From Grosvenor et al. 1987.) **(B)** Graphical representation of spherical equivalent refraction, right eye, on the basis of measurements made each six months for a three-year period, for twenty-two girls wearing + 2.00 D add bifocal lenses. (From Grosvenor et al. 1987.)

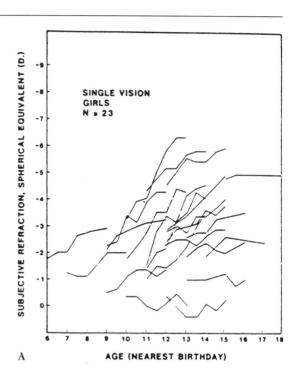

A

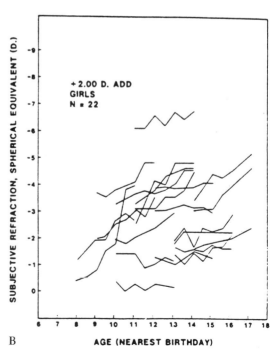

B

gested that pressure of the muscles on the eyeball during strong convergence was one of the factors leading to myopia. Greene (see Chapter 16) has proposed that myopia is brought about by a mechanical stretching of the sclera (scleral creep), which is due initially to pressure exerted on the globe by the medial rectus muscles, leading to an increase in vitreous chamber pressure which is transmitted to the back of the scleral shell. The use of base-in prisms has often been suggested as a method of myopia control to reduce the amount of convergence necessary for reading or other close work. Rehm (1975) has devised an instrument that allows a child to read without either accommodating or converging. However, the literature on myopia includes no reports of large-scale controlled clinical trials using base-in prisms for the control of myopia.

□ Summary of Bifocal Results

The results of all of the studies reported here are summarized in Table 20.2. The data presented in the right-hand column of this table (Mean Change) indicate that only the Miles (1962) and Oakley and Young (1975) studies demonstrated what might be considered a clinically significant difference (for example, 0.25 D per

Table 20.2.   Comparison of Results of Bifocal Studies

Study	Ages	Treatment	Mean change
Miles (1962)	6–14	Single vision	−0.75 D/year
	8–16	Bifocals	−0.40 D/year
Mandell (1959)	Mean 17.1	Single vision	(see below)*
	Mean 14.3	Bifocals	(see below)*
Roberts and Banford (1967)	<17	Single vision	−0.41 D/year
	<17	Bifocals	−0.36 D/year
Oakley and Young (1975)	6–21	Single vision	−0.37 D/year
(Native Americans)	6–21	Bifocals	−0.11 D/year
Oakley and Young (1975)	6–21	Single vision	−0.52 D/year
(Caucasians)	6–21	Bifocals	−0.02 D/year
Brodstein et al. (1984)	Not given	Single vision	−0.25 D/year
	Not given	Bifocals & atropine	−0.16 D/year
Goss (1986)	6–15	Single vision	−0.44 D/year
	6–15	Bifocals	−0.37 D/year
Grosvenor et al. (1987)	6–15	Single vision	−0.34 D/year
	6–15	+1.00 D add	−0.36 D/year
	6–15	+2.00 D add	−0.34 D/year

(From Grosvenor et al. 1987.)
*Mean changes in refraction were not reported, but it was concluded that bifocals did not eliminate or reduce the progression of myopia.

year or more) in rates of progression for bifocals and single-vision lenses. As already noted, the same patients served both as single-vision subjects and as bifocal subjects in the Miles study, being 2 years older when they wore bifocals than when they wore single-vision lenses. Therefore, for studies in which subjects were matched on the basis of sex, initial age, and initial amount of myopia, only the study reported by Oakley and Young shows a clinically significant difference in rates of progression between bifocal and single-vision lens wearers.

MINUS LENSES FOR DISTANCE USE ONLY

For amounts of myopia up to about 2.50 D, with little or no astigmatism or anisometropia, the accommodative demand for near work can be reduced by simply having the patient remove his or her glasses for prolonged near work: A 2.00 D myope who reads without glasses is wearing, in effect, a +2.00 D add. This form of treatment not only has the advantage of simplicity, but for young myopes who are esophoric at near the built-in add will tend to avoid symptoms of asthenopia. It also has the advantage that the patient is very much aware that his or her vision is quite adequate for near work, without glasses. Although many practitioners have used this form of management for many years, no controlled clinical studies have been reported.

CONTACT LENSES

Contact lenses have been advocated for two forms of myopia control: (1) to control the progression of myopia during childhood, and (2) to reduce the amount of existing myopia in adults, a procedure known as orthokeratology.

□ Contact Lenses for Myopia Control during Childhood

Whether contact lenses are effective in the control of myopia has been a matter of controversy ever since Morrison (1956) reported that he had fitted a large number of young myopes with contact lenses and that after a period of more than 2 years there was "no progression in any of the cases surveyed." His patients ranged in age from 7 to 19 years, and were fitted with polymethyl methacrylate (PMMA) lenses, fitted from 1.62 to 2.50 D flatter than the flattest corneal meridian. Morrison suggested that the lack of progression could have been due to a flattening effect on the cornea, an interference or effect on metabolism of the cornea, or other factors.

It was well known at that time that contact lenses fitted flatter than the flattest corneal meridian tended to cause corneal flattening, so Morrison's finding was not unexpected. If the axial length of the eye increased during the period of contact lens wear, the increase could have been more than offset by corneal flattening. However, in a later report, Morrison (1960) said that he was then using the alignment method of fitting (fitting the lenses essentially parallel to the flattest corneal meridian) and that he found that these lenses, too, kept myopia from progressing.

In response to the reports of Morrison and other practitioners, Bailey (1958) called attention to the following factors that may account for the apparent stabilization of myopia due to contact lens wear: (1) flattening of the cornea; (2) a possible reduction in anterior chamber depth due to corneal flattening, with a consequent decrease in the axial length of the eye; (3) overcorrection of the myopia due to the presence of photophobia during the initial and subsequent refractions while wearing the lenses; (4) settling of the lens on the cornea, reducing the tear layer thickness; (5) effective power error due to failure to take effective power into consideration when ordering contact lenses; (6) ophthalmometer error, caused by using an ophthalmometer (keratometer) to verify the finished lenses; and (7) the practitioner's tendency to overlook an overcorrection of myopia in follow-up examinations.

Of all the studies making use of PMMA lenses for myopia control, the most definitive was carried out by Stone and her colleagues. This study made use of a control group; an effort was made to match subjects in the experimental and control groups as to the initial amount of myopia. The age range of subjects was chosen to embrace the period of life when myopia is most likely to progress. The study was of sufficiently long duration, and the time of testing was specified in relation to the time of lens removal. As stated in Stone's first report (1973), the experimental group was made up of eighty-four contact lens wearers (fifty-three boys and thirty-two girls), and the control group was made up of forty spectacle wearers (eighteen boys and twenty-two girls). Members of the experimental group were fitted with lenses having a diameter of 9.2 mm or smaller and an optic zone width of 7.0 mm or smaller, fitted "just steeper than the flattest keratometer reading."

On completion of the 5-year study, Stone (1976) reported keratometric and refractive data taken immediately after lens removal. Inspection of her graphs (Figure 20.3) indicates that the mean increase in myopia for the contact lens wearers was 0.50 D (averaging the horizontal and vertical findings) for the 5-year period, or 0.10 D per year; whereas for the spectacle wearers, the mean increase in myopia was 1.75 D, or 0.35 D per year. The corneal changes were much less than the changes in refraction, mean corneal refracting power decreasing about 0.50 D for contact lens wearers and no more than 0.12 D for spectacle wearers during the 5-year period.

Figure 20.3. (A) Graphical representation of changes in corneal curvature and refraction for contact lens wearers. (From Stone 1976.) **(B)** Graphical representation of changes in corneal curvature and refraction for spectacle wearers. (From Stone 1976.)

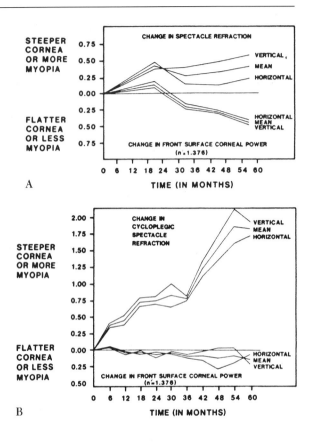

In discussing her results, Stone made the point that not all of the difference in progression of myopia for the last two groups could be accounted for by corneal flattening (that is, the difference in mean corneal flattening for the two groups was less than 0.50 D, whereas the difference in mean increase in myopia was 1.65 D). She concluded that since the effects of contact lenses on the progression of myopia cannot be due entirely to corneal flattening, it is possible that contact lenses may have an effect on the axial elongation of the eye. Unfortunately, axial length was not measured.

During the decade of the 1970s, the controversy concerning myopia control with contact lenses abated to a great extent, due to the popularity of hydrogel (soft) contact lenses. It is of interest that virtually nobody has claimed that soft contact lenses, which exert little if any mechanical pressure on the cornea, are effective in the control of myopia. However with the advent of gas permeable hard lenses, the controversy has been rekindled. Bailey (1984), a lecturer and publisher in the contact lens field, has made the comment that many practitioners believe that these lenses are not only effective in controlling myopia but also tend to reduce corneal astigmatism.

In spite of the progress made as a result of the studies of Stone and others, the following questions remained unanswered: (1) Are gas permeable hard lenses effective in the control of myopia? (2) Could the effectiveness of contact lenses in controlling the progression of myopia be due in part to a tendency of the contact lenses to control axial elongation of the eye? (3) How permanent are the stabilization effects of contact lenses on corneal curvature and myopia?

□ The Houston Contact Lens Myopia Control Study

In an attempt to answer these questions, a 3-year study was begun at the University of Houston in 1985. One hundred myopic children, 8 through 13 years of age, were fitted with Paraperm O_2+ silicone-acrylate gas-permeable contact lenses. Inclusion criteria for the study were myopia with no more than 2.00 D of astigmatism, normal binocular vision and normal ocular health, and no history of contact lens wear. The control group consisted of twenty single-vision spectacle lens wearers who had served as controls in the bifocal study. These subjects were matched with the contact lens wearers, as closely as possible, on the basis of initial age and initial amount of myopia.

Most subjects were fitted with lenses having a diameter of 9.0 mm and an optic zone width of 7.7 mm, although a few were fitted with lenses as large as 9.5 mm in diameter or as small as 8.5 mm. Secondary and peripheral curve radii and center thicknesses were those normally used by the manufacturer. Lenses were fitted by the alignment method, the criteria being (1) a "parallel fit" (as indicated by inspection under ultraviolet light after instillation of fluorescein) with a complete peripheral ring of pooling and an absesnce of a stagnant apical pool; and (2) a well-centered lens with about 2 mm of lag following a blink.

The study was conducted by two teams of researchers, an evaluation team and a patient care team. The evaluation team made baseline measurements consisting of conventional (manifest) refraction, keratometry and ultrasound measurement of axial length before each subject's enrollment in the study. These measurements were repeated at yearly intervals for the duration of the study, the testing being done on a Saturday morning before the subjects put on their lenses (having worn them on a full-time basis up to and including the day before the testing). Members of the patient care team supervised student clinicians in the contact lens fitting and follow-up care. Changes in lens power or in the physical parameters (base curve, diameter, etc.) were made, as needed, during the course of the study. Members of the evaluation team were unaware of any previous refractive or biometric findings or of any of the data collected by the patient care team, but members of the patient care team had access to both evaluation team data and patient-care team data.

At the end of the 3-year period, fifty-six of the original 100 subjects remained in the study. For these fifty-six subjects, the mean increase in myopia was 0.48

(±0.70) D for the 3-year period, or 0.16 D per year, whereas for the group of twenty spectacle-wearing control subjects the mean increase in myopia was 1.53 (±0.81) D, or 0.51 D per year (Grosvenor et al. 1989). These changes are illustrated in Figure 20.4: Comparing the two groups, the mean increase in myopia for the spectacle wearers was about 1.00 D more than the mean increase for the contact lens wearers. Distributions of 3-year changes in refractive error for the two groups are shown in Figure 20.5. As for corneal power and axial length changes for the contact lens wearers, there was a mean corneal flattening of 0.37 (±0.32) D and a mean axial length increase of 0.48 (±0.48) mm. Distributions of 3-year changes in keratometer findings and axial length are shown in Figure 20.6. Complete data concerning corneal and axial length changes were not available for the spectacle wearers; however, keratometry data on spectacle-wearing myopes published by Stone (1976) and by Fledelius (1982a) show that little if any change in corneal refracting power would be expected for myopes in this age range; and axial length data published by Fledelius (1982b) show that myopes whose progression was from 0.60 to 1.50 D between the ages of 10 and 18 years had a mean increase in axial length of 0.49 mm.

To find out what changes in myopia would occur if lens wear was discontinued, subjects still in the study at the end of 3 years were asked to give up contact lens wear during the summer vacation and to resume lens wear in the fall. In response to this request, twenty-three subjects discontinued wearing their lenses for an average of 2.5 months. During this period, there was a mean increase in myopia of 0.27 D and a mean corneal steepening of 0.25 D. However, when we compare the mean values of contact lens wearers and spectacle wearers, a contact lens

---

Figure 20.4. Mean annual progression of myopia for contact lens wearers and spectacle wearers. (From Perrigin et al. 1990.)

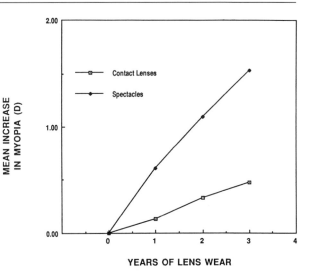

Figure 20.5. (A) Distribution of 3-year changes in refractive error for contact lens wearers. (From Perrigin et al. 1990.) **(B)** Distribution of 3-year changes in refractive error for spectacle wearers. (From Perrigin et al. 1990.)

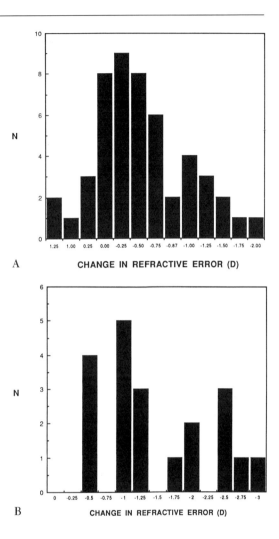

A CHANGE IN REFRACTIVE ERROR (D)

B CHANGE IN REFRACTIVE ERROR (D)

wearer whose myopia increased the mean amount during the 3-year period of lens wear (0.48 D) and during the period when the lenses were not worn (0.27 D) would still have a smaller amount of progression than mean amount for spectacle wearers during the 3-year period (1.53 D). As a result of these findings, Grosvenor et al. (1990) concluded the following:

1. *Progression of myopia.* When mean values are considered, Paraperm O_2+ lenses controlled the progression of myopia by a clinically significant amount, as mean progression was 1.00 D less for contact lens wearers than for spectacle wear-

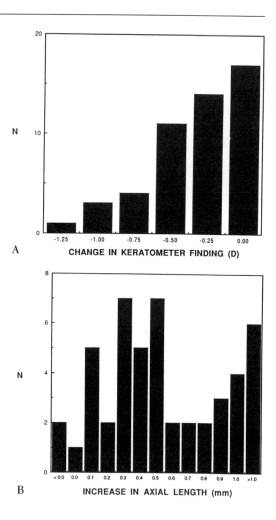

Figure 20.6. **(A)** Distribution of 3-year changes in keratometer findings for contact lens wearers. (From Grosvenor et al. 1989.) **(B)** Distribution of 3-year changes in axial length for contact lens wearers. (From Grosvenor et al. 1989.)

ers. For a given patient, however, it would not be possible to predict the effect of contact lenses in controlling myopia because of the large standard deviations for both groups.

2. *Corneal flattening.* Somewhat less than half of the effect of the contact lenses in controlling myopia progression could be attributed to corneal flattening (as measured by the keratometer). A tentative explanation is that the corneal flattening takes place primarily in the axial portion of the cornea, which the keratometer does not measure, and only secondarily in an annulus having a chord diameter of about 3 mm, which the keratometer does measure.

3. *Permanency.* The effect of the lenses in controlling the progression of myopia was present only as long as the lenses continued to be worn; however, when lens wear was resumed, the lenses continued to be effective in controlling the progression.

☐ Orthokeratology

A number of procedures have been advocated for fitting contact lenses to reduce the amount of existing myopia. One commonly used procedure is to fit successively flatter PMMA contact lenses to try to reduce the myopia through a gradual flattening of the cornea. Once the practitioner believes that a maximum amount of flattening (along with a maximum amount of reduction of myopia) has occurred, the patient's wearing time is gradually reduced with the intention that the reduction in myopia will persist with the reduced wearing schedule. Although the ideal outcome would be for the reduction in myopia to persist after discontinuation of lens wear, in most cases "retainer" lenses must be worn, on a reduced wearing schedule, in order for the reducion in myopia to persist.

Even though the stated aim of orthokeratology is to reduce the amount of myopia, the practitioner usually evaluates the success of the procedure in terms of improvement in unaided visual acuity. Although there is a large body of literature on the subject, much of it is made up of reports by practitioners who were obviously biased toward orthokeratology (or toward their own particular variation of orthokeratology). However, two large scale clinical trials have been reported.

Kerns (1976, 1977, 1978) reported on a study in which he took an objective position, not advocating the use of orthokeratology but investigating it on a scientific but clinically-oriented basis. Subjects were conventional contact lens wearers (twenty-six eyes) and experimental (orthokeratology) wearers (thirty-six eyes). The experimental wearers were fitted with larger, thicker, and flatter lenses to initiate orthokeratology changes. After somewhat more than a year, mean changes for the experimental group were:

Refraction in the horizontal meridian: 1.06 D less myopia (SD ±0.98 D).

Refraction in the vertical meridian: 0.68 D less myopia (SD ±0.09 D).

Refractive astigmatism (with-the-rule): 0.42 D increase (SD ±0.74 D).

The mean changes were such as to bring about a reduction in myopia, but with induced with-the-rule astigmatism. Kerns pointed out that the standard deviations were so high that it would not be possible to predict that changes comparable to the mean changes would occur with any given patient. Even the patient typified by the mean values would have approximately 1.00 D less spherical error at the end of the study, but 0.50 D more astigmatism than before the study began. Kerns reported that the limiting factor in inducing corneal flattening was the "sphericalization" of the cornea, which occurs when the corneal apex has become sufficiently flat so that it has the same radius of curvature as the periphery. No data were given about the permanence of the orthokeratology changes.

In another large scale clinical trial, Polse et al. (1983) fitted eighty subjects (forty experimental subjects and forty controls) with contact lenses and followed them for 18 months. Experimental (orthokeratology) subjects were fitted with larger and thicker lenses, and were fitted flatter than control subjects. This study was a randomized clinical trial, in which even the subjects did not know which group they were in. Mock lens changes were made for members of the control group (and real changes were made for members of the experimental group). For the experimental subjects, myopia was found to reduce by an average of 1.00 D as compared to 0.50 D for the control subjects. Polse et al. did not find the with-the-rule astigmatism reported by Kerns, and commented that this was because they monitored lens fit, making sure the lenses were well centered on the wearers' corneas rather than "riding high." They found that the reduction in myopia was not permanent, requiring the use of retainer lenses to perpetuate the effect. In addition, vision was variable from day to day. There were no clinically significant adverse effects, but the orthokeratology patients required more visits because of complications, than did the control subjects.

On the basis of the results of these studies, we may conclude that for a low myope, orthokeratology may bring about sufficient reduction in myopia so that contact lenses would not need to be worn on a full-time basis; however, they will usually have to be worn as retainers for several hours each day to maintain the reduction in myopia and improvement in visual acuity.

CAN WE PREDICT WHO WILL BECOME MYOPIC?

The suggestion was made earlier in this chapter that the lack of a significant effect of bifocals on the progression of myopia may be due to the fact that once the eye has begun to elongate, the scleral tissue may be stretched and thinned to the extent that it has lost much of its resiliency and will continue to elongate, even in the presence of lower intraocular pressure. If this is the case, methods of myopia control based on reducing the demand on accommodation (visual training, the use of bifocals, minus lenses for distance use only) might be more successful if they were begun before the eye began to elongate. To accomplish this, it would be necessary to be able to predict, in advance, which eyes will become myopic.

One possible method of predicting the onset of myopia would be on the basis of a genetic component for myopia: Although a genetic component has not yet been isolated, modern techniques of molecular genetics may eventually permit identification of the responsible gene(s) and their product(s) (Raviola and Wiesel 1988). Another possibility, already noted, is that any child who has no more than 0.50 D of hyperopia at 5 to 6 years of age may be at risk for the development of myopia, particularly if he or she also has against-the-rule astigmatism (Hirsch 1964). A third possible avenue for predicting who will become myopic may be based on measurements of the resting state of accommodation. Although much more work is needed in this area, a number of investigations (many of which are reviewed in Chapter 19) have shown that the resting state of accommodation for myopic subjects differs significantly from that for emmetropic and hyperopic subjects.

Still another possible method of predicting the onset of myopia involves the relationship between the axial length of the eye and the corneal radius: the axial length/corneal radius ratio. It has been shown that emmetropic Melanesian children examined in Vanuatu (Garner et al. 1988) had relatively short eyes and flat corneas, which should have led to hyperopia; whereas emmetropic children examined in England by Sorsby and Leary (1970) had significantly longer eyes as compared to the corneal radii (that is, significantly greater axial length/corneal radius ratios (Grosvenor 1988).)

Once it is possible to predict which children are at risk for the development of myopia, it will then be possible to institute myopia control procedures (for example, visual training, prescribing bifocals or contact lenses) when only a minimum of scleral stretching has occurred. Until then, practitioners can continue to base their management of myopia on the prevailing conventional wisdom (Grosvenor 1989). In all cases, prescribe minus lenses to provide good distance acuity. In addition (1) prescribe visual training or bifocals when their use is indicated for problems involving the relationship between accommodation and accomodative convergence; (2) for low myopia uncomplicated by astigmatism or anisometropia, there may be some merit in instructing the patient to wear glasses for distance vision only (most of these patients do not have to be told that they have good vision for near work without their lenses); (3) for those children who would like to wear contact lenses, rigid lenses seem to have a tendency to reduce the rate of progression, at least for some children.

REFERENCES

Bailey NJ. Possible factors in the control of myopia with contact lenses. Contacto 1958; 2:114–117.

Bailey NJ. Personal communication, 1984.

Baldwin WR, West D, Jolly J, Reid W. Effects of contact lenses on refractive corneal and axial length changes in young myopes. Am J Optom Arch Am Acad Optom 1969;46: 903–911.

Balliet R, Clay A, Blood K. The training of visual acuity in myopia. J Am Optom Assoc 1982;53:719–724.

Bates WH. Perfect Sight without Glasses. New York: Central Fixation Publ Co, 1920.

Betts EA. An evaluation of the Baltimore Myopia Project, Part A: Experimental procedures. J Am Optom Assoc 1947;18:681–695.

Berman PE, Levinger SI, Massoth NA, et al. The effectiveness of biofeedback visual training as a viable method of treatment and reduction of myopia. J Optom Vis Develop 1985; 16:17–21.

Betts EA, Doris V. Maintaining visual acuity in the navy. Optom Weekly 1948;39:691–692.

Bier N. Myopia controlled by contact lenses, a preliminary report. Optician 1958;135:427.

Brodstein RS, Brodstein DE, Olson RJ, et al. The treatment of myopia with atropine and bifocals. Ophthalmology 1984;91:1373–1379.

Corbett MD. How To Improve Your Sight. New York: Bonanza Books, 1953.

Cornsweet TN, Crane HD. Experimental study of visual accommodation (NASA Contractor Report CR-2007). Washington, DC: National Aeronautics and Space Administration, 1972.

Coulombre AJ. The role of intraocular pressure in the development of the chick eye. J Exp Zool 1956;133:211–225.

Donders FC. On the Anomalies of Accommodation and Refraction of the Eye. London: New Sydenham Society, 1864 (Boston: Milford House, 1972, reprint).

Eberl M. The Baltimore Myopia Project (editorial). Am J Optom Arch Am Acad Optom 1946;23:222–225.

Ewalt WH Jr. The Baltimore Myopia Project. J Am Optom Assoc 1946;17:167–185.

Fledelius HC. Ophthalmic changes from age of 10 to 18 years III. Acta Ophthalmol 1982a; 60:393–402.

Fledelius HC. Ophthalmic changes from age of 10 to 18 years IV. Acta Ophthalmol 1982b; 60:403–411.

Flom MC, Takahashi E. The AC/A ratio and undercorrected myopia. Am J Optom Physiol Opt 1962;39:305–312.

Gallaway M, Pearl SM, Winkelstein AM, Scheiman M. Biofeedback training of visual acuity and myopia: a pilot study. Am J Optom Physiol Opt 1987;64:62–71.

Garner LF, Kinnear RF, McKellar M, Klinger J, Hovander S, Grosvenor T. Refraction and its components in Melanesian school children in Vanuatu. Am J Optom Physiol Opt 1988;65:182–189.

Giglio EJ. Visual acuity under special circumstances. Am J Optom Arch Am Acad Optom 1952;29:647–655.

Goss DA. Overcorrection as a means of slowing myopic correction. Am J Optom Physiol Opt 1984;61:85–93.

Goss DA. Effect of bifocal lenses on the rate of childhood myopia progression. Am J Optom Physiol Opt 1986;63:135–141.

Goss DA, Winkler RL. Progression of myopia in yough: age of cessation. Am J Optom Physiol Opt 1983;60:651–658.

Greene PR. Mechanical considerations in myopia: relative effects of accommodation, convergence, intraocular pressure, and the extraocular muscles. Am J Optom Physiol Opt 1980;57:902–914.

Grosvenor T. High axial length/corneal radius ratio as a risk factor in the development of myopia. Am J Optom Physiol Opt 1988;65:689–696.

Grosvenor T. Myopia: what can we do about it clinically? Optom Vis Sci 1989;66:415–419.

Grosvenor T, Perrigin DM, Perrigin J, et al. The Houston Myopia Control Study, a randomized clinical trial: Part II. Final report by the patient care team. Am J Optom Physiol Opt 1987;64:482–498.

Grosvenor T, Perrigin J, Perrigin D, Quintero S. The use of silicone-acrylate contact lenses for the control of myopia: results after two years of lens wear. Am J Optom Physiol Opt 1989;66:41–47.

Grosvenor T, Perrigin D, Perrigin J, Quintero S. Rigid gas-permeable contact lenses for myopia control: effects of discontinuation of lens wear 1990; (manuscript in preparation).

Hackman RB. An evaluation of the Baltimore Myopia Control Project, Part B. Statistical procedure. J Am Optom Assoc 1947;18:416–426.

Hirsch MJ. Sex differences in the various grades of myopia. Am J Optom Arch Am Acad Optom 1953;30:135–138.

Hirsch MJ. Predictability of refraction at age 14 on the basis of testing at age 6 — Interim report from the Ojai longitudinal study of refraction. Am J Optom Arch Am Acad Optom 1964;41:567–573.

Hirsch MJ. What you wanted to know about myopia but never dared ask. Can J Optom 1972;46:54–66.

Huxley A. The art of seeing. New York: Harper and Brothers, 1942.

Kelly TS. Myopia or expansion glaucoma. In: Fledelius HC, Alsbirk PH, Goldschmidt E, eds. Third International Conference on Myopia, Copenhagen, 1980 (Documenta Ophthalmologica Proceedings Series, vol 28). The Hague: Junk Publications, 1981; 109–116.

Kerns RL. Research in orthokeratology. J Am Optom Assoc 1976;47:1047–1051, 1275–1285, 1505–1515, 1977;48:227–238, 345–359, 1134–1147, 1541–1543, 1978;49:308–314.

Mandell RB. Myopia control with bifocal correction. Am J Optom Arch Am Acad Optom 1959;36:662–668.

Marg E. "Flashes" of clear vision and negative accommodation with reference to the Bates method of visual training. Am J Optom Arch Am Acad Optom 1952;29:167–184.

Maurice DM, Mushin AS. Production of myopia in rabbits by raised body temperature and increased intraocular pressure. Lancet 1966;Nov:1160–1162.

Miles PW. A study of heterophoria and myopia in children, some of whom wore bifocal lenses. Am J Ophthalmol 1962;54:111–114.

Morrison RJ. Contact lenses and the progression of myopia. Optom Weekly 1956;47:1487–1488.

Morrison RJ. The use of contact lenses in adolescent myopic patients. Am J Optom Arch Am Acad Optom 1960;37:165–168.

Moss HI. Corneal contact lenses and myopia. Optom Weekly 1966;57:22–23.

Nolan JA. Progress of myopia and contact lenses. Contacto 1964;8:25–26.

Oakley KH, Young FA. Bifocal control of myopia. Am J Optom Physiol Opt 1975;52:758–764.

Peppard HM. Sight Without Glasses. Garden City, NY: Nelson Doubleday, 1936.

Perrigin J, Perrigin D, Quintero S, Grosvenor T. Silicone-acrylate contact lenses for myopia control: 3-year results. Optom Vis Sci 1990; (in press).

Polse KA, Brand RJ, Schwalbe JS, Vastine DW, Keener R. The Berkeley orthokeratology study, Part II: efficacy and duration. Am J Optom Physiol Opt 1983;60:187–198.

Prebble D. Visual training in myopia — a case report. Am J Optom Arch Am Acad Optom 1948;25:545–547.

Rehm D. The myopter viewer: an instrument for treating and preventing myopia. Am J Optom Physiol Opt 1975;52:347–350.

Raviola E, Wiesel TN. The mechanism of lid-suture myopia. Myopia Workshop. Acta Ophthalmol (Suppl) 1988;185:91–92.

Rengstorff RH. Variations in corneal curvature measurements: an after-effect observed with habitual wearers of contact lenses. Am J Optom Arch Am Acad Optom 1967;44:45–51.

Rengstorff RH. Diurnal variations in myopia after the wearing of contact lenses. Am J Optom Arch Am Acad Optom 1969a;46:812–815.

Rengstorff RH. Relationship between myopia and corneal curvature changes after wearing contact lenses. Am J Optom Arch Am Acad Optom 1969b;46:357–361.

Rengstorff RH. Diurnal variations in corneal curvature after the wearing of contact lenses. Am J Optom Arch Am Acad Optom 1971;48:239–244.

Rigby BJ, Hirai N, Spikes JP, Eytring H. J Gen Physiol 1959;43:265.

Roberts WL, Banford RD. Evaluation of bifocal correction technique in juvenile myopia. Optom Weekly 1967;58(38):25–31; 58(39):21–30; 58(40):23–28; 58(41):27–34; 58(43):19–24.

Shepard CF. The Baltimore project. Optom Weekly 1946;37:133–135.

Stone J. Contact lens wear in the young myope. Br J Physiol Opt 1973;28:90–134.

Stone J. The possible influence of contact lenses on myopia. Br J Physiol Opt 1976;31:89–114.

Trachtman JN. Biofeedback of accommodation to reduce myopia: a review. Am J Optom Physiol Opt 1987;64:639–643.

Woods AC. Report from the Wilmer Institute on the results obtained in treatment of myopia by visual training. Trans Am Acad Ophthalmol Otolaryngol 1945;49:37–65.

Young FA. The development and control of myopia in human and subhuman primates. Contacto 1975;19:16–31.

Young FA. Intraocular pressure dynamics associated with accommodation. In: Fedelius HC, Alsbirk PH, Goldschmidt E, eds. Third International Conference on Myopia, Copenhagen, 1980 (Documenta Ophthalmologica Proceedings Series, vol 28). The Hague: Junk, 1981;171–176.

Young FA, Leary GA, Grosvenor T, Maslovitz B, Perrigin DM, Perrigin J, Quintero S. Houston myopia control study: a randomized clinical trial. Part 1. Background and design of the study. Am J Optom Physiol Opt 1985;62:605–613.

21

Management of Myopia: Pharmaceutical Agents

Hanne Jensen and Ernst Goldschmidt

☐

This chapter considers recent studies of therapeutic approaches to prevent development of myopia and presents a pilot study on treatment with timolol maleate 0.25% eye drops, twice daily for 12 months.

A number of theories advanced to explain the development of myopia have led to many different types of therapy, particularly based on the assumption that exogenous factors may be important in causing progression of this condition. In the middle of the nineteenth century, Donders (1864) used cycloplegics in the treatment of pseudomyopia, and since then this type of treatment has been used for other forms of myopia. Animal experimentation by Young (1965), McKanna and Casagrande (1981), Raviola and Wiesel (1985) and others provided support for the opinion that cycloplegics could be effective in the treatment of myopia. In animal models, such as monkeys and tree shrews, myopia has been produced by a number of methods. Young (1965) kept monkeys in a near-point visual environment; and McKanna and Casagrande (1981) carried out eyelid sutures on tree shrews, as did Raviola and Wiesel (1985) on monkeys, with the common result that an increased axial length occurred and, as a consequence, myopia. For one species of monkey, Raviola and Wiesel (1985) found that if the animals were given atropine, lid-suture myopia was prevented. However, it is difficult to make a direct comparison with humans.

In addition to cycloplegics, mydriatics and antiglaucoma medication have also been tested (see Table 21.1). However the majority of studies using pharmaceutical agents have involved the use of cycloplegics; the other agents have never been widely used. Summaries and critical reviews have been published previously by Inkles (1976), Goss (1982), Curtin (1985), and others.

A survey follows of studies carried out during the past 20 years, in particular regarding the use of cycloplegics. None of these studies has been randomized, although a number have contained control groups.

Table 21.1.   Drugs Used for the Control of Myopia

Cycloplegic agents	Adrenergic agents	Antiglaucoma agents
Atropine	Phenylephrine	Pilocarpine
Scopolamine	Epinephrine	Adrenaline
Tropicamide		Acetazolamide
Cyclopentolate		Timolol
		Labetalol

■
CYCLOPLEGIC AGENTS

☐ Tropicamide

The use of tropicamide is based on the theory that accommodation primarily results in an increased, but reversible, amount of refractive power of the lens, and secondarily leads to permanent changes in the lens and eventually to an increased axial length of the eye. If tropicamide is given at night, the ciliary spasm is relaxed and the tension in the lens is reduced, and there are no complaints during the day as a result of the cycloplegic medication.

The results of studies making use of tropicamide are shown in Table 21.2. Tropicamide 1% was used by Abraham (1966), who found that the treatment was effective in reducing the rate of progression. Treated children progressed an average of 0.44 D during the observation period, whereas those in the control group progressed about twice as much (boys, 0.92 D; girls, 0.77 D). However, it is difficult to draw definite conclusions from Abraham's data because all children who were not treated, regardless of the reason, were placed in the control group. In addition, the author calculated the change in myopia for variable periods of observation rather than in terms of annual changes.

In a study in which 1% tropicamide was used in the evening by thirty-two myopes, Rosenthal (1970) evaluated the results subjectively and concluded that 68% of the subjects had good results. The duration of observation varied considerably, from 1 month to 2 years, and there was no control group. The study included all degrees of myopia, and it is impossible to draw any definite conclusions.

Curtin (1970) carried out a pilot study in which twenty-one subjects used two drops of 1% tropicamide in one eye in the evening, using a placebo in the other eye. He found three cases in which the highest rate of progression was in the control eye, nine with the highest rate in the treated eye, and nine with equal

Table 21.2. Studies Using Tropicamide 1% for the Control of Myopia

Author (year)	No. subjects	Age (yrs)	Follow-up (months)	Drop outs (T)	Results
Abraham (1966)	68 T* 82 C†	12.1 T 12.2 C	T 18.6 mo C 17.5 mo		0.44 D increase 0.77 to 0.92 D increase
Rosenthal (1970)	32 T	3–18 T	T 1–24 mo	23%	Good results for 68%
Curtin (1970)	21 T 21 C‡	8–16 T	T 8–30 mo C 8–30 mo		No effect demonstrated

*T, Treatment group.
†Control group.
‡Fellow eye as control.

progression in both eyes. It was thus impossible to demonstrate an effect of the tropicamide in this study.

□ Atropine

The use of atropine, a considerably stronger cycloplegic than tropicamide, is also based on the theory that accommodation plays an important role in the development of myopia. Some authors have considered that accommodation produces initial changes in the shape of the lens, as mentioned earlier; others believe it causes a pressure gradient between the anterior chamber and the vitreous chamber, with a subsequent rise in vitreous chamber pressure causing an increase in the axial length of the eye. Still others think that accommodation causes an increased intraocular pressure due to the zonular fibers clumping and blocking the passage of aqueous.

Studies making use of 1% atropine have been carried out by Gimbel (1973), Kelly et al. (1975), Gruber (1978), Bedrossian (1979), Brodstein et al. (1984), and Brenner (1985) — all of whom reported that the progression of myopia decreases after application. Curtin (1970) and Sampson (1979), on the other hand, were more skeptical about their results with atropine, but did not go so far as to state that the treatment had no beneficial effect. Curtin (1970) carried out a pilot study, instilling one drop of 1% atropine in one eye, in the evening, and no treatment for the other eye, to determine if the progression was delayed over a period of 6 months. In addition, he kept the children under observation for an additional 6 months after cessation of treatment. At the conclusion of the study, he found a mean difference of only 0.05 D between the two eyes. Data from the atropine studies are summarized in Table 21.3.

The effect of one drop of 1% atropine in both eyes was studied by Gimbel (1973). He began the study with a large experimental group (279 subjects) and a large control group (572 subjects). Refraction was determined under cycloplegia, and an attempt was made to determine whether the treatment had been carried

Table 21.3. Studies Using Atropine 1% for the Control of Myopia

Author (year)	No. subjects	Age (yrs)	Follow-up (months)	Drop outs (T)	Results
Curtin (1970)	10 T* 10 C†‡		T 6 C 12 PT§ 12		Mean difference of 0.05 D between T and C groups
Gimbel (1973)	279 T 572 C	5–15 T 5–15 C	T 12–36 C ?–72	53%	Difference in progression only after 1 year
Kelly (1975)	38 T 143 C	see text see text	T 6 C 12–48		No progression for 97% of T group‖
Gruber (1978)	100 T 100 C	5–16 T 5–15 C	T 12–24 C 24–250 PT 12–84	12%	T 0.11 D/yr progression C 0.28 D/yr progression PT 0.46 D/yr progression
Sampson (1979)	112 T	7–14 T	T 12 PT 6–12	11%	Change in refraction of −0.25 to +1.00 D
Bedrossian (1979)	62 T 62C⁺	8–13 T 8–13 C	T 12 C 12		0.17 to 0.29 D progression 0.81 to 0.99 D progression
Dyer (1979)	265 T 86 C	6–15 T 6–15 C	T 24–96 C 67 PT 12–48	68%	63% < 2.00 D progression 10% < 2.00 D progression
Brodstein (1984)	435 T 146 C	6–18 T 6–18 C	T 1–107 C 12–212 PT 1–110	42%	0.010 D/mo progression 0.028 D/mo progression
Brenner (1985)	79 T	6–13	T 7–84	6%	

*T, Treatment group.
†C, Control group.
‡Fellow eye used as control.
§PT, Post-treatment.
‖Used noncycloplegic refraction before treatment and cycloplegic refraction after treatment.

out according to instructions. The ages ranged from 5 to 15 years in both groups, but the children in the control group were on average 1 year older than those in the experimental group. The drop-out rate was 53%, with 30% discontinuing the treatment either from a lack of desire or discomfort. At the end of 1 year, ninety-seven children remained in the study, fifty-three after 2 years, and only sixteen at the end of 3 years. The difference in the progression rate for experimental and control groups was found to be significant only after the first year. Gimbel concluded that there was at least a short-term effect (1 year), but that a long-term effect had not been demonstrated.

Kelly et al. (1975) reported their experience with various treatment regimens, including atropine and phenylephrine (Tables 21.3 and 21.4), varying these regimens according to whether they achieved success with the individual child. A control group was included, and the refraction was determined according to a definite plan. Initially, an attempt was made with 1% atropine, three drops each day for 7 days, followed by bifocal glasses and one drop of 5% phenylephrine in the evening. If this treatment was not effective, then it was changed to one or two drops of 1% atropine daily. Those children treated with atropine continuously were under observation for 6 months. During this period, 97% of the children showed no progression, but this could have been a result of the fact that the degree of myopia was determined before treatment without the use of a cycloplegic but afterward with atropine cycloplegia.

The control group in the Kelly et al. (1975) study was well defined, with an initial age of 10 or 13 years, and they were examined after 1, 2, and 4 years. The initial age of the treatment group was described as equal to or less than 11 years or greater than 11 years, and it is difficult to determine whether these two groups were comparable with regard to age. Similarly, it is difficult to conclude whether daily use of atropine had an effect, as this treatment was given to a group of children who had previously been subjected to another form of treatment (phenylephrine). Kelly et al. concluded that the progression of myopia can be arrested in 50% of the subjects and delayed in the remainder, provided the treatment is initiated in time.

A study making use of atropine was reported by Gruber (1978) at the International Ophthalmological Congress in Kyoto. Atropine 1% was used daily, with an experimental group of 100 subjects and a control group of the same size. The study was based on patients in a general ophthalmology practice, who were followed for as long as 21 years, although the children in the treatment group were followed for a shorter time (varying from a few days up to 7.5 years). After the treatment had been discontinued, the children were kept under observation for as long as 7 years. Gruber found a difference between the two groups, inasmuch as the control group showed progression at a mean rate of 0.28 D per year as compared to 0.11 D per year for the experimental group. However, after cessation of treatment, the experimental group progressed at a mean rate of 0.46 D per year. It was concluded that if atropine is to delay the progression of myopia, it must be started early and continued for a period of 5 to 10 years. It is not clear from the report on what basis the children were selected for the experimental group or the control group.

Sampson (1979) used one drop of 1% atropine daily in combination with bifocal glasses for reading, using 112 subjects, but with no control group. For periods of observation no longer than 12 months, he found changes in myopia with the use of atropine of −0.25 to +0.50 D for 79% of subjects, +0.75 and +1.00 D for 15% of subjects, and more than +1.00 D for 6%. After treatment had been discontinued, the children were observed for a period of 6 to 12 months, during which period a rapid rate of progression was immediately observed (more than 1.00 D in 17%). Sampson concluded that even though atropine can delay progression, it does not stop the tendency for progression, and that progression continues when the treatment is discontinued. Sampson commented on the risks entailed in prolonged treatment with atropine. As with other studies, one must object to the short duration of the study and to the fact that there was no control group.

A cross-over study was reported by Bedrossian (1979), in which one eye was treated for a period of 12 months followed by treatment of the other eye for 12 months. With this experimental design, each eye was alternately the experimental eye and the control eye. He found that myopia increased in the control eye at a rate of 0.81 to 0.99 D per year, whereas myopia decreased in the treated eye at a rate of 0.17 to 0.29 D per year. However, it can be seen from a previous study carried out by Bedrossian (1964) that atropine drops cause the degree of myopia to be reduced rapidly when the treatment is first begun, but it increases again when the treatment is stopped. Consequently, the effect is not as pronounced as it would appear to be (Figure 21.1).

Figure 21.1.
Differences in degree of myopia when changing atropine from test eyes to control eyes. (From Bedrossian 1979. Reprinted by permission.)

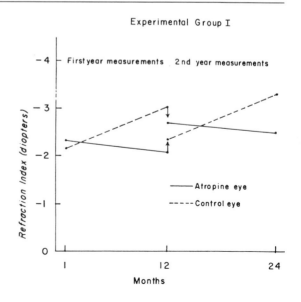

Dyer (1979) reported a study in which one drop of 1% atropine was used daily for 2 to 8 years, with an observation time of at least 1 year after the treatment had been discontinued. His experimental group contained 265 subjects, with a control group of 115 subjects; and the next year (1980) he published the results for an additional fifty-eight subjects. After an observation period of 24 to 96 months for the experimental group and 67 months for the control group, Dyer found the following changes in the degree of myopia:

Less than 1.00 D: 15% (treatment group); 1% (control group)

1 to 1.75 D: 48% (treatment group); 9% (control group)

2 to 2.75 D: 13% (treatment group); 24% (control group)

More than 3.00 D: 24% (treatment group); 66% (control group)

It is difficult to compare the two groups directly because the children in the treatment group were on average 1 year older than those in the control group, and the period for which the progression was measured varied from one subject to another. Nor is it possible to understand how the degree of myopia in the control group was distributed at the start of the investigation. The author concluded that atropine is effective, but there was a very high drop-out rate which may have had an effect on the conclusions.

In a study by Brodstein et al. (1984), in which both atropine and bifocals were used, the monthly progression rate was found to be 0.010 D during atropine treatment compared to 0.028 D for the control group. This difference was found to be statistically significant. Brodstein et al. (1984) concluded that the younger and the more myopic the patient, the more likely that atropine delays the progression of myopia; however, the rate of progression increased again when treatment was discontinued. Conclusions are uncertain: The degree of myopia and the placement of subjects in the two groups were not randomized; the control group included a number of children who were not willing to undergo the atropine treatment; and there was a very high drop-out rate.

Finally, Brenner (1985) initially carried out an investigation using one drop of 1% atropine daily, later changing to two to three times per week. He surveyed the problem of compliance, and concluded that the study could provide only indefinite trends. The initial mean refraction was -0.87 D, and after a period of 9 years had risen to -2.73 D. There was no control group for comparison; therefore, the figures provide little information.

In the atropine studies, there was a high drop-out rate, often an age difference in the treated subjects and the control group, and in several cases the control groups included children who could not be included in the treatment group. All of these factors make it difficult to draw definite conclusions. On the other hand, there remains the possibility that an effect can be obtained from the use of atropine in some children. It is interesting to note that Sampson (1979) concluded that the most satisfied children were those who had discontinued the atropine medication; that is, the discomfort caused by the cycloplegic was considerably important to the child. It can also be stated that because the amount of solar radiation falling on the retina is proportional to the area of the pupil, the retinas of the children treated with atropine will receive about twenty-five times the normal amount of solar energy. Experimental studies have shown that this amount is noxious to the animal retina; children under atropine treatment, therefore, have been advised to wear sunglasses.

___■___

ADRENERGIC AGENTS

As already noted, Kelly (1975) started with 7 days of atropine treatment, measured the refraction, and then gave bifocal correction combined with 5% phenylephrine. After 1 year, he found no progression in 60% of the treated subjects as compared to only 15% of the subjects in the control group. However, it is difficult to compare the age distributions of the two groups, and there was a high drop-out rate.

According to Curtin (1985), studies conducted in Japan by Toki (1960) and Ooka (1964) have demonstrated that 5% phenylephrine at night is effective in preventing a low degree of myopia, especially the so-called *pseudomyopia*. This expression is particularly common in the Japanese literature, but it is unknown to us whether pseudomyopia is quite different from early myopia or is the early stage of genuine myopia. Epinephrine was used by Wiener (1931) and later by Macdiarmid (1964) with some success, mainly in children under 7 years of age.

Table 21.4. Studies Using Phenylephrine 5% for the Control of Myopia

Author (year)	No. subjects	Age (yrs)	Follow-up (months)	Drop outs (T)	Results
Kelly	89 T*	T < 11	T ?–24	50%	†
(1975)	86 C‡	C > 11	C 12–48	(both age groups)	
	71 T	T < 11	T ?–24		
	78 C	C > 12	C 12–48		

*T, treatment group.
†No progression for 60% of T group compared to 15% of C group.
‡C, Control group.

ANTIGLAUCOMA AGENTS

The use of pilocarpine is described mainly in Japanese literature. The rationale behind this treatment is possibly based on a reduction of intraocular pressure or an increase in the subnormal accommodation (Obata 1985). To date, the more potent antiglaucoma drugs have been used only in adults with progressive high myopia.

Hosaka (1982) has treated children having pseudomyopia with the β-blockers, labetalol, and timolol, expecting that the β-adrenergic blocking action of these drugs might lead to relaxation of the ciliary muscle (Table 21.5). He found that labetalol produced an improvement greater than 0.38 D in 75.8% of the eyes, with no change or a worsening in 24.2%. Either timolol or the use of a placebo produced an improvement in 28% of subjects. This was a short-term study, and Hosaka did not take into account the long-term effect of the drug's hypotensive action on the intraocular pressure.

TIMOLOL STUDY

We have performed a pilot study with children, using the pressure-reducing effect of 0.25% timolol, based on the assumption that raised pressure in the posterior chamber can cause increased axial length. Our main objectives were to determine whether children could tolerate timolol, whether there were serious side effects

Table 21.5. Studies Using Antiglaucoma Agents for the Control of Myopia

Drug	No. of subjects	Age (yrs)	Follow-up (months)	Results
Labetalol ½ or ¼%	50 T* 16 eyes C†	6–14 T	T 2–4	>0.38 D less myopia in 76% of T group
Timolol ¼%	20 T 16 eyes C	7–14 T	T 2	Less myopia for 28%‡

(From Hosaka 1982.)
*T, Treatment group.
†C, Control group.
‡Less myopia was also found for 28% when a placebo was used.

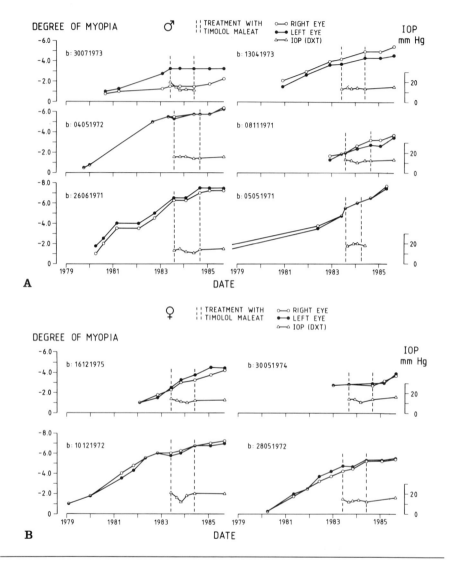

Figure 21.2. **A and B, Myopia progression and intraocular pressure during study on treatment of myopia with timolol maleate eye drops, 0.25%.**

from the treatment, and whether the intraocular pressure would be reduced. Subjects in this pilot study were ten children (four girls and six boys) between the ages of 7 and 12 years. The inclusion criteria, in addition to the age limits, were (1) strongly progressive myopia (minimum of 1.00 D per year) during the period before entering the trial, and (2) a strong disposition to myopia, such that the family was highly motivated to participate in the study.

Each child was examined by a pediatric specialist, and a complete ophthalmologic examination was performed. Oral and written information was given to the parents detailing the project and the possible side effects from treatment with timolol eye drops. The children were treated with 0.25% timolol twice daily, and all were examined every third month by both an ophthalmologist and a pediatrician. The treatment was completed after 12 months, and an eye examination was performed similar to that performed before treatment. Data on myopia progression and intraocular pressure are shown in Figure 21.2, including data taken before treatment and 12 months after completion of the treatment.

The study has shown that children tolerate quite well treatment with β-blocking drugs, administered as eye drops, and that the local side effects were negligible. None of the children complained of weakness during physical exercise. Any periods of tiredness were recorded, but all were attributed by family to influenza or other illness. One child developed asthma, and should not have been included originally in the study, but the parents had unfortunately forgotten about an attack of asthma that had occurred during infancy.

Figure 21.2 depicts the progression for all ten children before, during, and 1 year after treatment. The progression curves illustrate just how difficult it is to determine whether treatment has been successful. It appears that progression diminished during treatment for a few of the subjects and tended to remain so after the treatment had been stopped. Treatment had very little effect on the intraocular pressure, although there is probably a tendency for those children responding to the eye drops, with a lower tension, to show some inhibition in the development of myopia. We concluded that further studies are necessary, including a larger sample, longer observation time, and a control group. Such a study has just been completed, comprising fifty-one children in the treatment group and fifty-one children in the control group, but the preliminary results do not suggest that timolol maleate is able to reduce the rate of progression.

■
CONCLUSIONS

Before accepting the results on any investigation or before planning an investigation of the use of a particular drug in influencing the development of myopia, the following points should be taken into consideration: (1) Are the children selected representative? (2) Is there a control group comparable with the treatment group, and are the ages and degrees of myopia of the two groups well defined? (3) Are their environments (including diet and close work) similar? (4) Is the observation period sufficient? (5) Are the methods of measurement well defined and unambiguous, or is investigational bias possible? (6) Is there sufficient cooperation of both the family and the child to insure a high level of compliance and a low drop-out rate? All of these are essential aspects, and must be considered before documentation of efficacy of a drug can be reported.

Although there does not appear to be any simple method by which we can delay or reduce the rate of progression of myopia, this does not imply that we should give up on research in this field. In our opinion, it is of very limited value to reduce the final amount of myopia from 4.00 D to 3.00 D, especially if the reading capability or binocularity of the child is negatively influenced by the drug. However, it is important to attempt to avoid the development of pathologic myopia with its well-known complications.

■

REFERENCES

Abraham SV. Control of myopia with tropicamide. A progress report. J Pediatr Ophthalmol 1966;3:10–22.

Bedrossian RH. The effect of atropine on myopia. Lecture. First International Conference on Myopia. New York, Sept 10–13, 1964.

Bedrossian RH. The effect of atropine on myopia. Ophthalmology 1979;86:713–717.

Brenner RL. Further observations on use of atropine in the treatment of myopia. Ann Ophthalmol 1985;17:137–140.

Brodstein RS, Brodstein DE, Olson RJ, et al. The treatment of myopia with atropine and bifocals. Ophthalmology 1984;91:1373–1379.

Curtin BJ. Myopia: a review of its etiology, pathogenesis and treatment. Surv Ophthalmol 1970;15:1–17.

Curtin BJ. The management of myopia. Trans Pa Acad Ophthalmol Otolaryngol 1972; 25:117–123.

Curtin BJ. The Myopias. Basic Science and Clinical Management. Philadelphia: Harper & Row, 1985.

Donders FC. On the Anomalies of Accommodation and Refraction of the Eye. London: The New Sydenham Society, 1864.

Dyer JA. Role of cycloplegics in progressive myopia. Ophthalmology 1979;86:692–694.

Dyer JA. Medical treatment of myopia: an update. Contact Intraocular Lens Med J 1980; 6:405–406.

Gimbel HV. The control of myopia with atropine. Can J Ophthalmol 1973;8:527–532.

Goss DA. Attempts to reduce the rate of increase of myopia in young people — a critical literature review. Am J Optom Physiol Opt 1982;59:828–841.

Gruber E. The treatment of myopia with atropine: a clinical study. In: Shimizu ET, Oosterhuis JA, eds. Ophthalmology. Proc International Congress, Kyoto 1978. Amsterdam: Excerpta Medica, 1979; 1212–1216.

Hosaka A. Topical use of labetalol in the treatment of pseudomyopia. Lecture. II International Conference on Myopia, San Francisco, October 28–30, 1982.

Inkles DM. Myopia prophylaxis — a review. Ophthalmic Semin 1976;1:197–226.

Kelly TS-B, Chatfield C, Tustin T. Clinical assessment of the arrest of myopia. Br J Ophthalmol 1975;59:529–538.

Macdiarmid DC, Hamilton N. The treatment of myopia. N Z Med J 1964;16:66.

McKanna JA, Casagrande VA. Atropine affects lid-suture myopic development. Experimental studies of chronic atropinization in tree shrews. Doc Ophthalmol 1981;28: 187–192.

Obata S. Pilocarpine cure of myopia and pseudomyopia. Acta Soc Ophthalmol Jpn 1944; 48:241. (Cited from Curtin BJ. The Myopias. Philadelphia: Harper & Row, 1985.)

Ooka R, Kawai T, Morikawa K. Effect of a mydriatic (neosynesine) in cases of suspected pseudomyopia. J Clin Ophthalmol Jpn 1964;18:1259. (Cited from Curtin BJ. The Myopias. Philadelphia: Harper & Row, 1985.)

Raviola E, Wiesel TN. An animal model of myopia. N Engl J Med 1985;312:1609–1615.

Rosenthal JW. Medical treatment of myopia. Contacto 1970;14:28–30.

Sampson WG. Role of cycloplegia in the management of functional myopia. Ophthalmology 1979;86:695–697.

Toki T. Treatment of myopia with local use of neosynephrine hydrocloride. Jpn J Clin Ophthalmol 1960;14:248. (Cited from Curtin BJ. The Myopias. Philadelphia: Harper & Row, 1985.)

Wiener M. The use of epinephrine in progressive myopia. Am J Ophthalmol 1931;14: 520–522.

Young FA. The effect of atropine on the development of myopia in monkeys. Am J Optom Arch Am Acad Optom 1965;42:439–449.

22

Management of Myopia: Classification of Surgical Methods

George O. Waring III

☐

■

TERMINOLOGY

Most specialized fields develop their own technical terminology or jargon. Corneal surgery is no exception. The penchant for professional shorthand has produced jargon such as *keratorefractive surgery,* a Greek-Latin hybrid that flows easily from the tongue and pen of those enamored by neologisms. Some surgeons have become keratotomists, and their patients are keratotomized. Words have been invented, such as *lenticle,* instead of the correct term, *lenticule* — the piece of tissue or synthetic material used to change corneal shape. Commercial trademark terms have appeared; the donor lenticule used in epikeratoplasty has been dubbed Kerato-Lens.™ Eponyms abound. Common use of some colloquial terms has fixed them in our vocabulary. For example, some say "myopic keratomileusis" (Is the keratomileusis myopic?) instead of the more precise designation, keratomileusis for myopia. Thus far we have been spared "myopic radial keratotomy."

To clarify the language we use in this rapidly changing surgical area, I propose a classification of refractive corneal surgery, which I hope is broad enough to include all corneal procedures that have a major refractive component, systematic enough to organize our present knowledge, flexible enough to accommodate new developments, and precise enough to decrease the proliferation of jingly "keratospeak."

The study reported here was supported by National Eye Institute Grant EY03751 and supported in part by an unrestricted grant to the Department of Ophthalmology from Research to Prevent Blindness, Inc., New York.

TYPES OF REFRACTIVE SURGERY

Refractive surgery is any operation intended to alter the refractive state of the eye (Barraquer 1967). Thus, radial keratotomy, cataract extraction with implantation of an intraocular lens, and scleral reinforcement to treat degenerative myopia are all forms of refractive surgery. Refractive corneal surgery refers to operations on the cornea, which are intended to alter the refractive state of the eye. This type of surgery is popularly referred to as *refractive keratoplasty*, an appropriate term, since keratoplasty means "to mold the cornea."

CLASSIFICATION OF REFRACTIVE CORNEAL SURGERY

I propose a classification based on surgical technique. It describes basic techniques that can be applied to many refractive errors, such as keratomileusis for both myopia and hyperopia. It accommodates new techniques that are modifications of previously used ones, such as epikeratoplasty as a modification of keratomileusis. It requires only one description of a technical procedure that is used in different refractive operations, such as the use of a microkeratome in keratomileusis, keratophakia, and keratokyphosis.

This classification specifies first the surgical technique, then the refractive disorder being treated; for example, keratomileusis for myopia. Of course, precision demands appropriate modifiers — such as alloplastic keratophakia for aphakia, using a hydrogel lenticule — which unfortunately makes the terminology more cumbersome.

Some of the techniques can be applied to scleral surgery intended to modify refraction, such as a limbal sclerectomy to steepen the flat axis of the cornea, but I have limited the classification to corneal surgery.

□ Lamellar Refractive Keratoplasty

Lamellar refractive keratoplasty involves the placement of a lenticule on or within the cornea to alter its refractive power, usually by changing its anterior curvature. There are four lamellar refractive keratoplasty techniques: (1) keratomileusis (Barraquer 1981) ("carving the cornea") in which a disk of the patient's anterior cornea is removed with a microkeratome, ground into a new shape on a cryolathe, and sutured back into place (Figure 22.1); (2) epikeratoplasty (Friedlander et al. 1983) ("graft on top of the cornea") in which a human donor lenticule — either lyophilized or fresh — is ground into a new shape on a cryolathe and is sutured to a groove in the deepithelialized surface of the cornea (Figure 22.2); (3) keratophakia ("lens in the cornea") in which a human donor (Taylor et al. 1981) or synthetic

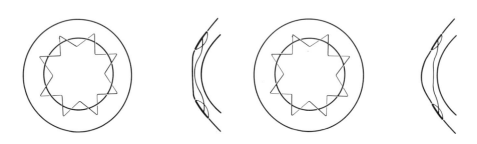

Figure 22.1. Keratomileusis. For myopia (left), keratomileusis involves the excision of a lamellar disk of the patient's cornea with a microkeratome, carving the disk on a cryolathe to form a concave lenticule, and suturing the disk back on to the cornea. This flattens the cornea and decreases the refractive power. For aphakia (right), keratomileusis also involves excision of a lamellar disk of the cornea with a microkeratome, but the disk is carved on a cryolathe to form a convex lenticule, which is resutured onto the cornea, steepening the cornea and increasing the refractive power. Waring GO, Making sense of "keratospeak." A classification of refractive corneal surgery. Arch Ophthalmol 1985;103:1472–1477.

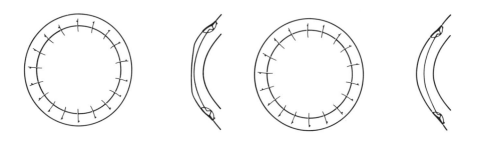

Figure 22.2. Epikeratoplasty. For myopia (left) epikeratoplasty involves removal of a lamellar disk from a donor cornea, carving it on a cryolathe to form a concave lenticule, placing it on the surface of the deepithelialized recipient cornea, and suturing it onto a peripheral circumferential groove, which flattens the central corneal curvature and decreases the refractive power. For aphakia (right) epikeratoplasty involves a similar process using a convex donor lenticule that steepens the corneal curvature, increasing the refractive power. Waring GO, Making sense of "keratospeak." A classification of refractive corneal surgery. Arch Ophthalmol 1985;103:1472–1477.

plastic lenticule (Beekhuis et al. 1986) is placed within the corneal stroma (Figure 22.3); and (4) lamellar keratoplasty (Richard 1978) and epikeratoplasty in which a lenticule that has no refractive power is used to diminish the myopia and irregular astigmatism of keratoconus or of some peripheral corneal thinning disorders (Figure 22.4) (Schanzlin et al. 1983). New techniques will have new appellations, such as those that use a mold to shape the corneal bed or the lenticule as they are cut with a microkeratome, including keratokyphosis (Hoffmann et al. 1982) ("a protrusion of the cornea").

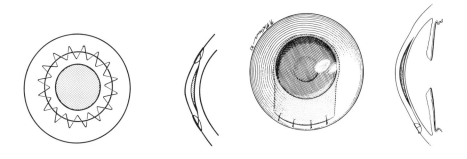

Figure 22.3. Keratophakia. Keratophakia involves placement of a lenticule within the corneal stroma to change the refraction of the cornea. If the lenticule is designed to change the curvature of the anterior surface of the cornea, excision of a lamellar disk of the cornea with a microkeratome is necessary (left). Then the lenticule of human donor cornea or hydrogel material is placed in the lamellar bed and the disk of recipient cornea resutured into its original position. If the donor lenticule has a different index of refraction, thereby changing the refraction of the cornea, it can be placed in a deep lamellar pocket (right). Waring GO, Making sense of "keratospeak." A classification of refractive corneal surgery. Arch Ophthalmol 1985;103:1472–1477.

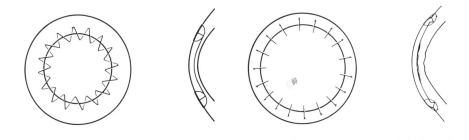

Figure 22.4. Lamellar keratoplasty. A lamellar keratoplasty (left) and epikeratoplasty (right) can use donor lenticules without power to diminish the myopia and irregular astigmatism in keratoconus.

□ Keratotomy

Keratotomy ("cutting the cornea") involves making a partial-thickness incision into the cornea to flatten it and reduce its refractive power in that meridian (Figures 22.5 through 22.7). A description of the pattern of the incisions usually modifies the term (Franks and Binder 1985), such as radial (Waring et al. 1983, Waring 1985), trapezoidal incisions (Lavery and Lindstrom 1985) (four transverse incisions between two semiradial ones), T incisions (transverse incisions adjacent to a radial incision), L incisions (three to five longitudinal incisions parallel to one radial incision), or crescentic keratotomy (relaxing incision) (Troutman 1973, Sugar and Kirk 1983). Removing a tight suture from a corneal or limbal incision acts like a keratotomy because it usually flattens the cornea in that meridian (Kozarsky and Waring 1985). As technologies advance, other descriptive terms will likely be

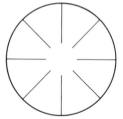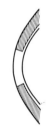

Figure 22.5. Radial keratotomy for myopia. Equally spaced radial incisions made deeply into the corneal stroma flatten the central cornea and decrease its refractive power, reducing the refractive error in myopia. Waring GO, Making sense of "keratospeak." A classification of refractive corneal surgery. Arch Ophthalmol 1985;103:1472–1477.

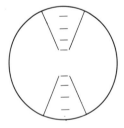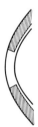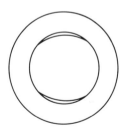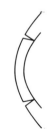

Figure 22.6. Keratotomy for astigmatism. Trapezoidal keratotomy (left) consists of two semiradial incisions and four nonconnecting transverse incisions that flatten the corneal curvature and decrease its refractive power in the axis of surgery. A crescentic keratotomy (relaxing incision, right) consists of deep incisions into the healed scar in the steepest axis that flatten that axis and reduce the astigmatism that can occur after penetrating keratoplasty.

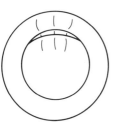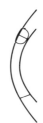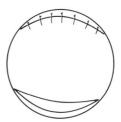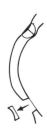

Figure 22.7. Keratotomy for astigmatism. A crescentic wedge resection (left) can reduce astigmatism after a penetrating keratoplasty by removing a piece of tissue from the corneal scar in the flat axis and resuturing the wound together, which steepens the axis and increases the refracting power of the cornea. A crescentic lamellar keratoctomy (right) can help manage thinning disorders of the peripheral cornea by strengthening the thin areas and by steepening the flat axis of the central cornea. Waring GO, Making sense of "keratospeak." A classification of refractive corneal surgery. Arch Ophthalmol 1985;103:1472–1477.

added, such as radial keratotomy with an excimer laser (Gotliar et al. 1985) or radial keratotomy using the "XYZ" formula (Sanders 1985).

□ Keratectomy

A keratectomy ("excision of a piece of cornea") to change the refraction of the cornea involves the removal of a crescentic piece of stroma and suturing the wound, which steepens the cornea and increases its power in that axis. Keratectomy procedures are usually described by the pattern of the tissue excised, such as a wedge resection for astigmatism after a penetrating keratoplasty (Krachmer and Fenzl 1980) or a crescentic lamellar resection for Terrien's marginal degeneration (Caldwell et al. 1984). Revising and resuturing a slipped or separated corneal or limbal wound acts like a keratectomy if it steepens the cornea in the meridian of surgery (Cravy 1983, van Rij and Waring 1984).

□ Penetrating Keratoplasty

The major reason for performing penetrating keratoplasty is to replace the central portion of a scarred or distorted cornea by clear regular donor tissue. Between 1940 and 1980, the major clinical challenge was to maintain a clear graft. However, now that grafts remain clear in approximately 85% of cases (Bourne 1981, Volker-Dieben et al. 1982), control of the refractive effect of the donor has become increasingly important (Figure 22.8), especially when an intraocular lens is used, as in a combined penetrating keratoplasty, cataract extraction, and intraocular lens insertion (triple procedure). The surgeon not only must control factors that affect

Figure 22.8. Penetrating keratoplasty (refractive aspects). The residual astigmatism in a penetrating keratoplasty can be diminished by careful attention to wound configuration, suture pattern, and trephine size. In eyes that contain an intraocular lens, the spherical power of the corneal graft should correlate appropriately with that of the intraocular lens and of the axial length of the globe to achieve the desired final refraction. Waring GO, Making sense of "keratospeak." A classification of refractive corneal surgery. Arch Ophthalmol 1985;103:1472–1477.

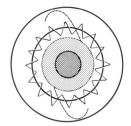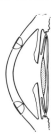

Figure 22.9. Thermokeratoplasty. Controlled application of heat can shrink and scar the underlying stromal collagen, which flattens the cornea in the area of heating and helps treat disorders such as keratoconus. Waring GO, Making sense of "keratospeak." A classification of refractive corneal surgery. Arch Ophthalmol 1985;103:1472–1477.

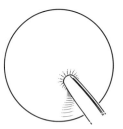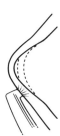

the spherical and cylindrical power of the graft (for example, wound configuration, suture pattern, donor size), but also must select an intraocular lens power that appropriately matches the final refractive power of the graft and the axial length of the globe (Crawford et al. 1984).

☐ Thermokeratoplasty

The application of heat from various sources (thermal probe, laser, radiofrequency current) shrinks the corneal stromal collagen and flattens the cornea in the area of heat application (Aquavella et al. 1976). It has been used to treat keratoconus (Figure 22.9).

□ Other Classification Systems

There are other approaches to the classification of refractive corneal surgery. One is to use the ametropia being treated (Binder 1985) — myopia, hyperopia, aphakia, or astigmatism — as the basis; but this requires repeated description of similar surgical techniques for each refractive error, such as keratomileusis for myopia and for aphakia. A more abstract classification is based on the type of alteration of the cornea (Barraquer 1967): resection of tissue (for example, keratomileusis, wedge resection), relaxation of the tissue (for example, radial keratotomy, suture removal), addition of tissue (for example, keratophakia, epikeratoplasty), substitution of tissue (for example, penetrating keratoplasty, keratomileusis using a donor cornea), retraction of tissue (for example, thermokeratoplasty), and compression of tissue (for example, tight sutures, epikeratoplasty for keratoconus). One may also classify refractive corneal surgery in bioengineering terms: changes in corneal volume, thickness, surface area (Troutman et al. 1980), and, in the future, even stress-strain forces. Meanwhile, a classification based on surgical technique (Table 22.1) will enhance communication and understanding among those interested in refractive surgery.

TERMINOLOGY USED IN TRANSPLANTATION

The fields of genetics, tissue transplantation, and refractive corneal surgery share a common language that seems to remain in flux, creating confusion about words that contain the Greek prefixes *auto-*, *iso-*, *syn-*, *allo-*, *homo-*, *xeno*, and *hetero-*. Consensus among the three fields is emerging (Stites et al. 1984, Bellanti 1978) for the usage outlined in Table 22.2.

An autograft involves tissue from the host, as in keratomileusis. An allograft involves tissue from a donor of the same species who has a different genetic makeup, as in a penetrating keratoplasty, epikeratoplasty, and both keratophakia and keratomileusis using a human donor cornea. The term *alloplastic* refers to use of synthetic donor material as in keratophakia using a hydrogel lenticule. Unfortunately, there is confusion here, as an allograft with donor tissue is sometimes colloquially referred to as an "alloplasty." In a xenograft, the donor tissue comes from a different species than the host. No xenografts give good clinical results in human corneal surgery.

Table 22.1. Classification of Refractive Corneal Surgery

Type of refractive corneal surgery	Surgical technique	Other terms	Refractive error treated
Lamellar	Keratomileusis Use of mold with microkeratome	Barraquer technique	Myopia, hyperopia, aphakia (astigmatism)*
	Epikeratoplasty	Keratokyphosis Epikeratophakia, Onlay lamellar graft	(Myopia, hyperopia, aphakia astigmatism) Aphakia, myopia, keratoconus, (astigmatism)
	Keratophakia Human donor Synthetic lenticule	Barraquer technique Intracorneal lens, Alloplastic keratophakia	Aphakia, hyperopia
	Hydrogel High index of refraction	e.g. Polysulfone	Aphakia (Myopia) Aphakia Myopia
	Lamellar keratoplasty Central Crescentic		Keratoconus Terrien's or pellucid marginal degeneration

Keratotomy	Radial		Myopia, astigmatism
	Combined radial and transverse	Trapezoidal-Ruiz, L, T, half-T, etc.	Astigmatism
	Crescentic	Relaxing incision	Astigmatism after penetrating keratoplasty
	Suture removal	Acts like keratotomy	Astigmatism
Keratectomy	Crescentic wedge	Wedge resection	Astigmatism after penetrating keratoplasty
	Crescentic lamellar		Terrien's or pellucid marginal degeneration
	Repair wound slip or dehiscence		Astigmatism after cataract or corneal surgery
Penetrating keratoplasty (refractive aspects)	Donor cornea alone	Corneal transplant, Corneal graft, Allograft	Corneal opacity or distortion (goal: minimal residual ametropia)
	With intraocular lens	Triple procedure, IOL insertion or exchange	Cataract, aphakia
	Infant donor, oversized donor button		Aphakia
Thermokeratoplasty			Keratoconus

*Items in parentheses indicate techniques or indications not yet used in humans.

Table 22.2. Types of Grafts Used in Refractive Corneal Surgery

Type of graft	Synonym	Source of tissue	Genetic identity of donor	Examples from human corneal surgery
Autograft (G. Autos, self)*	Autoplastic procedure	Host	Identical (Autogeneic)	Keratomileusis Penetrating keratoplasty donor from opposite eye
Isograft (G. Isos, equal)	None	Monozygotic twin	Near identical (Isogeneic, syngeneic)	Penetrating keratoplasty donor from identical twin
Allograft (G. Allos, another — in the sense of another person)	Homograft (G. Homos, same — in the sense of same species) Homoplastic procedure	Another member of same species	Dissimilar (Allogeneic, homogeneic)	Keratomileusis or keratophakia with human donor Epikeratoplasty Penetrating keratoplasty Lamellar keratoplasty
Alloplastic (G. Allos, another — in the sense of another material)	Synthetic or inert implant, intracorneal lens	Nonbiologic material	None	Keratophakia with plastic implant
Xenograft (G. Xenos, foreign)	Heterograft (G. Heteros, different)	Member of different species	Very dissimilar (Xenogeneic, heterogeneic)	None

*G, Word of Greek origin.

REFERENCES

Aquavella JV, Smith RS, Shaw EL. Alterations in corneal morphology following thermo-keratoplasty. Arch Ophthalmol 1976;94:2082–2085.

Barraquer JI. Basis of refractive keratoplasty. Arch Soc Am Oftal Optom 1967;6:21–68.

Barraquer JI. Keratomileusis for myopia and aphakia. Ophthalmology 1981;88:701–722.

Beekhuis WH, McCarey BE, Waring GO, et al. Hydrogel keratophakia: a microkeratome dissection in the monkey model. Br J Ophthalmol 1986;70:192–198.

Bellanti JA. Immunology II. Philadelphia: WB Saunders Company, 1978; 82.

Binder PS. The current and future status of refractive surgery. CLAO J 1985;11:358–375.

Bourne WM. Current techniques for improved visual results after penetrating keratoplasty. Ophthalmic Surg 1981;12:321–327.

Bourne WM, Davison JA, O'Fallon WM. The effects of oversize donor buttons on post-operative intraocular pressure and corneal curvature in aphakic penetrating keratoplasty. Ophthalmology 1982;89:242–246.

Caldwell DR, Insler MS, Boutros G, Hawk T. Primary surgical repair of severe peripheral marginal ectasia in Terrien's marginal degeneration. Am J Ophthalmol 1984;97:332–336.

Cravy TV. Modification of postcataract astigmatism by wound revision. In: Binder PS, ed. Refractive Corneal Surgery: The Correction of Astigmatism, vol. 23. Boston: Little, Brown & Co, 1983;111–126.

Crawford GJ, Van Meter WS, Waring GO, Stulting RD, Wilson LA. Prediction of intra-ocular lens power in the triple procedure. Ophthalmology (Suppl) 1984;91:88.

Franks JB, Binder PS. Keratotomy procedures for the correction of astigmatism. J Refractive Surg 1985;1:11–17.

Friedlander MH, Safir A, McDonald MB, Kaufman HE, Granet N. Update on epikerato-phakia. Ophthalmology 1983;90:365–368.

Gotliar AM, Schubert HD, Mandel ER, et al. Excimer laser radial keratotomy. Ophthalmology 1985;92:206–208.

Hoffmann F, Jessen K, Pahlitzsch TH, Buchen R. Hypermetropic and myopic keratoky-phosis — a new method of refractive keratoplasty. I. Effect of a synthetic lens on intra-ocular pressure. Cornea 1982;1:137–141.

Kozarsky AM, Waring GO. Photokeratoscopy in the management of astigmatism following keratoplasty. Dev Ophthalmol 1985;11:91–98.

Krachmer JH, Fenzl RE. Surgical correction of high postkeratoplasty astigmatism: relaxing incisions versus wedge resection. Arch Ophthalmol 1980;98:1400–1402.

Lavery GW, Lindstrom RL. Clinical results of trapezoidal astigmatic keratotomy. J Refractive Surg 1985;1:70–74.

Pfister RR, Breaud S. Aphakic refractive penetrating keratoplasty using newborn donor corneas. Ophthalmology 1983;90:1207–1212.

Richard JM, Paton D, Gasset AR. A comparison of penetrating keratoplasty and lamellar keratoplasty in the surgical management of keratoconus. Am J Ophthalmol 1978;86:807–811.

Sanders DR. Computerized radial keratotomy predictability programs. J Refractive Surg 1985;1:109–117.

Schanzlin DJ, Sarno EM, Robin JB. Crescentic lamellar keratoplasty for pellucid marginal degeneration. Am J Ophthalmol 1983;96:253–254.

Stites DP, Stobo JD, Fudenberg HH, Wells JV. Basic and Clinical Immunology, 5th ed. Los Altos, CA: Lange Medical Publications, 1984;763–773.

Sugar J, Kirk AK. Relaxing keratotomy for postkeratoplasty high astigmatism. Ophthalmic Surg 1983;14:156–160.

Taylor DM, Stern AL, Romanchok KG, Keilson LR. Keratophakia. Clinical evaluation. Ophthalmology 1981;88:1141–1150.

Troutman RC. Microsurgical control of corneal astigmatism in cataract and keratoplasty. Trans Am Acad Ophthalmol Otolaryngol 1973;77:563–567.

Troutman RC, Gaster RN, Swinger C. Refractive keratoplasty. In Symposium on Medical and Surgical Disease of the Cornea: Transactions of the New Orleans Academy of Ophthalmology. St. Louis: CV Mosby, 1980;428–449.

Van Rij G, Waring GO. Changes in corneal curvature induced by sutures and incisions. Am J Ophthalmol 1984;98:773–783.

Volker-Dieben HJ, Kok-van Alphen CC, Lansbergen Q, Persijn G. Different influences on corneal graft survival in 539 transplants. Acta Ophthalmol 1982;60:190–202.

Waring GO III. Changing status of radial keratotomy for myopia: Part II. J Refractive Surg 1985;1:119–137.

Waring GO III, Moffitt SD, Gelender H, et al. Rationale for and design of the National Eye Institute Prospective Evaluation of Radial Keratotomy (PERK) Study. Ophthalmology 1983;90:40–58.

23

Management of Myopia: Post-RK Vision Care

Theodore Grosvenor

☐

Radial keratotomy (RK) was first described by Sato et al. in 1953, but the procedure was abandoned for almost 30 years before being reintroduced by Fyodorov and Durnev (1979). Although as recently as 1980 the National Eye Advisory Council had grave doubts concerning the procedure (AOA News, July, 1980) radial keratotomy has become increasingly popular during the past decade. The degree to which it has become an accepted procedure is due, in large part, to the Prospective Evaluation of Radial Keratotomy (the PERK study), conducted by Waring and his coworkers (1985).

THE PERK STUDY

The PERK study was designed to investigate the safety, efficacy, predictability, and stability of a single standardized surgical technique of RK (Waring et al. 1985). The study was a nine-center clinical trial involving 435 patients ranging in age from 21 to 35 years, having bilateral physiologic myopia from 3.00 to 8.00 D (equivalent sphere) and refractive astigmatism no greater than 1.50 D. The surgical procedure involved the use of eight radial incisions and provided a clear zone of 4.0 mm for eyes having from 2.00 to 3.12 D of myopia, 3.5 mm for eyes having 3.25 to 4.37 D of myopia, and 3.0 mm for eyes having myopia of 4.50 D or more. RK was performed on only one eye of each subject.

The results of the PERK study reported by Waring et al. (1985, 1986) and by Rowsey et al. (1988) may be summarized in terms of postsurgical spherical refractive error, visual acuity, astigmatism, complications, and changes in corneal topography.

□ Postsurgical Spherical Refractive Error and Acuity

One year after surgery, both residual spherical refractive error and uncorrected visual acuity indicated that the lower the presurgical myopia, the greater the possibility of a successful outcome (Table 23.1). Depending on the presurgical refractive error group, at the end of 1 year, from 22 to 57% of subjects had a spherical equivalent refraction between + 0.50 and − 0.50 D; and from 26% to 71% of subjects had uncorrected visual acuity of 6/6 (20/20). Three years after surgery, the results differed little from the 1-year results (Table 23.2); somewhat fewer subjects in the low refractive error group had spherical equivalent refractions between + 0.50 and − 0.50 D at 3 years than at 1 year, and the percentage of subjects having 6/6 (20/20) uncorrected acuity was somewhat higher at 3 years than at 1 year.

□ Postsurgical Astigmatism

Combining all three presurgical groups, at the end of 1 year uncorrected astigmatism was found to change no more than 0.25 D (as compared to the presurgical amount) for 55% of subjects, but with a range extending from a decrease of 2.25 D to an increase of 2.25 D. Uncorrected astigmatism appeared to change little between the 1-year and 3-year postsurgical examinations; combining all three presurgical groups, during this period astigmatism was found to change no more than 0.25 D for 53% of subjects, with a range extending from a decrease of 1.25 D to an increase of 2.75 D.

□ Complications

In the 1-year report (Waring et al. 1985), both transient and persistent complications were reported. Transient complications included postsurgical pain (sometimes severe) lasting from 12 to 48 hours after surgery; mild to moderate photophobia due to mild stromal inflammation and iridocyclitis, disappearing after 1 to 3 weeks; and diurnal fluctuation of vision, becoming less noticeable between 3 months and 1 year for some patients but still persistent at the end of 1 year for others.

Persistent complications included a decrease in best-corrected acuity, with 13% of eyes losing one to two acuity lines; reports of glare (compared to presurgical baseline data) for 15% of patients; and epithelial erosions, experienced by four subjects (1%) occurring from 1 to 7 months after surgery.

Table 23.1. PERK Study Refractive and Visual Acuity Results at the End of 1 Year*

	Results at the end of 1 year		
Presurgical refraction	Percentage +0.50 to −0.50 D	Percentage +1.00 to −1.00 D	Range	Percentage having visual acuity of 6/6 (20/20) or better
−2.00 to −3.12 D	57%	84%	+3.12 to −3.00 D	71%
−3.25 to −4.37 D	33%	62%	+3.12 to −3.00 D	49%
−4.25 to −8.00 D	22%	38%	+3.12 to −4.25 D	26%

(From Waring et al. 1985.)
*All refractions are expressed as equivalent sphere.

Table 23.2. PERK Study Refractive and Visual Acuity Results at the End of 3 Years*

	Results at the end of 3 years		
Presurgical refraction	Percentage +0.50 to −0.50 D	Percentage +1.00 to −1.00 D	Range	Percentage having visual acuity of 6/6 (20/20) or better
−2.00 to −3.12 D	45%	76%	+4.00 to −3.00 D	74%
−3.25 to −4.37 D	38%	62%	+4.00 to −3.00 D	50%
−4.25 to −8.00 D	20%	39%	+4.00 to −4.62 D	33%

(From Waring et al. 1987.)
*All refractions are expressed as equivalent sphere.

☐ Changes in Corneal Topography

CorneaScope photographs of PERK study subjects' corneas were taken before surgery and at various periods of time after surgery (Rowsey et al. 1988). Comparison of photographs taken 6 months after surgery to the presurgical photographs showed a marked flattening in the central portion of the cornea, with a smaller amount of flattening in the periphery. For the more highly myopic subjects, the optical zone of the cornea flattened by an average of 0.72 mm after surgery. Rowsey et al. calculated a conversion factor of 0.166 mm for each diopter of refractive change obtained by surgery: This would indicate that the average refractive change, due to corneal flattening, was 0.72/0.166, or 4.33 D. It was found that the smaller the RK optical zone, the greater the central corneal flattening. Comparing younger and older subjects, it was found that the corneas of older subjects experienced more central and peripheral flattening for all optical zones.

___■_____

OTHER RADIAL KERATOTOMY STUDIES

One- and 2-year follow-up results for a group of 142 RKs were reported by Arrowsmith and Marks (1987). One year after surgery, 49% of the eyes had uncorrected visual acuity of 6/6 (20/20) or better, but 2 years after surgery the percentage of eyes having acuity of 6/6 (20/20) or better had decreased to 39%. Postoperative complaints 2 years after surgery included reports of glare (9%), fluctuating vision (11%), and ghost images (4%).

Follow-up results at 18 months and 3 years were reported on a group of 198 consecutive RKs (Sawelson and Marks 1987). They found that the mean spherical equivalent refraction was −0.78 D at 18 months, reducing to −0.53 D at 3 years. The frequency of complaints such as glare, foreign body sensation, and monocular diplopia decreased markedly from the 18-month examinations to the 3-year examinations.

___■_____

EVALUATION OF RK RESULTS

A controversy has arisen among RK surgeons as to whether uncorrected visual acuity should be used as a criterion for success. Comparing his own data to that of the PERK study, Neumann (1986) noted that uncorrected vision is often unexpectedly better than residual refractive error would indicate and recommended that uncorrected visual acuity should be used as a criterion for success. Responding to Neumann's remarks, Waring (1986) argued that uncorrected visual acuity could be misleading, as those PERK study subjects who had uncorrected visual acuity of 6/6 (20/20) 1 year after surgery had refractive errors ranging from −1.50 D to +3.00 D. Waring also noted that 25% of the subjects who had 6/6 (20/20) acuity were overcorrected by 0.62 to 3.00 D.

□ Fluctuations of Refractive Error and Vision

Data on diurnal variations in refractive error, keratometric findings, and visual acuity were reported for forty-six PERK study subjects who complained of fluctuating vision 1 year after surgery (Schanzlin et al. 1985). During the 12-hour period from 7:00–8:00 A.M. to 7:00–8:00 P.M., these authors found a mean increase in myopia of 0.42 D, a mean corneal steepening of 0.42 D, and a mean acuity loss of 5.3 letters (about one line of letters).

Two ophthalmologists who had undergone RK described, in separate reports, their own diurnal variations in refractive error. In one of these reports (Wyzinski and O'Dell 1987), the surgery had been bilateral with the intention of producing a monovision effect: Surgery on the right eye was intended to correct that eye for distance vision, whereas surgery on the left eye was intended to produce an undercorrection of about 1.25 D (for use in near vision). In what the authors described as typical measurements, taken on the thirty-ninth postoperative day, spherical equivalent refraction for the right eye was +1.87 D on awakening, decreasing to +0.50 D after 1 hour, to +0.12 D after 4 hours, and to −0.37 D by 15 hours after awakening. An interesting observation made by Wyzinski and O'Dell was that by refracting the subject before and after an afternoon nap, it was found that hyperopia was present on awakening just as it had been when awakening in the morning. They commented that this subject had found, as others had reported, that a short nap before going out in the evening seemed to improve night vision!

In a report of radial keratotomy "as seen through operated eyes," Richmond (1987) noted that his moderate myopia (about 4.00 D, each eye, preoperatively) was well corrected in the left eye but was overcorrected by approximately 3.00 D in the right eye. He estimated diurnal variation in corneal curvature and refractive error to be about 1.25 D, and noted that the fluctuation in refraction varied not only from morning to night but from day to day. He suggested that three factors may be involved in the diurnal variation: (1) lid and orbital pressure due to convergence of the eyes in reading, (2) corneal edema occurring during the night, and (3) rapid changes in introacular pressure.

□ Undercorrection and Overcorrection

Noting that undercorrection and overcorrection are the most frequently encountered optical complications of RK, Binder (1986) reported that undercorrection occurs with a much greater frequency than overcorrection, particularly in eyes with myopia greater than 6.00 D. He does not consider undercorrection a significant handicap to the patient, although 30 to 40% of eyes will require vision correction in the form of contact lenses or glasses.

In the 3-year PERK study results, Waring et al. (1987) reported that 16% had an overcorrection of more than 1.00 D, whereas 26% had an undercorrection of more than 1.00 D. They commented that overcorrection was an undesirable outcome as it hastened the occurrence of symptoms of presbyopia; whereas undercorrected patients were often pleased that they could perform some visual functions (at near) without the need for glasses or contact lenses. Waring et al. commented that, unfortunately, there was no way to identify, preoperatively, those patients who will be undercorrected or overcorrected.

□ Postoperative Anisometropia

The RK literature contains a large number of reports of postoperative anisometropia. For example, one of the surgeons who reported on his own variations in refractive error (Richmond 1987) reported anisometropia amounting to approximately 3.00 D. In the 3-year results of the PERK study, Waring et al. (1987) reported that of the patients who had undergone RK on both eyes, 41% had a residual anisometropia of 1.00 D after 6 months. This may be compared to a prevalence of anisometropia in an unselected population of no more than 10%.

Refractive data on four patients with anisometropia as a result of RK were reported by Duling and Wick (1988). For two patients, having postoperative anisometropia of 2.75 D and 2.12 D, respectively, both eyes had been operated. For the other two patients, only one eye had been operated. One of these patients, after having RK performed on the right eye, declined to have the left eye operated because of glare induced by the RK scars; this patient had a resulting anisometropia of 9.50 D. The other patient had approximately 1.00 D of myopia before surgery; after RK on the right eye resulted in more than 7.00 D of hyperopia, she was so unhappy with the result that she declined to have surgery on the left eye.

□ Prediction of a Successful Outcome

On the basis of the PERK study results, Lynn and Waring (1987) addressed the problem of predictability of outcome of RK. Limiting their attention to subjects whose preoperative spherical equivalent refraction was between -3.25 and

−4.37 D (whose surgery resulted in a clear zone diameter of 3.5 mm), these authors calculated that for a sample size greater than 30, they could predict with 90% success a mean postoperative reduction in myopia of 3.41 D with a standard deviation of 1.91 D. For a 4.00 D myope, they could predict with a 90% certainty that refraction after 1 year would be between −2.50 D and +1.32 D.

□ Postoperative Keratitis

The late development of keratitis in radial keratotomy scars has been documented in two separate reports. Mandelbaum et al. (1986) described three cases of ulcerative keratitis that developed from 7 to 30 months after uncomplicated RK. All ulcers occurred along keratotomy scars. In one case, the ulcer appeared spontaneously; the second patient may have sustained an unrecognized corneal injury; and the third patient was wearing extended-wear soft contact lenses for the correction of residual myopia. With treatment, all three ulcers healed without reducing visual acuity.

Shivitz and Arrowsmith (1986) described three episodes of delayed keratitis in two RK patients. The three episodes occurred 9 months, 35 months, and 45 months after surgery. One of the patients had experienced repeated episodes of pain postoperatively, which were thought to be due to recurrent corneal erosions within the radial incisions. Thirty-five months after surgery, she had a sudden onset of pain, decreased vision, and redness of the eye: Cultures were positive for *Pseudomonas aeruginosa*, and 6/6 (20/20) acuity gradually returned with treatment. The second patient experienced pain, photophobia, and redness 9 months postoperatively, due to an ulceration at the intersection of a radial and a transverse incision. *Staphylococcus* and *Moraxella* species were cultured, and the patient responded to treatment, with 6/6 (20/20) unaided acuity. The authors concluded that the likely cause of the episodes of keratitis was delayed wound healing and epithelial inclusion cysts within the RK incisions.

□ Effects of Postoperative Trauma

Concern has often been expressed about the ability of a post-RK eye to withstand trauma. Forstot and Damiano (1988) reported on a series of eight cases of trauma occurring after RK. The trauma in three cases was to the orbit and globe due to a tennis ball, in one case due to a softball, in one case due to a tire-iron striking the orbital-globe area, in one case due to a war-game pellet, and in two cases due to the patient leaning over and inadvertently striking the globe with a solid object. In two of the cases, a single radial incision was opened by the trauma, and the wounds healed with the use of bandage therapeutic lenses. The authors noted that histopathologic studies show that corneal wound healing may be delayed after RK, possibly not being complete until 66 months after surgery; they warned that those having undergone RK should exercise care to avoid trauma.

Simons et al. (1988) reported that a patient who had undergone RK had subsequently suffered rupture of the globe as a result of blunt trauma. On the twenty-fourth day after uneventful RK, the patient stated that he was struck with an elbow in the eye and noted an immediate decrease in vision. On examination the patient was found to have a ruptured globe; this was primarily repaired, but the blind, painful eye was subsequently enucleated. Simons et al. made the point that this case demonstrates that the integrity of the RK operated eye may be compromised, and they suggested that, "at the very least, patients undergoing RK should be advised of this potential complication and further that they use protective eyewear" (P. 34). They commented that if it should subsequently be shown that the corneal wounds never regain their tensile strength (as in the case of the skin), it would be prudent for patients to always wear protective eyewear — but this would defeat the purpose of the surgery, which is to avoid the encumbrance of eyewear.

■

MANAGEMENT OF POST-RK REFRACTIVE PROBLEMS

The dramatic increase in the number of RK surgeries in recent years has been accompanied by an increasing demand for postsurgical vision correction. Glasses are seldom seriously considered as a viable option for this purpose, both because of the fluctuations in refraction and because the universal reason for the surgery is to rid oneself of visual appliances. Therefore, with some exceptions, contact lens fitting is usually the treatment of choice.

☐ The Effect of RK on Corneal Topography

To understand the problems involved in fitting a contact lens to a post-RK cornea, it is helpful to consider the changes in corneal topography produced by this procedure. On the basis of the analysis of CorneaScope photographs taken before and after surgery, Fleming (1986) reported the change in corneal refracting power for each of the twelve keratoscope rings, as a result of surgery. As shown in Table 23.3, for six eyes in which surgery resulted in a 3.0 mm clear zone, mean preoperative corneal refracting power was 44.24 D for ring 3 (which corresponds to the positions of the measuring points on a keratometer mire), reducing to 42.55 D for ring 12 (which is just inside the limbus); whereas 1 year postoperatively, mean corneal refracting power was 39.60 D for ring 3 and 42.51 D for ring 12. Therefore, as a result of the surgery, there was a mean flattening of 4.64 D for the central cornea (ring 3), with essentially no change in the peripheral cornea (ring 12). Fleming noted that whereas the normal cornea flattens from the center to-

Table 23.3. Refracting Power for CorneaScope Rings Preoperatively and 1 Year Postoperatively: 3.0 mm Optical Zone, Mean for 6 Patients

Ring	Preoperative mean	Postoperative mean	Mean change
3	44.24 D	39.60 D	−4.65 D
6	43.85	41.63	−3.33
9	43.60	42.91	−0.69
12	42.55	42.51	−0.04

(From Fleming 1986.)

ward the periphery, 1 year postoperatively the cornea *steepens* from the center toward the periphery.

□ Recommended Fitting Procedures

In discussing the fitting of postsurgical contact lenses, Ebling (reported by Sposato (1987) suggested that this procedure requires one to be a master psychologist, as many RK patients have tried contact lenses before surgery and are apprehensive about wearing them again. His experience was that patients tend to be ecstatic during the period immediately after surgery, but may seek refractive error correction after about 1 year. He commented that although he has not seen a serious problem with soft lenses, he normally fits rigid gas-permeable lenses for daily wear; however, patients who were unable to wear rigid lenses before surgery are usually not able to wear them post-surgery. Ebling made the following suggestions:

1. The presurgical keratometry readings should be used.
2. A large, Korb-type lens should be fitted to obtain lateral centration.
3. Due to the steep lens-corneal relationship, the power of the lens required in the over-refraction will be about the same as that required to correct the refractive error before surgery.
4. The fluorescein pattern should be used to evaluate lens fit.
5. Adequate movement should be present to ensure tear-pumping.
6. The practitioner should not worry about the fact that the lenses are 3.00 to 4.00 D steep.
7. Heavy bearing on transverse incisions should be avoided.

Mallinger (1986) recommends the Korb technique of fitting a high-riding rigid lens with a larger-than-normal optic zone and with flatter-than-normal peripheral curves. He proposed that (1) for a postsurgical refractive error change up to 2.00 D, the preoperative flattest meridian is used as the base curve radius, whereas (2) for a postoperative change of 2.00 to 4.00 D, the base curve is the preoperative flattest meridian to 1.00 D flatter than that meridian, and (3) for a change of 4.00 to 6.00 D, the base curve is the preoperative flattest meridian to 2.00 D flatter than that meridian. His recommended lens diameters and optic zones were 9.5/8.0 mm for the first group, 9.8/8.3 mm for the second group, and 10.0/8.5 mm for the third group.

☐ Evaluation of Post-RK Contact Lens Wear

In a prospective study of 1,100 consecutive RK patients, Shivitz et al. (1986) reported that forty-four eyes (4%) had significant postoperative refractive errors and were fitted with contact lenses. Fitting was done no earlier than 6 months after surgery. All patients were fitted by a trial lens method, the initial trial lens being determined on the basis of preoperative keratometry readings. Of the forty-four eyes, twenty-four were undercorrected by the surgery, resulting in from 0.25 D to 3.01 D of myopia; nineteen were overcorrected, resulting in from 0.25 D to 8.25 D hyperopia; and one eye had induced astigmatism of 3.75 D. Daily-wear rigid gas-permeable lenses were fitted for 58% of the subjects, while daily-wear soft lenses were fitted for 42%. The only complication was corneal vascularization, occurring in 61% of the eyes fitted with soft lenses. This neovascularization was always located superficially within the radial incisions, and developed from 4 to 12 months after surgery. None of the eyes fitted with rigid gaspermeable lenses developed neovascularization.

After failing in an attempt to reduce residual myopia in post-RK patients by fitting rigid gas-permeable lenses, Edwards and Schaffer (1987) found by accident that soft contact lenses were effective in reducing residual myopia by flattening the cornea. They reported on ten eyes for which CSI soft lenses had been fitted postoperatively in an attempt to reduce residual myopia. The amount of change in myopia ranged from a decrease of 2.75 D to an increase of 0.25 D, with a mean of 0.83 D reduction. The time of fitting of the lenses ranged from 5 days to 13 months postoperatively, and the period of time the lens was worn before the subsequent reported refraction ranged from 4 days to 14 months. The authors postulated that the corneal flattening after radial keratotomy was due to the effect of stromal edema at the radial keratotomy incision sites, and that the effect of wearing a soft contact lens may have been due to the lens causing the cornea to heal in a flatter shape induced by the lens. Suggesting that the effect may be permanent, the authors warned against the fitting of soft contact lenses in cases of *overcorrection* of myopia due to radial keratotomy.

□ Case Reports Involving Anisometropia

In the report cited above in the discussion of induced anisometropia, Duling and Wick (1988) described the management of four patients who had postoperative anisometropia. Because anisometropia induced by RK is refractive, rather than axial, contact lenses are the obvious treatment for this condition. However, since many people who undergo radial keratotomy do so because they have not been successful with contact lenses, this form of treatment is not always a viable option.

Two of Duling and Wick's patients, who had undergone RK on both eyes, were not interested in wearing contact lenses with the result that glasses were prescribed for both. Patient 1 was a law student who had to do a large amount of reading, and complained of asthenopia while reading with the glasses that had been prescribed after surgery. Training was recommended, but he was not interested because of a lack of time. Eikonic lenses were designed on the basis of eikonometer findings; these lenses were worn with reasonable comfort, but the patient was bothered by the image movement (due to anisophoria) that occurred on movement on the eyes. Patient 2 complained of fluctuating vision with the right eye. Eikonic lenses were prescribed, but the lenses had to be changed after 1 month because of a change in refraction to 1.00 D.

The remaining two patients had had RK for one eye only. Patient 3 had worn soft contact lenses in both eyes before surgery. Her problem was solved by wearing a contact lens in the left (unoperated) eye, with no correction for the right eye. Patient 4, who had only about 1.00 D of myopia before surgery, had a refractive error of $+7.25$ DS -2.50 DC $\times$ 80, right eye, after surgery. Rigid gas permeable lenses, fitted for both eyes, were worn successfully.

THE STATUS OF RADIAL KERATOTOMY

The status of RK — including its safety, efficacy and stability — was discussed in a symposium chaired by Guyton (1987). In the introduction to the symposium, Guyton stated that eighteen reviewers had been unable to agree on a consensus document on RK, even after nine revisions. In this symposium, Smith (1987) made the point that myopia is not a disease state, and can be corrected with glasses or contact lenses; whereas 99% of the myopes who wear glasses or contact lenses can be corrected to 6/6 (20/20), 30% of RK patients must have the assistance of glasses or contact lenses in order to achieve 6/6 (20/20) visual acuity. He questions why a ± 2.00 D range is considered acceptable for RK, and made the following additional points: (1) glare is reported by roughly 26% of RK patients but by only 5% of patients wearing glasses or contact lenses; (2) fluctuating vision occurs in 18% of RK patients; (3) progressive hyperopia occurs in 18% of RK patients but does not occur in wearers of glasses or contact lenses; (4) a decrease in best corrected visual acuity occurs in about 8% of RK patients but does not occur in wearers of glasses or contact lenses (with the exception of "spectacle blur" for some contact lens wearers); (5) structural complications, such as infectious keratitis, corneal ulcers, cataracts, endophthalmitis, retinal detachment, optic atrophy, epithelial ingrowth, and rupture of incisions, occur in eyes whose myopia has been corrected by RK but not (with the exception of occasional keratitis and corneal ulcers in contact lens wearers) in eyes corrected with glasses or contact lenses. Smith made the additional point that the risk of having RK should not be compared to the risk of procedures such as intraocular lens implantation but to the risks of wearing glasses or contact lenses.

Expressing more optimistic views of radial keratotomy were Salz (1987) and Deitz (1987), who also participated in the symposium. Salz (1987) reported that of 1653 eyes submitted to RK (973 of which were included in the PERK study and 680 seen in private practices of himself and other surgeons) the only vision-threatening complications were three cases of late-onset bacterial keratitis from the PERK study, two of which were related to soft contact lens wear. Deitz (1987) reported that he had not lost an eye or seen irreparable harm in any of his own 1520 cases.

In an article entitled "What's the rush with RK?" Abraham (1986) suggested that 10 to 20 years could pass before we know the tolerance of operated eyes to future surgery, and questioned the use of the human eye as an "experimental model." He made the point that the best RK results are for patients having 3.00 D of myopia or less, noting that patients with this amount of myopia enjoy the use of their eyes at near without glasses or other aids. Abraham ended his commentary by asking "How many doctors . . . will permit radial keratotomy on themselves," noting that only a handful of U.S. ophthalmologists had opted for this procedure.

■

REFERENCES

Abraham SV. What's the rush with RK? Cont Lens Spectrum 1986;1:54–55.

Arrowsmith PN, Marks RG. Visual, refractive and keratometric results of radial keratotomy: a two-year follow-up. Arch Ophthalmol 1987;105:76–80.

Binder PS. Optical problems following refractive surgery. Ophthalmology 1986;93:739–745.

Deitz MF, Sanders DR. Progressive hyperopia with long-term follow-up of radial keratotomy. Arch Ophthalmol 1985;103:782–784.

Deitz MR. Symposium on RK. Predictability and stability of radial keratotomy. J Refractive Surg 1987;3:191–193.

Duling K, Wick B. Binocular vision complications after radial keratotomy. Am J Optom Physiol Opt 1988;65:215–223.

Edwards DA, Schaffer MK. Corneal flattening associated with daily wear soft contact lenses following radial keratotomy. J Refractive Surg 1987;3:54–58.

Fleming JF. Corneal topography and radial keratotomy. J Refractive Surg 1986;2:249–254.

Forstot SL, Damiano RE. Trauma after radial keratotomy. Ophthalmology 1988;95: 833–835.

Fyodorov SN, Durnev VV. Operation of dosage dissection of corneal circular ligament in cases of myopia of mild degree. Ann Ophthalmol 1979;12:1885–1890.

Guyton DL. Symposium on RK. Introduction: radial keratotomy in perspective. J Refractive Surg 1987;3:186.

Kremer FB, Steer RA. Stability of refraction following radial keratotomy over 4 years. J Refractive Surg 1986;2:217–220.

Lynn MJ, Waring GO. Symposium on RK. Response by Michael J. Lynn, MS, and George O. Waring III, MD, FACS. J Refractive Surg 1987;3:193–196.

Mallinger JC. Post-RK: a contact lens fitting methodology. Cont Lens Spectrum 1986;1: 43–46.

Mandelbaum S, Waring GO, Forster RK, et al. Late development of ulcerative keratitis in radial keratotomy scars. Arch Ophthalmol 1986;104:1156–1160.

Neumann AC. Editorial: Interpreting PERK, present and future data. J Refractive Surg 1986;2:198–200.

O'Day D. Symposium on RK. Response by Denis O'Day, MD. J Refractive Surg 1987; 3:189–190.

Richmond RD. Special report: radial keratotomy as seen through operated eyes. J Refractive Surg 1987;3:22–27.

Rowsey JJ, Balyeat HD, Monlux R, et al. Prospective evaluation of radial keratotomy: photokeratoscope corneal topography. Ophthalmology 1988;95:322–333.

Salz JJ. Symposium on RK. How safe is radial keratotomy? J Refractive Surg 1987;3: 188–189.

Sato T, Akiyama K, Shibata H. A new surgical approach to myopia. Am J Ophthalmol 1953; 36:823–829.

Sawelson H, Marks RG. Three-year results of radial keratotomy. Arch Ophthalmol 1987; 105:81–85.

Schanzlin DJ, Santo VR, Waring GO, et al. Diurnal change in refraction, corneal curvature, visual acuity, and intraocular pressure after radial keratotomy in the PERK study. Ophthalmology 1985;93:167–175.

Shivitz IA, Arrowsmith PN. Delayed keratitis after radial keratotomy. Arch Ophthalmol 1986;104:1153–1155.

Shivitz IA, Russell BM, Arrowsmith PN, Marks RG. Optical correction of postoperative radial keratotomy patients with contact lenses. CLAO J 1986;12:59–62.

Simons KB, Linsalata RP, Zaragosa AM. Ruptured globe secondary to blunt trauma following radial keratotomy. J Refractive Surg 1988;4:132–135.

Smith RE. Symposium on RK. Status of radial keratotomy. J Refractive Surg 1987;3:187.

Sposato P. Report from the Institute for Contact Lens Research. Contact Lens Spectrum 1987;2:58–69.

Waring GO, Lynn MJ, Gelender H, Laibson PR, Lindstrom RL, Myers WD, Obstbaum

SA, Rowsey JJ, McDonald MB, Schanzlin DJ, Sperduto RD, Borque LB. Results of the prospective evaluation of radial keratotomy (PERK) study one year after surgery. Ophthalmology 1985;92:177–208.

Waring GO. Editorial: PERK director responds. J Refractive Surg 1986;2:201–205.

Waring GO, Lynn MJ, Culbertson W, Laibson PR, Lindstrom RD, McDonald MB, Myers WD, Ostbaum SA, Rowsey JJ, Schanzlin DJ. Three-year results of the prospective evaluation of radial keratotomy (PERK) study. Ophthalmology 1987;94:1339–1353.

Wyzinski P, O'Dell W. Diurnal cycle of refraction after radial keratotomy. Ophthalmology 1987;94:120–124.

24

Management of Myopia: Excimer Laser Surgery

Theodore Grosvenor

☐

The first suggestion that the argon-fluoride excimer laser might be useful in refractive surgery was made by Trokel et al. (1983). During the period in which the chapters for this volume were outlined, written, assembled, and edited, excimer laser refractive surgery has grown from an idea to a procedure that appears to hold promise in the management of myopia and is now being used on human volunteers in blind eye clinical trials. The driving force for the development of excimer laser surgery has been the desire for a noninvasive form of refractive surgery that is more reliable and has fewer potential complications than current forms of refractive surgery such as radial keratotomy.

Although radial keratotomy has become established as an acceptable procedure in the management of myopia, many problems remain to be solved. A major problem is the lack of predictability. As noted in the previous chapter, PERK study results indicated that only 22 to 57% of the subjects (depending on the presurgical refractive error) had a postsurgical spherical equivalent refraction between +0.50 and −0.50 D, whereas 38 to 84% had a postsurgical spherical equivalent refraction between +1.00 and −1.00 D (Waring et al. 1985). This lack of predictability is due largely to the fact that it is not possible to control the depths of the incisions accurately. Other unsolved problems, also noted in the previous chapter, are glare, diurnal fluctuations in vision, a decrease in best-corrected visual acuity, a high prevalence of postoperative anisometropia, and the risk of postoperative keratitis and other severe consequences.

In a discussion of the use of steel and gemstone knives for corneal surgery, Trokel (1989) described a knife as a wedge, which generates an enormous pressure at the cutting edge, resulting in both cutting and shearing actions. As a scalpel cuts, it displaces tissue both away from and at right angles to the incision, with the result that it is impossible to create an incision to a predetermined depth or to create a perfectly smooth cut surface. Marshall (1989) made the point that once the blade touches the corneal surface, the surface is indented; the depth of the cut depends on the speed of movement, the sharpness of the blade, the rotational aspects of the tissue, and the elastic constants of the tissue. He concluded that the depth of a cut can be predicted with an accuracy no greater than 10 to 12%. Studies of surgically created surfaces have shown that they are invariably rough and irregular, corneal healing being accompanied by variable amounts of scarring and surface irregularity (Trokel 1989).

THE EXCIMER LASER

The development of excimer laser corneal surgery has been an international effort, much of the early work having been performed by Dr. Stephen Trokel and his colleagues at Columbia University in New York and by Professor John Marshall and his colleagues at the Institute of Ophthalmology in London. The following description is excerpted from a lecture given by Marshall (1989), at a meeting of the British Contact Lens Association, Marshall described the excimer laser as a chamber in which an inert gas (argon) combines, under extreme pressure and high voltage, with a halogen (fluorine). Once the argon fluoride molecule is formed, it breaks up and emits an extremely high energy photon of ultraviolet radiation, having a wavelength of 193 nm. The pulse duration of the emitted laser radiation is about 10 to 20 nsec, and the pulses are emitted at the rate of 1 to 100 per second.

Noting that the carbon-carbon bonds of human tissue require an energy of three electron volts "to keep them together," Marshall (1989) stated that the individual 193 nm wavelength excimer laser photon has an energy of 6.4 electron volts, sufficient to cause any biologic macromolecule that absorbs the photon to literally fall apart, a process known as *photoablation*. The photon penetrates about 1 μm into a biological surface. When a surface is irradiated, only the molecules that absorb energy are capable of undergoing change; when a photon is absorbed, the molecule expands, and molecular fragments are expelled from the surface. A pseudomembrane is formed at the surface, resulting in a smooth surface. The excimer laser beam is sufficiently broad, having a rectangular cross section of about 20×10 mm, so that with a suitable optical system (consisting of a cylindrical lens and a circular aperture) the beam can be made into a disk having a diameter of 3 mm. With this energy source, a very small depth of tissue removal will achieve a large dioptric change. Removal of tissue to a depth of 25 μm, using the 3 mm diameter disk, will produce a change of 10.00 D in corneal refraction (Marshall 1989).

Early excimer laser experiments, described by Trokel (1989), showed that this new modality could be used for refractive surgery in either of two ways: (1) to create narrow, linear incisions, emulating the knife incisions used in radial keratotomy; or (2) to remove tissue directly from the anterior corneal surface (with a wide beam, as described earlier), thus reshaping or "sculpturing" the cornea.

Trokel commented that the most striking and unique feature of the 193 nm laser ablation is the extreme smoothness of the surfaces after ablation and the parallel nature of the edges when a trough of tissue was removed. He described the pseudomembrane as having many of the characteristics of a true membrane: It serves as a template for reepithelialization during healing, and serves as a barrier to water transport preventing postoperative swelling. In previous corneal surgical procedures, it has been considered necessary to preserve Bowman's layer; however, in excimer laser reshaping, Bowman's layer is lost and does not reform, although the basement layer of the epithelium does reform during reepithelialization.

EXCIMER LASER
RADIAL KERATOTOMY

Studies of the use of the excimer laser to reduce myopia by the use of radial incisions, as in radial keratotomy, have been reported by several teams of investigators. Berns et al. (1988) reported on a study in which 193 nm ultraviolet radiation from an argon fluoride laser was used to produce radial incisions in the corneas of rabbits. Two ranges of energy densities were used, 1.0 to 2.1 J/cm^2 and 200 to 700 mJ/cm^2 per pulse. The results of the surgery were determined by histologic and electron microscopic examination of the corneas after enucleation. The eyes that had been submitted to the higher energy density exposures were found to show ridging on the corneal surface along the edges of the cuts, micropitting of the stroma inside the cuts, and denudation of the endothelium under the ablation zone; whereas the eyes submitted to the lower energy density exposures did not exhibit significant surface ridging or endothelial loss, but exhibited significant stromal swelling during the laser exposure. This stromal swelling made it difficult to produce incisions of a precisely controlled depth.

Aron-Rosa et al. (1988) reported on the results obtained on two eyes of volunteer subjects that were scheduled for enucleation because of choroidal melanoma. Excimer laser radial keratotomy was performed on each of the two eyes on three occasions: 21 days, 14 days, and 1 day before enucleation. Postoperative keratometer findings were found to be flatter by 3.00 D for one subject and by 1.75 D, in one principal meridian only, for the other subject. Subjective refraction before and after the surgery could not be measured because the eyes were blind; changes in retinoscopy findings or in objective refraction by other means were not reported. In discussing their results, the authors commented that holding the eye steady during the time of the laser application was found to be extremely difficult for the patients, and that precise laser photoablation was disturbed by the small eye movements induced by breathing and the choroidal pulse. They also reported that the cuts were broader than expected, being similar in slit-lamp appearance to cuts made with a diamond knife; and that all cuts were shallower than programed, never exceeding 85% of the programed depth.

In order to address the problem of controlling the depth of the radial incisions, Stern et al. (1989) conducted experimentation with what they called "femtosecond optical ranging" for noninvasive measurement of excimer laser incision depth during the ablation process. They described this procedure as an optical analog of ultrasonic pachymetry, explaining that they measured the time required for a femtosecond (fsec) laser pulse to make a round trip between the corneal surface and the bottom of an incision. The laser source for the measurements produced a train of 65 fsec pulses at 625 nm. Unsolved problems with this technique according to Stern et al. are the following: (1) Femtosecond ranging of incision depth must be performed on a relatively dry eye, (2) the eye must be carefully positioned so that the probe beam is perpendicular to the corneal surface, and (3) the eye must be stationary during measurement. They noted that in larger area surface ablation, as in corneal sculpturing, the high transverse resolution of femtosecond ranging is not required; measurement techniques such as photokeratoscopy are probably more useful.

CORNEAL SCULPTURING WITH THE EXCIMER LASER

Trokel (1989) has listed the following advantages of direct laser corneal sculpturing: (1) The laser beam removes tissue to a predetermined depth, with an accuracy of a fraction of a micron; (2) the tissue is removed without conductive damage in the remaining tissue; (3) the tissue is smoothly surfaced by a pseudomembrane, which (as already noted) serves as a template for reepithelialization and acts as a barrier to water transmission.

□ Instrumentation and Technique

In his discussion of the use of the excimer laser beam for corneal sculpturing in a myopic eye, Trokel (1989) described the use of a circular aperture to control the diameter of a uniform laser beam that falls on the cornea (Figure 24.1): "By progressively narrowing the diameter of the ablated cornea, a new optical surface is created in a controlled manner. Because each ablated step removes 0.25 μm of tissue, the surface is smooth to optical standards and the steps are not visible by optical techniques."

The instrumentation and technique for excimer laser corneal sculpturing have been described by L'Esperance et al. (1989). The 10 × 20 mm laser beam is

Figure 24.1. Corneal sculpturing with the excimer laser. If the beam has more energy centrally (left), the cornea will be flattened and reduced in doptric power. Steepening of the cornea can be achieved (right) by removing more corneal tissue from the periphery than from the central zone. (From Trokel 1989. Reprinted by permission.)

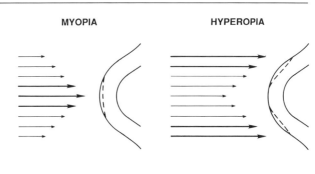

expanded by the use of prisms into a 20 × 20 mm square rotating beam. This rotating beam is passed successively through a series of apertures mounted in one of three aperture wheels, one wheel being used for myopia, one for hyperopia, and one for astigmatism. The aperture wheel used for myopia (Figure 24.2, left) has a series of apertures of decreasing diameter, the wheel used for hyperopia has annular apertures of decreasing radial width, and the wheel used for astigmatism has a series of slit-shaped apertures of varying width. The ablation profile is illustrated schematically, to an exaggerated scale (Figure 24.2, right) before regrowth

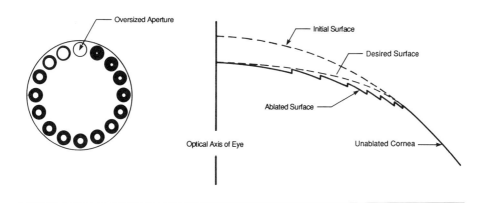

Figure 24.2. The aperture wheel used for myopia allows the laser beam to ablate the central cornea more deeply than the peripheral cornea. The right-hand diagram shows an exaggerated representation of the stepped profile ablation of the cornea to reduce myopia. (From L'Esperance et al. 1989. Copyright 1989, American Medical Association. Reprinted by permission.)

of the epithelium. L'Esperance et al. (1989) describe the apparatus as being designed to correct a refractive error of at least 6.00 D over an ablated area having a diameter of 5.5 mm; they state that later models will allow 12.00 D of correction over a 7 mm diameter. A digital keratoscope is incorporated into the laser beam delivery system to provide measurements of the topography of the cornea before and after the ablation. Before the surgical procedure, the eye is immobilized with a limbal retention ring held against the cornea and sclera with a gentle vacuum, while the patient is supine. After anesthesia by retrobulbar and peribulbar injection, the epithelium is removed with a "hockey stick" blade to a distance of approximately 1 mm outside of the proposed ablation site, creating a denuded area 5 to 8 mm in diameter, depending on the intended keratectomy zone size. These authors described a typical procedure as requiring from 25 to 30 seconds to create an ablation to a depth of 50 to 70 μm in the anterior stroma of the patient's cornea, the diameter of the impact area ranging from 3 to 5.5 mm.

□ Results on Human Volunteers

L'Esperance et al. (1989) have described the results obtained on eleven human volunteers enrolled in the first phase of their study, authorized by the U.S. Food and Drug Administration. Of the eleven subjects, four had eyes that were scheduled for enucleation or corneal transplantation, and seven had eyes that were blind from long-standing glaucoma, retinal detachment, or retinal artery occlusion. The purpose of the treatment was not to alter the subjects' refractive errors, but "to study the morphologic and histopathologic changes that occurred to have the ability to eventually proceed judiciously with reconstructive lameller keratectomy or refractive lamellar keratectomy in selected patients" (P. 138). The authors reported that all of the eyes reepithelialized completely and normally within 60 to 72 hours, and that over the short term (up to 12 days postoperatively) the eyes showed little or no histopathologic disturbance of epithelial, stromal, or endothelial cells and, on gross and biomicroscopic examination, showed clear corneas. They added, however, that "a fine fibrillar haze was observed in eyes under slit-lamp examination with magnification over the long term, although they appeared clinically clear on gross examination."

The first study in which the excimer laser was used on human eyes for the purpose of corneal reshaping to reduce myopia was reported by Taylor et al. (1989). Ten blind eyes of volunteer subjects were submitted to corneal flattening ablations within the central 3.0 to 5.2 mm of the cornea. Depths of the ablated areas ranged from 40 to 113 μm. Preoperative and postoperative keratometric findings were taken with a Bausch and Lomb keratometer; preoperative and postoperative refraction was measured by static retinoscopy. For subjects 1 through 4, no attempt was made to create a change in refractive error, but for subjects 6 through 10 a change in the direction of less myopia or more hyperopia was attempted by making a series of 15 gradual steps from the periphery to the center of the cornea, with the center receiving the greatest exposure. After the surgery, all eyes reepithelialized by the second or third postoperative day. Of seven eyes that were observed for prolonged periods, all eyes appeared to be clear in the area of the ablation when viewed without magnification; however, slit-lamp examination showed an edematous haze in the ablated area for the first 2 weeks, which was gradually replaced by a mild speckled interface between the epithelium and the stroma.

The presence of opaque media made it impossible to obtain keratometry and retinoscopy findings on three of the six eyes on which myopia reduction was attempted. For the three eyes on which these findings were available, there was a postoperative corneal flattening followed after 2 or more weeks by a steepening, and a postoperative change in refraction in the direction of less myopia (or more hyperopia) followed after 2 or more weeks by a change either in the myopic or the hyperopic direction. On the basis of the data reported by Taylor et al. (1989) the following changes were found:

Subject 6: Postoperative corneal flattening of 5.00 D, followed by 3.00 D of corneal steeping by 36 weeks; postoperative increase in hyperopia of 12.00 D, followed by a further increase of 2.00 D by 36 weeks.

Subject 7: Postoperative corneal flattening of 4.00 D, followed by 1.50 D of corneal steepening by 24 weeks; postoperative change (from low myopia to moderate hyperopia) of 4.50 D, followed by a decrease in hyperopia of 2.50 D by 24 weeks.

Subject 10: Postoperative corneal flattening of 1.50 D, followed by a steepening back to the original finding by 23 weeks; postoperative increase in hyperopia of 0.75 D, followed by a further increase in hyperopia of 1.75 D by 12 weeks.

The authors commented that the tendency to lose some of the contouring effect as the eye healed was due to a progressive "filling in" of the defect, by some 30 to 50 μm over the first 4 to 6 months. They concluded that the filling in was due, in part, to epithelial hyperplasia over the excavated areas and to new collagen and ground substance formation directly under the epithelium. As the authors observed, postoperative changes in keratometer findings were not consistent with the consequent changes in refractive error determined by retinoscopy. A possible explanation is that the area of ablation, although it corresponds to the area of the cornea through which light passes when static retinoscopy is performed, does not correspond to the area (a chord diameter of about 3 mm) measured by the keratometer.

The first case in which excimer laser sculpturing was performed on a sighted eye was reported by McDonald et al. (1989). This report concerned a subject enrolled in a blind-eye trial, who was considered to be blind in the right eye, but whose blindness was apparently functional. Before surgery, the subject's uncorrected visual acuity in the right eye was minimal light perception, with a refractive error of -5.75 $+2.00$ × 95. Excimer laser surgery was performed, designed to eliminate the 4.75 D (spherical equivalent) of myopia, the ablated area having a diameter of 5 mm. Seven weeks after the treatment, the patient had an uncorrected visual acuity in the right eye of 20/25, with a refractive error of -0.50 $+1.50$ × 90. Three months after treatment, the uncorrected visual acuity was 20/20, with a very small residual refractive error. The authors concluded that the patient had suffered from functional blindness after the removal of a pituitary tumor, some years previous to the excimer surgery, and that after the surgery the patient's hysteria resolved and she regained her vision. The authors commented that this was the first report, to their knowledge, of a good visual result in a human eye from excimer laser photoablation surgery.

THE FUTURE OF EXCIMER LASER SURGERY

As this volume goes to press, little data are available on the results of excimer laser surgery for the management of myopia. However, the weight of the evidence appears to show that direct corneal sculpturing, or reshaping, holds more promise than indirect reshaping by the use of radial incisions. Marshall (1989) has commented that the use of the excimer laser for making corneal incisions is "a very expensive scalpel." As already noted, Trokel (1989) listed the advantages of direct corneal sculpturing as predictability of ablation depth, a lack of damage to remaining tissue, and the formation of the pseudomembrane.

However, even the results that have been reported for direct corneal sculpturing are not particularly encouraging. Statements about the accuracy with which laser ablations can be made seem to have given way to the reality that the ablated area "fills in" following surgery, tending to reduce or even eliminate the change in refractive error; and the fact that postoperative corneas, although grossly clear when viewed without magnification, show clouding or other opacities on slit-lamp examination, remains to be explained.

Finally, there is the matter of the cost of the new technology. Lichter (1988), in an editorial entitled "The Medical-Industrial Complex and the Excimer Laser," estimated that the cost of an excimer laser in a commercial model run would be between $150,000 and $200,000, and he commented that the price tag may be such that some ophthalmologists may not be able to afford the instrument — although those same individuals may find that they can ill afford not to have it, especially if it is seen as a practice builder. Lichter made the observation that the time may come when government, other third parties, and even patients will decide that costs will preclude some of the technological advances in medicine; and that "the excimer laser may be a good test of this conundrum" (P. 422).

------ ■ ------

REFERENCES

Aron-Rosa DS, Boerner CF, Gross M, Timsit J-C, Delacour M, Bath PE. Wound healing following excimer laser radial keratotomy. J Cataract Refractive Surg 1988;14:173–179.

Berns MW, Liaw LH, Oliva A, Andrews JJ, Rasmussen RE, Kimel S. An acute light and electron microscope study of ultraviolet 193-nm excimer laser corneal incisions. Ophthalmology 1988;95:1422–1433.

L'Esperance FA, Warner JW, Telfair WB, Yoder PR, Martin CA. Excimer laser instrumentation and technique for human corneal surgery. Arch Ophthalmol 1989;47:131–139.

Lichter PR, The medical-industrial complex and the excimer laser. Ophthalmology 1988; 95:421–422.

McDonald MB, Kaufman HE, Frantz JM, Shofner S, Salmeron B, Klyce SD. Excimer laser ablation in a human eye. Arch Ophthalmol 1989;107:641–642.

Marshall J. The potential of lasers in refractive surgery. Trans Br Contact Lens Assoc 1989; 11:63–67.

Stern D, Lin W-Z, Puliafito CA, Fujimoto JG. Femtosecond optical ranging of corneal incision depth. Invest Ophthalmol Vis Sci 1989;30:99–104.

Taylor DM, L'Esperance FA, Del Poro RA, Roberts AD, Gigstad JE, Klintworth G, Martin CA, Warner J. Human excimer laser lamellar keratectomy. Ophthalmology 1989; 96:654–664.

Taylor DM, L'Esperance FA, Warner JW, Del Pero RA, Roberts AD, Gigstad JE, Martin C. Experimental corneal studies with the excimer laser. J Cataract Refractive Surg 1989; 15:384–389.

Trokel S, Srinivasan R, Braren B. Excimer laser surgery of the cornea. Am J Ophthalmol 1983;96:710–715.

Trokel S. Evolution of excimer laser corneal surgery. J Cataract Refractive Surg 1989; 15:373–383.

Waring GO, Lynn MJ, Gelender H, et al. Results of the prospective evaluation of radial keratotomy (PERK) study one year after surgery. Ophthalmology 1985;92:177–208.

INDEX